Platelet Immunology:
Fundamental and Clinical Aspects

Immunologie plaquettaire :
aspects fondamentaux et cliniques

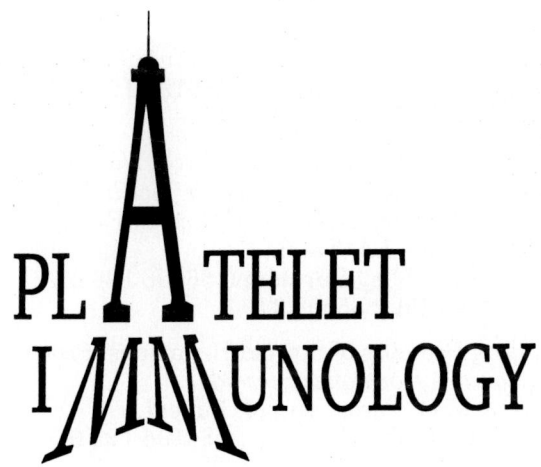

Colloques INSERM
ISSN 0768-3154

Other *Colloques* published as co-editions by John Libbey Eurotext and INSERM

133 Cardiovascular and Respiratory Physiology in the Fetus and Neonate. *Physiologie Cardiovasculaire et Respiratoire du Fœtus et du Nouveau-né.*
Scientific Committee : P. Karlberg, A. Minkowski, W. Oh and L. Stern;
Managing Editor : M. Monset-Couchard.
ISBN : John Libbey Eurotext 0 86196 125 0
INSERM 2 85598 340 1

134 Porphyrins and Porphyrias. *Porphyrines et Porphyries.*
Edited by Y. Nordmann.
ISBN : John Libbey Eurotext 0 86196 087 4
INSERM 2 85598 281 2

137 Neo-Adjuvant Chemotherapy. *Chimiothérapie Néo-Adjuvante.*
Edited by C. Jacquillat, M. Weil and D. Khayat.
ISBN : John Libbey Eurotext 0 86196 125 0
INSERM 2 85598 340 1

139 Hormones and Cell Regulation (10th European Symposium). *Hormones et Régulation Cellulaire (10ᵉ Symposium Européen).*
Edited by J. Nunez, J.E. Dumont and R.J.B. King.
ISBN : John Libbey Eurotext 0 86196 125 0X
INSERM 2 85598 340 1

147 Modern Trends in Aging Research. *Nouvelles Perspectives de la Recherche sur le Vieillissement.*
Edited by Y. Courtois, B. Faucheux, B. Forette, D.L. Knook and J.A. Tréton.
ISBN : John Libbey Eurotext 0 86196 126 0X
INSERM 2 85598 340 1

149 Binding Proteins of Steroid Hormones. *Protéines de liaison des Hormones Stéroïdes.*
Edited by M.G. Forest and M. Pugeat.
ISBN : John Libbey Eurotext 0 86196 125 0
INSERM 2 85598 340 1X

151 Control and Management of Parturition. *La Maîtrise de la Parturition.*
Edited by C. Sureau, P. Blot, D. Cabrol, F. Cavaillé and G. Germain.
ISBN : John Libbey Eurotext 0 86196 125 0
INSERM 2 85598 340 1

Suite page 323

Platelet Immunology: Fundamental and Clinical Aspects

Immunologie plaquettaire : aspects fondamentaux et cliniques

Proceedings of the first European Symposium on platelet immunology held in Paris, Palais du Luxembourg (France), March 1-2, 1990

Under the patronage of the Sénat, INSERM, INTS and Assistance Publique-Hôpitaux de Paris

Edited by

Cécile Kaplan-Gouet
Nicole Schlegel
Charles Salmon
John McGregor

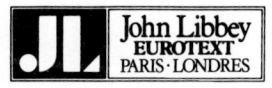

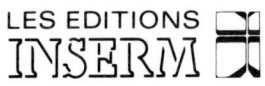

British Library Cataloguing in Publication Data
Platelet immunology
1. Man. Blood. Platelets
I. Tittle
612.117

ISBN 0 86196 285 0
ISSN 0768-3154

First published in 1991 by

Editions John Libbey Eurotext
6 rue Blanche, 92120 Montrouge, France. (1) 47 35 85 52
ISBN 0 86196 285 0

John Libbey & Company Ltd
13 Smiths Yard, Summerley Street, London SW18 4HR, England.
(1) 947 27 77

Institut National de la Santé et de la Recherche Médicale
101 rue de Tolbiac, 75654 Paris Cedex 13, France.
(1) 45 84 14 41
ISBN 2 85598 439 4

ISSN 0768-3154

© 1991 Colloques INSERM/John Libbey Eurotext Ltd,
All rights reserved
Unauthorised publication contravenes applicable laws

In memory of Aron Kaplan

En mémoire de Aron Kaplan

Acknowledgements

The First European Symposium on Platelet Immunology was held in Paris, on the 1st and 2nd of March 1990, to present new data and review the substantial progress made in platelet immunology. Participants to this meeting came from laboratories in Europe, Israel and North America.
The members of the scientific committee for this meeting were :
- C. Kaplan, Paris
- J. McGregor, Lyon
- C. Mueller-Eckhardt, Giessen
- A. von dem Borne, Amsterdam
- K. Clemetson, Berne
- Ch. Salmon, Paris

The meeting was organized by :
- C. Kaplan, Paris
- J. McGregor, Lyon
- N. Schlegel, Paris

The First European Symposium presided by Professor Ch. Salmon and opened by Professor J. Caen took place at the Palais du Luxembourg. We are greatly indebted to the Sénat President, Alain Poher, for allowing this first European meeting to take place in such a prestigious setting. Morever, we would like to thank the mayor of Paris for receiving the participants of the symposium in the Town Hall.

The meeting was held under the patronage of the Sénat, INSERM, INTS and Assistance Publique-Hôpitaux de Paris. The publication of this book was sponsored by the Institut National de la Santé et de la Recherche Médicale (INSERM). We would also like to thank : Baxter, Becton-Dickinson, Behring, Bioart, Biotransfusion, Cerg, Choay-Sanofi, Coultronics, Diagnostic-Transfusion, Eurobio, IBM, Immuno-France, Immunotech, Kabi, Mérieux, Ortho Diagnostic Systems, Rhône-Poulenc, Stago, Zeiss, for sponsoring this symposium.

Remerciements

Le premier Symposium Européen sur l'immunologie plaquettaire s'est tenu à Paris les 1 et 2 mars 1990. Son objectif était de présenter les nouvelles données et les progrès substantiels accomplis dans le domaine de l'immunologie plaquettaire. Les participants à ce congrès venaient des laboratoires d'Europe, d'Israël et d'Amérique du Nord.
Les membres du comité scientifique étaient :
- C. Kaplan, Paris
- J. McGregor, Lyon
- C. Mueller-Eckhardt, Giessen
- A. von dem Borne, Amsterdam
- K. Clemetson, Berne
- Ch. Salmon, Paris

La réunion était organisée par :
- C. Kaplan, Paris
- J. McGregor, Lyon
- N. Schlegel, Paris

Ce premier Symposium Européen était présidé par le Professeur Ch. Salmon et a été ouvert par le Professeur J. Caen. Il s'est tenu au Palais du Luxembourg et nous sommes grandement redevables au Président du Sénat, Alain Poher, d'avoir permis que le premier Symposium Européen ait lieu dans un cadre si prestigieux. Nous voudrions également remercier Monsieur le Maire de Paris d'avoir reçu les participants du symposium dans les salons de l'Hôtel de Ville.

La réunion s'est tenue sous l'égide du Sénat, de l'INSERM, de l'INTS et de l'Assistance Publique-Hôpitaux de Paris. La publication de ce livre a été réalisée avec le soutien de l'Institut National de la Santé et de la Recherche Médicale (INSERM). Nous voudrions remercier également : Baxter, Becton-Dickinson, Behring, Bioart, Biotransfusion, Cerg, Choay-Sanofi, Coultronics, Diagnostic-Transfusion, Eurobio, IBM, Immuno-France, Immunotech, Kabi, Mérieux, Ortho Diagnostic Systems, Rhône-Poulenc, Stago, Zeiss, d'avoir apporté leur soutien à ce symposium.

Preface

During this past decade substantial progress have been made in basic platelet research as well as clinical practice in platelet immunology. The First European Symposium on Platelet Immunology covered the most recent advances in fundamental aspects of the platelet membrane at both the cellular and molecular levels, monoclonal antibodies and current developments in the clinical management of autoimmune and alloimmune thrombocytopenias.

This book has been organized into 4 sections. The first section is devoted to cellular and molecular biology of the platelet glycoproteins. The next section deals with the effects of the monoclonal antibodies on the platelet receptors and the regulation of platelet-vessel wall interactions. The third section looks at recent aspects of inherited thrombopathies with special emphasis on Glanzmann thrombasthenia. In the fourth section the potential clinical implications of platelet immunology are considered and extensive coverage is given to auto and allo-immunity.

C. Kaplan
N. Schlegel
J. McGregor

Préface

Au cours de cette dernière décennie, de substantiels progrès ont été obtenus dans le domaine de l'immunologie plaquettaire, tant sur le plan de la recherche fondamentale sur les plaquettes que sur celui de ses applications cliniques. Le premier symposium européen sur l'immunologie plaquettaire a traité des avancées les plus récentes dans l'étude fondamentale de la membrane plaquettaire aux niveaux cellulaire et moléculaire, des anticorps monoclonaux et des développements actuels dans le traitement clinique des thrombocytopénies auto- et allo-immunes.

Ce livre a été divisé en quatre parties. La première est consacrée à la biologie cellulaire et moléculaire des glycoprotéines plaquettaires. La seconde traite des effets des anticorps monoclonaux sur les récepteurs plaquettaires et la régulation des interactions plaquette-paroi vasculaire. La troisième partie est consacrée aux aspects récents des thrombopathies héréditaires plus particulièrement à la thrombasthénie de Glanzmann. Dans la quatrième et dernière partie, les applications cliniques potentielles de l'immunologie plaquettaire sont examinées et les phénomènes d'auto- et d'allo-immunité sont largement traités.

C. Kaplan
N. Schlegel
J. McGregor

List and addresses of contributors
Liste et adresses des auteurs

Beardsley D.S., Pediatric Hematology Division, Yale University School of Medicine, 333 Cedar Street, PO Box 3333, New Haven, Connecticut 06510-8064, USA.

Bellucci S., INSERM U 150, CNRS UA 334, Hôpital Lariboisière, 2, rue Ambroise Paré, 75010 Paris, France.

Boukerche H., INSERM U 331, Faculté de Médecine Alexis Carrel, 8, rue Guillaume Paradin, 69372 Lyon Cedex 08, France.

Breton-Gorius J., INSERM U 91, Hôpital Henri Mondor, 51, av. du Maréchal de Lattre de Tassigny, 94010 Créteil, France.

Bussel J.B., New York Hospital, Cornell Medical Center, Division of Pediatrics N-740, 525 East 68th Street, New York, NY 10021, USA.

Clemetson K.J., Theodor Kocher Institute, University of Bern, Freiestrasse 1, CH-3012 Bern, Suisse.

Clezardin P., INSERM U 331, Laboratoire d'Hémobiologie, Faculté de Médecine Alexis Carrel, 8, rue Guillaume Paradin, 69372 Lyon Cedex 08, France.

Daffos F., Institut de Puériculture, 26, bd Brune, 75014 Paris, France.

Dessaint J.P., Centre d'Immunologie et de Biologie Parasitaire, Unité Mixte INSERM U 167 – CNRS 624, Institut Pasteur, 1, rue du Pr A. Calmette, BP 245, 59019 Lille Cedex, France.

Forestier F., Institut de Puériculture, 26, bd Brune, 75014 Paris, France.

Kaplan-Gouet C., Service d'Immunologie Leuco-Plaquettaire, Institut National de Transfusion Sanguine, 6, rue Alexandre Cabanel, 75015 Paris, France.

Kiefel V., Klinikum Der Justus-Liebig Universität, Institut für Klinische, Immunologie und Transfusions Medizin, Langhansstrasse 7, 6300 Giessen, Allemagne.

Lecompte T., Laboratoire Central d'Hématologie, Hôtel-Dieu, 1, place du Parvis-Notre-Dame, 75004 Paris, France.

Mac Ever R.P., Department of Medicine, University of Oklahoma Health Sciences Center, 825 NE 13th Street, Oklahoma City, OK 73104 USA.

Mac Gregor J.L., INSERM U 331, Laboratoire d'Hémobiologie, Faculté de Médecine Alexis Carrel, 8, rue Guillaume Paradin, 69372 Lyon Cedex 08, France.

Morel-Kopp M.C., Biochimie Plaquettaire, Institut National de Transfusion Sanguine, 6, rue Alexandre Cabanel, 75015 Paris, France.

Mueller-Eckhardt C., Klinikum Der Justus-Liebig Universität, Institut Für Klinische Immunologie und Transfusions Medizin, Langhansstrasse 7, 6300 Giessen, Allemagne.

Nurden A.T., Pathologie Cellulaire de l'Hémostase, Hôpital Cardiologique, avenue de Magellan, 33604 Pessac, France.

Parmentier S., INSERM U 331, Faculté de Médecine Alexis Carrel, 8, rue Guillaume Paradin, 69372 Lyon Cedex 08, France.

Rabiet M.J., INSERM U 217, Unité de Recherches sur l'Hémostase Cellulaire et Moléculaire, avenue des Martyrs, 38041 Grenoble Cedex, France.

Rosa J.P., INSERM U 150, Hôpital Lariboisière, 2, rue Ambroise Paré, 75010 Paris, France.

Santoso S., Klinikum der Justus-Liebig Universität, Institut für Klinische, Immunologie und Transfusions Medizin, Langhansstrasse 7, 6300 Giessen, Allemagne.

Schafer A.I., Medical Service, Veterans Affairs Medical Center, 2002 Holcombe Boulevard, Houston, Texas 77030, USA.

Schlegel N., Laboratoire d'Hématologie, Hôpital Robert Debré, 48, bd Sérurier, 75019 Paris, France.

Seligsohn U., Ichilow Hospital, 6 Weizman Street, Tel Aviv, Israel.

Sonnenberg A., Central Laboratory of the Netherlands, Red Cross Blood Transfusion Service Plesmanlaan 125, 1066 CX Amsterdam, PO Box, 9190, 1006 AD Amsterdam, Pays-Bas.

Tchernia G., Laboratoire d'Hématologie, Hôpital Antoine Béclère, 157, rue de la Porte-de-Trivaux, 92140 Clamart, France.

Uzan G., INSERM U 217, Unité de Recherches sur l'Hémostase Cellulaire et Moléculaire, av. des Martyrs, 38041 Grenoble Cedex, France.

Von dem Borne A., Department of Immunologic Haematology, Central Laboratory of the Netherlands Red Cross Blood Transfusion Service, Plesmanlaan 125, PO Box 9190, 1066 CX Amsterdam, Pays-Bas.

Waters A.H., St Bartholomew's Hospital, Department of Haematology, West Smithfield, London EC 1A 7BE, Grande-Bretagne.

List and addresses of participants
Liste et adresses des participants

Aakhus A.M., Research Institute for Internal Medicine, Rikshospitalet, 0027 Oslo 1, Norvège.

Algiman M., Laboratoire d'Hématologie, Hôpital Cochin, 27, rue du Faubourg-Saint-Jacques, 75014 Paris, France.

Allebes W.A., University Transfusion Service, Transplantation Serology, Geert Grooteplein Zuid 12, 6525 GA Nijmegen, Pays-Bas.

Allen D.L, National Blood Transfusion Service, John Radcliffe Hospital, Headington, Oxford OX3 9DU, Grande-Bretagne.

Armitage S., National Blood Transfusion Service, North London Blood Transfusion Centre, Colindale Avenue, London NW9 5BG, Grande-Bretagne.

Avenard G., Bio Transfusion, Z.A. Courtabeuf, BP 99, 91943 Les Ulis Cedex A, France.

Bardet M.C., Diagnostics Transfusion, 3, bd Raymond Poincaré, BP 20, 92430 Marnes-La-Coquette, France.

Baruch D., INSERM U 143, Hôpital de Bicêtre, 78, rue du Général Leclerc, 94270 Le Kremlin-Bicêtre, France.

Berrebi A., Hematology Unit, Kaplan Hospital, 76100 Rehovot, Israël.

Bertolini F., Ospedale Maggiore, Via Francesco Sforza 35, 20122 Milan, Italie.

Bettaieb A., CDTS Val de Marne, HLA, Hôpital Henri Mondor, 51, av. du Maréchal de Lattre de Tassigny, 94010 Créteil Cedex, France.

Bierling P., CDTS Val de Marne, HLA, Hôpital Henri Mondor, 51, av. du Maréchal de Lattre de Tassigny, 94010 Créteil Cedex, France.

Blanchard D., CRTS, Allée Charles Mirallié, BP 349, 44011 Nantes Cedex 01, France.

Blot P., Hôpital Robert Debré, 48, bd Sérurier, 75019 Paris, France.

Boccara J.-F., Hôpital Saint-Vincent de Paul, 74, av. Denfert Rochereau, 75014 Paris, France.

Boizard-Boval B., CTS Lariboisière, 2, rue Ambroise Paré, 75010 Paris, France.

Bolot P., Hôpital Saint-Michel, Pédiatrie, 33, rue Olivier de Serres, 75730 Paris Cedex 15, France.

Bonghton B., Queen Elizabeth Hospital, Edgbaston Birmingham B15 2TH, Grande-Bretagne.

Bonnet M.C., Institut Mérieux, Division Immunologie, 1541 av. Marcel Mérieux, 69280 Marcy-l'Etoile, France.

Borzini P., Centro Transfusionale e laboratorio di Ematologia, Ospedale San Gerardo, Via Solferino 16 I-20052 Monza MI, Italie.

Bouillenne C., CTS Liège, Laboratoires des Groupes Sanguins et de Transfusion, rue dos Fanchon 41, 4020 Liège, Belgique.

Boulanger M.D., CRTS, Histocompatibilité, 2, bd Tonnellé, 37044 Tours, France.

Buchs J.-P., Central Laboratory of Haematology, University of Bern, Inselspital, 3010 Bern, Suisse.

Caen J., Institut des Vaisseaux et du Sang, 6, rue Guy Patin, 75010 Paris, France.

Caillet R., Hôpital Saint-Camille, 2, rue des Pères Camilliens, 94366 Bry-sur-Marne Cedex, France.

Canepa S., CRTS, bd Tonnellé, 37020 Tours Cedex, France.

Cartron J., Hôpital Necker, 149, rue de Sèvres, 75015 Paris, France.

Cartron J.-P., INTS-INSERM U76, 6, rue Alexandre Cabanel, 75015 Paris, France.

Cavalier J., CDTS Essonne, 30, rue Boissière, 75116 Paris, France.

Cesbron Vergracht A., CRTS Nantes, Allée Charles Mirallié, BP 349, 44011 Nantes Cedex 01, France.

Coadou Y., Bureau des Colloques et Conférences, Mission de l'Information et Communication, INSERM, 101, rue de Tolbiac, 75654 Paris Cedex 13, France.

Collet C., Laboratoire d'Hématologie, CDT, BP 59, 78302 Poissy Cedex, France.

Combe S., Pharmuka, 31, rue de Fleurus, 75006 Paris, France.

Couillault G., Pédiatrie I, Oncologie Hématologie, Hôpital d'Enfants, 10, bd du Maréchal de Lattre de Tassigny, 21034 Dijon Cedex, France.

Copplestone A., Plymouth health authority, Derriford Hospital, Derriford Road, Plymouth, Devon PL6 8DH, Grande-Bretagne.

Cox A., Royal Free Hospital School of Medicine, University of London, Haemophilia Centre and Haemostasis Unit, Academic Dept of Haematology, Rowland Hill Street, London NW3 2PF, Grande-Bretagne.

Crespo A., Rhône-Poulenc Santé, Centre de Recherches, 13, quai Jules-Guesde, 94403 Vitry-sur-Seine Cedex, France.

Crespo B., 66, av. Foch, 94120 Fontenay-sous-Bois, France.

Criel A., Laboratory of Hematology, A.Z. St. Jan, Ruddershove 10, B 8000 Bruges, Belgique.

Darke C., Blood Transfusion Service, Blood Transfusion Centre, Rhydlafar, Cardiff CF 56XF, Royaume-Uni.

Deckmyn H., Center for Thrombosis and Vascular Research, K4 Leuven Campus Gasthuisberg, Herestraat 49, B 3000 Leuven, Belgique.

Dehecq E., Service d'hématologie, CHR Hôpital Calmette, rue du Pr J. Leclercq, 59000 Lille, France.

Delobel J., Laboratoire d'Hématologie, CHR Amiens, Place Victor Pauchet, BP 3006, 80030 Amiens Cedex, France.

Demetriadou K., CTS, Hôpital A. Fleming, 14, 25 Martiou Melissia, GR 15127 Athens, Grèce.

De Vries H.R., Red Cross Bloodbank, Postbox 567, 7500 An Enschede, Pays-Bas.

Doinel C., INTS 6, rue Alexandre Cabanel, 75015 Paris, France.

Dreyfus M., Hématologie, Hôpital Antoine Béclère, 157, rue de la Porte-de-Trivaux, 92140 Clamart, France.

Dubernard V., INSERM U 150, VA 334 CNRS, Hôpital Lariboisière, 8, rue Guy Patin, 75010 Paris, France.

Elias M., Red Cross Blood Bank Gronigen-Drenthe, PO Box 1191, Groningen 9701 BD, Pays-Bas.

Emonds M.-P., CTS, O.L. Urovwstraat 42, B 3000 Leuven, Belgique.

Fabris F., Istituto di Semeiotica Medica, Universita di Padova, Via Ospedale 105, 35100 Padova, Italie.

Favier R., Hôtel-Dieu, place du Parvis-Notre-Dame, 75181 Paris Cedex 04, France.

Favre-Gilly J., Service d'Hématologie Clinique, CHU Lyon-Sud, Hôpital Jules Courmont, 69310 Pierre-Bénite, France.

Felber E., Dept of Clinical Immunology, Institute of Immunology, Goethestrasse 31, 8000 Munich 2, Allemagne.

Fiat A.M., Laboratoire des Protéines, CNRS UA 11 88, 45, rue des Saints-Pères, 75270 Paris Cedex 06, France.

Finlay Louden B., Department of Haematology, St George's Hospital Medical School, Cranmer Terrace, London SW17 ORE, Grande-Bretagne.

Fournier M., Hôpital Huriez, Hématologie, place de Verdun, 59037 Lille, France.

Frachet P., INSERM U 217, Département de Recherche Fondamentale, Laboratoire d'Hématologie, CENG 85 X, 38041 Grenoble Cedex, France.

Freedman J., St Michael's Hospital, 30 Bond street, Toronto, Ontario M5B IW8, Canada.

Fromont P., CDTS Val de Marne, HLA, Hôpital Henri Mondor, 51, av. du Maréchal de Lattre de Tassigny, 94010 Créteil Cedex, France.

Gaudeau Toussaint M.F., Centre Hospitalier, Service de Biologie Médicale, 8, av. Lisse, 52000 Chaumont, France.

Goldschmeding R., Central Laboratory of the Netherlands Red Cross Blood Transfusion, Plesmanlaan 125, PO Box 9190, 1006 CX Amsterdam, Pays-Bas.

Goudemand J., Laboratoire d'Hématologie, Hôpital Claude Huriez, place de Verdun, 59037 Lille Cedex, France.

Goudemand M., CRTS, 21, rue Camille Guérin, 59012 Lille Cedex, France.

Gouin I., Central d'Hématologie, 1, place du Parvis-Notre-Dame, 75004 Paris, France.

Gozin D., Génie Cellulaire, INTS, 6, rue Alexandre Cabanel, 75015 Paris, France.

Gruel Y., Hématologie, Hôpital Trousseau, 29, bd Tonnelé, 37044 Tours Cedex, France.

Grunnet N., Regional Centre for Blood Transfusion and Clinical Immunology, Aalborg Hospital, PO Box 561, DK 9100 Aalborg, Danemark.

Gulowsen A.C., Universitetet I Oslo, Rikshospitalet, University Hospital, 0027 Oslo 1, Norvège.

Han Z.C., INSERM U 150, Hôpital Lariboisière, 8, rue Guy Patin, 75010 Paris, France.

Hardisty R.-M., Royal Free Hospital School of Medicine, Pond street, London NW3 2QG, Grande-Bretagne.

Hatzidimitriou-Papazaharia K., Blood Transfusion Service, Evangelismos Hospital, Himitou 119, Pagrati 116 - 33 Athens, Grèce.

Hegde U.M., Ealing Hospital, Uxbridge Road, Southall. Middx, UB1 3EU London, Grande-Bretagne.

Hourdille P., Hôpital Cardiologique, Laboratoire d'Hémobiologie, 33604 Pessac, France.

Hovig T., JNST. Pathology, Rikshospitalet, Oslo 1, Norvège.

Hurtaud M.F., Hôpital Robert Debré, 48, bd Sérurier, 75019 Paris, France.

Jansz A., Bloedbank Midden Brabant, Hilvarenbeekseweg 60, 5022 GC Tilburg, Pays-Bas.

Janvier D., Hôpital Saint-Louis, Hémobiologie, 9, rue Taylor, 75010 Paris, France.

Jude B., Laboratoire d'Hématologie, Hôpital Calmette, rue du Pr. J. Leclercq, 59000 Lille Cedex, France.

Kahf S., Biotest Ag, Landsteinerstrasse 5, 6072 Dreieich, Allemagne.

Kekomaki R., Medical Services, Finnish Red Cross Blood Transfusion Service, Kivihaantie 7, SF 00310 Helsinki, Finlande.

Kehrel B., Medizinische Klinik, Experimentelle Hamostase Forschung, Domagkstr 3, 4400 Munster, Allemagne.

Kohl J., Medizinische Hochschule Hannover, Institut für Medizinische Mikrobiologie, Konstanty Gutschowstr. 8, 3000 Hannover 61, Allemagne.

Kontopoulou G.I., RTC Hippokration General Hospital, 114 Vas Sophias St, 115 27 Athens, Grèce.

Kretzschmar T., Medizinische Hoschule Hannover, Institut für Medizinische Mikrobiologie, Konstanty Gutschowstr.8, 3000 Hannover 61, Allemagne.

Kroll H., Klinikum der Justus Liebig Universität, Institut für Klinische, Immunologie und Transfusions Medizin, Langhansstrasse 7, 6300 Giessen, Allemagne.

Kronenberg A., Medizinische Klinik A, Experimentelle Haemostasiologie, Domagkstr. 3 Altbau, 4400 Munster, Allemagne.

Krusius T., Medical Services, Finnich Red Cross Blood Transfusion Service, Kivihaantie 7, SF 00310 Helsinki, Finlande.

Kuijpers R.W.A.M., Centr. Lab. of Netherlands, Red Cross Blood Transfusion Service, Plesmanlaan 125, 1066 CX Amsterdam, Pays-Bas.

Lafay M., Laboratoire de Biochimie-Hormonologie, Hôpital Robert Debré, 48, bd Sérurier, 75019 Paris, France.

Lalau Keraly C., INSERM U 313, Hôpital Pitié-Salpêtrière, 91, bd de l'Hôpital, 75013 Paris, France.

Lamare O., Rhône-Poulenc Santé, Centre de Recherches, 13, quai Jules-Guesde, 94403 Vitry-sur-Seine Cedex, France.

Lambermont M., SVC Immunologie Transfusion, Hôpital Universitaire Erasme, 808 route de Lennik, 1070 Bruxelles, Belgique.

Laurent P.E., Laboratoires Lafon, 19, av. du Pr Cadiot, BP 22, 94701 Maisons-Alfort Cedex, France.

Lauwers S., Centraal Laboratorium, Frankryklei 67-69, B 2000 Antwerpen, Belgique.

Legrand C., INSERM U 150, Hôpital Lariboisière, 8, rue Guy Patin, 75010 Paris, France.

Legrand Y., Unité de Recherches sur les Vaisseaux et l'Hémostase, INSERM U 150, Hôpital Lariboisière, 6, rue Guy Patin, 75475 Paris Cedex 10, France.

Lenhard, Landsteinerstrasse 5, 6072 Dreieich, Allemagne.

Lubenko A., National Blood Transfusion Service, North London Blood Transfusion Centre, Colindale Avenue, London NW9 5BG, Grande-Bretagne.

Lucas G.F., Blood Group Reference Laboratory, Regional Transfusion Centre, Southmead Road, Bristol BS 10 SND, Grande-Bretagne.

Luo S. K., Hôtel-Dieu, 1, place du Parvis-Notre-Dame, 75004 Paris, France.

Magalhaes Brito S., North London Blood Transfusion Centre, Colindale Av., London, NW9 5BG Grande-Bretagne.

Manbelbrot L., Hôpital Cochin, Maternité Port Royal, 123, bd Port-Royal, 75014 Paris, France.

Matthieu F., Service de Transfusion, Keizcrlyk Plein 45, Alost 9300, Belgique.

Mayr W.R., Institut für Transfuzionsmedizin der Medizinischen Einrichtungen der Rhein Westf Techn Hochschule Aachen, Pauwelsstrasse, 5100 Aachen, Allemagne.

Meenaghan M., South West Regional Transfusion Centre, Southmead Road, Bristol BS10 5ND, Grande-Bretagne.

Mercier P., Laboratoire d'Histocompatibilité, CTS, 149, bd Baille, 13392 Marseille Cedex 5, France.

Metzelaar M., Dept of Haematology, University Hospital Utrecht, Heidelberglaan 100, GO3.647 Utrecht, 3584 CX, Pays-Bas.

Meyer D., INSERM U 143, Hôpital de Bicêtre, 78, rue du Général Leclerc, 94270 Le Kremlin-Bicêtre, France.

Mibashan R.S., King's College School of Medicine and Dentistry of King's College London, Department of Haematological Medicine, Prenatal Diagnosis/Haemophilia Centre, Bessemer Road, London SE5 9PJ, Grande-Bretagne.

Montagnani G., Servizio Immunoematologia, Policlinico, Via del Pozzo 71, 41053 Modena, Italie.

Morell A., Medical department, Central Laboratory Blood Transfusion Service, Swiss Red Cross, Wankdorfstrasse 10, 3000 Bern 22, Suisse.

Muniz Diaz E., Servei d'Hemoterapia, Hospital de Sant Pau, C/Praga 4, 3º 4a, 08024 Barcelona, Espagne.

Murphy S., Thomas Jefferson University Hospital Cardeza, Foundation for hematologic Research, 1015 Walnut Street, Philadelphia, PA 19107, USA.

Murphy W., South East Scotland Blood Transfusion Service, Royal Infirmary of Edinburgh, Lauriston place, Edinburgh EH3 9HB, Royaume-Uni.

Muylle L., Centre de Transfusion, Wilrijk straat 8, B 2520 Edegem, Belgique.

Nieves Puig Alcaraz, Centro de Transfusion de la Comunidad Valenciana, Av del Cid 65, 46014 Valencia, Espagne.

Nordhagen R., Dept of Immunology, National Inst of Public Health(siff), Geitmyrsvein 75, 0462 Oslo 4, Norvège.

Oksenhendler, Service d'Immunologie Hématologie, Hôpital Saint-Louis, 1, av. Claude Vellefaux, 75475 Paris Cedex 10, France.

Oksman F., CRTS, CHU, Hôpital Purpan, Service d'immunologie, 31052 Toulouse Cedex, France.

Olsson I., Stockholm County Council, Blood Transfusion Service, Box 38100, S-100 64 Stockholm, Suède.

Oyonarte S., Laboratorio de Inmunohematologia, Centro Regional de Transfusion Sanguinea de Granada, c/ Dr Mesa Moles s/n, Granada 18012, Espagne.

Pamphilon D., South West Regional Transfusion Centre, Southmead Road, Bristol BS 10 5ND, Grande-Bretagne.

Parise P., Central d'Hématologie DMI, Centre Hospitalier Universitaire Vaudois, BH 18, 1011 Lausanne, Suisse.

Pedersen T.M., Research Institute for Internal Medicine, Rikshospitalet, 0027 Oslo 1, Norvège.

Peltier F., Bio Transfusion, Z.A. Courtabeuf, BP 99, 91943 Les Ulis Cedex A, France.

Perrier P., Laboratoire d'Immuno-hématologie, CRTS, 9-11, rue Lionnois, 54052 Nancy Cedex, France.

Poissonnier M.H., Hôpital Saint-Vincent de Paul, 74 av. Denfert Rochereau, 75014 Paris, France.

Poncelet P., Hématologie, Faculté de Pharmacie, 27, bd Jean Moulin, 13385 Marseille, France.

Poplovsky J.L., CTS, CHU du Sarttilman, 4000 Liège, Belgique.

Potron G., Hématologie, Hôpital Robert Debré, rue Alexis Carrel, 51092 Reims Cedex, France.

Prel L.I., Blood Bank of Lower Saxony, Institut Rotenburg/wn, Bothel, Duesterneichen 252, D 2725 Allemagne.

Qader C.L., Trent Regional Health Authority, Blood Transfusion Service, Longley Lane, Sheffield S5 7 JN, Grande-Bretagne.

Ribera A., Immunohematology dept, Blood Transfusion Center Vall d'Hebron, Alta de Pedrell 74 1er 3e, 08032 Barcelona, Espagne.

Romet-Lemone J.L., CNTS, 3, av. des Tropiques, 91943 Les Ulis, France.

Saelman E., Dept Hematology, University Hospital Utrecht, Heidelberglaan 100, G 0347 Utrecht, 3584 CX, Pays-Bas.

Saito N., INSERM U 150, Hôpital Lariboisière, 6, rue Guy Patin, 75475 Cedex 10, France.

Salmon C., INTS, 6, rue Alexandre Cabanel, 75015 Paris, France.

Samama M.M., Hôtel-Dieu, 1, place du Parvis-Notre-Dame, 75004 Paris, France.

Sartiaux C., Immunologie cellulaire et cytométrie flux, CRTS, 19-21, rue C. Guérin, BP 2018, 59012 Lille Cedex, France.

Schneider P., Croix Rouge Suisse, CTS, rue du Bugnon 27, 1005 Lausanne, Suisse.

Schwartz D., Institut für Blutgruppenserologie, Univ. Wien, Spitalg. 4, A-1090 Wien, Autriche.

Sciorelli, Societa Italiana Farmaceutici Ravizza, 77063 Isola A Mella Scala, Via Camagre, 41-43, Verona, Italie.

Scrobohaci M.L., INSERM U 150, Hôpital Saint-Louis, 2, place du Dr A. Fournier, 75475 Paris Cedex 10, France.

Sedivy P., Biologie Cardiovasculaire, Rhône-Poulenc Santé, Centre de Recherches de Vitry-Alfortville, 13, quai Jules-Guesde, BP 14, 91403 Vitry-sur-Seine Cedex, France.

Sellers J., Welsh Regional Blood Transfusion Centre, Rhydlafar, Cardiff South Glamorgan CF5 6XF, Royaume-Uni.

Sermasi G., Ospedale S. Orsola Centro Trasfus, Via Massarenti 9, 40138 Bologna, Italie.

Servais B., Diagnostics Transfusion, 3, bd Raymond Poincaré, B.P. 20, 92430 Marnes-La-Coquette, France.

Sklavou S., Hippokration General Hospital, Blood Bank, 114 Vas Sophias st, 115 27 Athens, Grèce.

Skogen B., Immunological Dept and Blood Bank, 9012 Regiosykehuset I Tromso, Norvège.

Spycher M., Central Laboratory, Blood Transfusion Service SRC, Wanktdorstrasse 10, CH-3000 Bern 22, Suisse.

Stenzinger W., Medizinische Universitätklinik, Abteilung A, Albert Schweitzer Str. 33, 4400 Munster, Allemagne.

Strada P., Ospedale Galliera Centro Trasfus, Mura Delle Cappuccine 14, 16128 Genova, Italie.

Sultan Y., Hémostase, Hôpital Cochin, 27, rue du Faubourg-Saint-Jacques, 75014 Paris, France.

Taylor P., Biochemistry Research Dept, Ciba-Geigy Pharmaceuticals, Wimblehurst Road, Horsham, West Sussex, RH 12 4AB, Grande-Bretagne.

Terrier E., Centre de Transfusion, Hôpital Broussais, 96, rue Didot, 75014 Paris, France.

Testi M., CNTS CRI, Via B. Ramazzini 15, 00151 Roma, Italie.

Thomson A., North London Blood Transfusion Centre, Colindale Av, London NW9 5BG, Grande-Bretagne.

Tongio M.-M., CTS, 10, rue Spielmann, 67085 Strasbourg, France.

Toulon P., Laboratoire d'Hématologie, Hôpital Cochin, 27, rue du Faubourg-Saint-Jacques, 75014 Paris, France.

Tsakiris D., Coagulation and Fibrinolysis Laboratory, Kantonsspital Basel, 4031 Basel, Suisse.

Uzan A., Rhône-Poulenc Santé, Centre de Recherches de Vitry-Alfortville, 90, rue Marcel Bourdarias, BP 118, 94143 Alfortville Cedex, France.

Valentin N., CTS Nantes, Allée Charles Miraillié, 44000 Nantes, France.

Van Agthoven A., Immunotech S.A., Case 915, Domaine de Luminy, 13268 Marseille, France.

Vanderplaj G., RC BloodBank Arnhem, PB 3151, 6802 Arnhem, Pays-Bas.

Vanhaesbroucke C., Service d'hémobiologie, Hôpital Cardiologique, Avenue Leclerq, 59000 Lille, France.

Van Hove L., Department of Haematology, University Hospital Leuven, Herestraat 49, 3000 Leuven, Belgique.

Van Vliet H.H.D.M., Hematological Laboratory, University Hospital Rotterdam-Dijkzigt, Dr Molewaterplein 40, 3015 GD Rotterdam, Pays-Bas.

Varga M., National Institute of Haematology and Blood Transfusion, 24, Daroczi út, 1502 Budapest, Hongrie.

Verhallen P.F.J., Scherin Ag, Herz Kreislauf Pharmakologie, Postfach 650311, D-1000 Berlin 65, Allemagne.

Vicariot M., Hôpital Augustin Morvan, Hématologie, 29279 Brest Cedex, France.

Von Felten A., Laboratory of Blood Coagulation, Room D-Lab 28, University Hospital, CH-8091 Zurich, Suisse.

Westerterp-Maas A., Red Cross Blood Bank Gronigen-Drenthe, PO Box 1191, Groningen 9701 BD, Pays-Bas.

Wikman A., Stockholm County Council, Blood Transfusion Service, Box 38100, S-100 64 Stockholm, Suède.

Wilmer M., Medizinische Klinik A, Experimentelle Haemostasiologie, Domagkstrasse 3 (Altbau), 4400 Munster, Allemagne.

Zupanska B., Laboratory for Platelet and Leucocyte Immunology, Institute of Haematology, 5 Chocimska Street, 00957 Warsaw, Pologne.

Contents
Sommaire

VII Acknowledgements
VIII *Remerciements*
IX   Preface
X   *Préface*
XI   List and addresses of contributors
     Liste et adresses des auteurs
XV   List and addresses of participants
     Liste et adresses des participants

CELLULAR AND MOLECULAR BIOLOGY
OF THE PLATELET GLYCOPROTEINS
*BIOLOGIE CELLULAIRE ET MOLECULAIRE
DES GLYCOPROTEINES PLAQUETTAIRES*

3   **N. Debili, W. Vainchenker, J. Guichard, L. Edelman, J. Breton-Gorius**
    Immunolocalization of platelet glycoproteins Ib, IIb-IIIa and IV during megakaryocyte differentiation
    Immunolocalisation des glycoprotéines plaquettaires Ib, IIb-IIIa et IV pendant la différenciation mégacaryocytaire

17 **Z. Han, S. Bellucci, D. Pidard, J.P. Caen**
    Coexpression in the same cell in marrow culture of antigens from erythroid and megakaryocytic lineage
    Coexpression, dans la même cellule médullaire en culture, d'antigènes des lignées érythroïde et mégacaryocytaire

19 **K.J. Clemetson, R.H. Wenger, J.M. Clemetson, J. Drouin**
    Biochemistry and molecular biology of the platelet membrane glycoprotein Ib complex and the Bernard-Soulier syndrome

Biologie moléculaire et biochimie du complexe membranaire plaquettaire GPIb et le syndrome de Bernard-Soulier

31 **G. Uzan, M.H. Prandini, M. Prenant, F. Martin, G. Marguerie**
Megakaryocyte specific expression of human platelet GPIIb gene
Expression du gène de la GPIIb dans la mégacaryocyte

41 **B. Catimel, S. Parmentier, L.K.K. Leung, J.L. McGregor**
Molecular and cellular biology of glycoprotein IIIb (GPIV, CD36)
Biologie moléculaire et cellulaire de la GPIIIb (GPIV, CD36)

55 **R.P. McEver**
GMP-140, an inducible receptor for leukocytes on platelets and endothelium
Structure et fonction de la glycoprotéine GMP-140, récepteur inductible sur les plaquettes et l'endothélium

63 **S. Parmentier, L. McGregor, J.L. McGregor**
A new family of cell-cell adhesion molecules : ELAM-1, GP90^{MEL-14} and GMP-140
Une nouvelle famille de molécules responsables de l'adhésion intercellulaire : ELAM-1, GP90^{MEL-14} et GMP-140

75 **A. Sonnenberg, P.W. Modderman, P. van der Geer, M. Aumailley, R. Timpl**
Structure and function of platelet glycoprotein IC-IIa (VLA-6)
Structure et fonction des glycoprotéines plaquettaires IC-IIa (VLA-6)

EFFECTS OF MONOCLONAL ANTIBODIES ON PLATELET RECEPTORS – REGULATION OF PLATELET-VESSEL WALL INTERACTIONS
EFFETS DES ANTICORPS MONOCLONAUX SUR LES RECEPTEURS PLAQUETTAIRES. REGULATION DES INTER-ACTIONS PLAQUETTE-PAROI CAPILLAIRE

99 **M.J. Rabiet, C. Boudignon, D. Gulino, J.J. Ryckewaert, A. Andrieux, G. Marguerie**
A monoclonal antibody against platelet GPIIb/IIIa interacts with a calcium binding site and induces fibrinogen binding and platelet aggregation
Un anticorps monoclonal dirigé contre les GPIIb/IIIa plaquettaires interagit avec un site de liaison du calcium et induit la liaison du fibrinogène et l'agrégation plaquettaire

109 **T. Lecompte, R. Favier, F. Potevin, M.-C. Morel, S.-K. Luo, C. Kaplan, M.M. Samama**
Anti-platelet monoclonal activating or inhibitory antibodies to probe the functions and regulations of the glycoprotein IIb-IIIa complex
Des anticorps monoclonaux antiplaquettaires activateurs ou inhibiteurs pour explorer les fonctions et les régulations des complexes glycoprotéiques IIb-IIIa

129 **A.I. Schafer**
Regulation of platelet-vessel wall interactions by the fibrinolytic system
Régulation des interactions plaquettes-paroi vasculaire par le système fibrinolytique

INHERITED THROMBOPATHIES
TROMBOPATHIES HEREDITAIRES

139 **A.T. Nurden, M. Pico, D. Fournier, V. Jallu, D. Lacaze, P. Hourdillé**
Glanzmann's thrombasthenia : a general introduction with comments on specific cases
Thrombasthénie de Glanzmann : introduction générale et commentaires sur des cas particuliers

153 **N. Schlegel, M.-C. Morel, T. Lecompte, M.-F. Hurtaud, C. Kaplan**
New cases of Glanzmann's thrombasthenia. Familial studies
Nouveaux cas de thrombasthénie de Glanzmann. Etudes familiales

161 **M.-C. Morel-Kopp, T. Lecompte, N. Schlegel, P. Hivert, C. Kaplan**
Use of murine monoclonal antibodies to study thrombopathies related to GPIIb-IIIa complexes
Utilisation d'anticorps monoclonaux murins pour étudier les thrombopathies liées au complexe GPIIb-IIIa

173 **I. Djaffar, D. Vilette, J.-L. Wautier, J.-P. Rosa**
Molecular aspects of Glanzmann's thrombasthenia
Aspects moléculaires de la thrombasthénie de Glanzmann

CLINICAL IMPLICATIONS OF PLATELET IMMUNOLOGY
IMPLICATIONS CLINIQUES DE L'IMMUNOLOGIE PLAQUETTAIRE

187 **J.-P. Dessaint, A. Tsicopoulos, V. Pancré, M. Joseph, J.-C. Ameisen, A.-B. Tonnel, A. Capron**
Platelets, IgE and allergy
Plaquettes, IgE et allergie

195 **P. Clezardin, E. Alfaro, J. Grange, C. Desgranges, C. Kaplan, P. Delmas, M. Dechavanne**
Thrombospondin binding by human osteosarcoma cells : relationship to platelet-aggregating activity of osteosarcoma cells
Liaison de la thrombospondine aux cellules humaines d'ostéosarcome : relation avec l'activité agrégante plaquettaire des cellules d'ostéosarcome

209 **H. Boukerche, O. Berthier-Vergnes, E. Tabone, J.L. Mc Gregor**
The role of cytoadhesins in mediating platelet-melanoma cell interaction and *in vivo* melanoma tumor growth
Le rôle des cyto-adhésines dans l'interaction plaquette-cellule de mélanome et dans la croissance in vivo *de la tumeur*

219 **A.E.G. Kr. von dem Borne, R.W.A.M. Kuijpers**
Platelet antigens, new aspects
Antigènes plaquettaires, nouveaux aspects

241 **S. Santoso, V. Kiefel, C. Mueller-Eckhardt**
Platelet glycoproteins IIa, IIIa and Ib carry blood group A and B determinants
Les glycoprotéines plaquettaires IIa, IIIa et Ib portent les déterminants des groupes sanguins A et B

249 **C. Mueller-Eckhardt, H. Kroll, V. Kiefel and the members of the European PTP Study Group**
Posttransfusion purpura
Le purpura post-transfusionnel

257 **F. Forestier. F. Daffos, Y. Solé, N. Catherine, P. Champeix, C. Kaplan**
Fetal primary hemostasis
Hémostase primaire fœtale

267 **C. Kaplan, F. Daffos, F. Forestier, M.C. Morel, N. Chesnel, G. Tchernia**
Current trends in neonatal alloimmune thrombocytopenia : Diagnosis and therapy

Thrombopénies néonatales allo-immunes : actualités thérapeutiques et diagnostiques

279 **A.H. Waters, R.S. Mibashan, K.H. Nicolaides, M.F. Murphy, R. Ireland, H.W.H. Pullon**
Management of fetal alloimmune thrombocytopenia : the place of intrauterine platelet transfusions
Traitement de la thrombocytopénie fœtale allo-immune : la place des transfusions plaquettaires intra-utérines

287 **J.B. Bussel**
Antenatal treatment of neonatal alloimmune thrombocytopenia with intravenous gammaglobulin
Traitement anté-natal de la thrombocytopénie néonatale allo-immune par l'injection intraveineuse de gammaglobulines

297 **V. Kiefel, S. Santoso, C. Mueller-Eckhardt**
Antibody detection in autoimmune thrombocytopenic purpura
Anticorps dans le purpura thrombopénique auto-immun

305 **D.S. Beardsley, B.Y. Thompson**
Autoimmune platelet destruction in pregnancy and its relationship to neonatal thrombocytopenia
Destruction plaquettaire auto-immune pendant la grossesse et corrélation avec la thrombopénie néonatale

315 **G. Tchernia, C. Kaplan, F. Daffos, G. Tertian, F. Forestier, M. Dreyfus, N. Catherine**
Autoimmune thrombocytopenic purpura and pregnancy : from threat to routine, a new danger ?
Purpura thrombocytopénique auto-immun et grossesse : de la menace à la routine : un nouveau danger ?

Cellular and molecular biology of platelet glycoproteins

Biologie cellulaire et moléculaire des glycoprotéines plaquettaires

Immunolocalization of platelet glycoproteins Ib, IIb-IIIa and IV during megakaryocyte differentiation

N. Debili, W. Vainchenker, J. Guichard, L. Edelman* and J. Breton-Gorius

INSERM U 91, Hôpital Henri Mondor, 94010 Créteil, France
* Institut Pasteur, 25, rue du Dr Roux, 75724 Paris cedex 15, France

INTRODUCTION

It is well established that platelet glycoproteins (Gp) play an essential role in platelet physiology. These Gps are synthesized by megakaryocytes (MK). Since MK represent less than 0.05% of all bone marrow cells and are difficult to purify in large quantities, the biosynthesis and processing of Gp Ib-IX (Lopez et al., 1987; 1988; Hickey et al., 1989) and Gp IIb-IIIa (Bray et al., 1987; Silver et al., 1987; Duperray et al., 1987, Rosa et al., 1988) have been recently studied with either a leukemic continuous cell line, HEL cells or from MK growing from peripheral blood progenitors obtained from patients with chronic myeloid leukemia. Only a few studies have been performed on normal maturing MK (Jenkis et al., 1986; Debili et al., 1990).

It was shown by immunofluorescence using monoclonal antibodies (MoAb) that Gp IIb-IIIa are expressed on the promegakaryoblast membrane very early during maturation at day 5 of culture, while Gp Ib appears later (Vinci et al., 1984). Recent studies have provided evidence that demarcation membranes (DM) of MK exhibit the same Gps as the cell membrane; however, Gps are present on the cell membrane before the production of DM (Debili et al., 1990).

Platelet Gp IV (also referred to as Gp IIIb) can be identified by several MoAbs characterized at the Fourth International Workshop on human leukocyte differentiation antigens (Knapp et al., 1989) and has now been designated as CD36. FA6-152 MoAb which was obtained by immunizing mice with fetal human red cells (Edelman et al., 1986) reacts with an 88 KDa cell surface Gp which is immunologically related to the platelet Gp IV (Kieffer et al., 1989). Using FA6-152 MoAb, it was shown that this Gp appears late in MK maturation since promegakaryoblasts were weakly labeled or unlabeled (Edelman et al., 1986).

The aim of the present work was to compare these results with the expression of membrane Gp Ib, IIb-IIIa and IV on MK maturing in liquid culture from normal bone marrow using double ultrastructural immunogold labeling. Furthermore, we examined the possibility that different growth factors might modulate this expression.

MATERIALS AND METHODS

Materials and cell culture

Bone marrow aspirates were obtained from normal adult donors for bone marrow transplantation. The method of cell culture was previously reported (Debili et al., 1990). Briefly, light-density cells were separated by density centrifugation on Ficoll-metrizoate (d = 1.077). Adherent cells were eliminated by adherence to plastic. The remaining cells were cultured in suspension in Iscove's modified Dubelcco's medium supplemented with 10% plasma from aplastic patients (AP). AP was prepared from heparinized blood of patients who had undergone a bone marrow transplantation and who were markedly thrombocytopenic at the time of blood collection. The results obtained with AP were compared to AP supplemented with rhIL3 (100 U/ml), rhGM-CSF (2 ng/ml) or rhEpo (2 U/ml). Beginning on day 6, adherent cells were eliminated by daily transfer of supernatants into new culture flasks. Cell culture was performed for 7 and 11 days in tissue culture flasks (Corning Glasswork Co., N.Y.) at 37° C in a 5% CO_2 fully humidified atmosphere.

Antibodies used: They are listed in Table 1.

Table 1

Antibody	Mouse monoclonal	Rabbit polyclonal	Specificity	Origin	
Anti-glycocalicin	-	+	Gp Ib	Wicki and Clemetson,	1985
Anti-Gp IIb-IIIa	-	+	Gp IIb-IIIa	Cramer et al.,	1990
FA6-152	+	-	Gp IV	Edelman et al.,	1986
				Kieffer et al.,	1989

Ultrastructural and immunogold staining

10^7 unfixed cells obtained on days 7 and 11 of culture were incubated for 1 h at 4° C with a mixture of the following antibodies (dilution 1/50):

1. A polyclonal antibody against glycocalicin and FA6-152
2. A polyclonal antibody against Gp IIb-IIIa and FA6-152

After two washes in cold buffer, a mixture of goat anti-rabbit IgG coupled to 5 nm gold particles and goat anti-mouse IgG coupled to 15 nm gold particles (Janssen Pharmateutica, Beerse, Belgium) was added for 1 h at 4° C.

The cells were then fixed with 1.25% glutaraldehyde for 10 min., incubated in diaminobenzidine (DAB) medium to detect platelet peroxidase (PPO) (Breton-Gorius et al., 1984), post-fixed with osmium tetroxide, dehydrated, and embedded in epon. Thin sections were examined with a Philips electron microscope CM10 after lead citrate staining.

Flow cytometry

Cultured cells were fixed for 20 minutes with 1% paraformaldehyde. A mixture of the polyclonal antibody against Gp IIb-IIIa and FA6-152 was applied as above. Cells were washed and incubated with goat IgG directed against rabbit IgG and coupled to phycoerythrine and sheep Fab'$_2$ against mouse IgG and coupled to fluorescein (Southern Biotechnology, Birmingham, Alab.) After washing the cells were analyzed with an ATC 3000 (Bruker, Wissembourg, France).

RESULTS

Ultrastructural immunolabeling of MK growing in the presence of AP alone or with AP supplemented with rhGM-CSF or rhEpo.

A minimum of twenty MK were examined for each condition of culture after double labeling using either the anti-glycocalicin polyclonal antibody and FA6-152 or the anti-Gp IIb-IIIa polyclonal antibody and FA6-152.

On day 7, in all conditions of culture, promegakaryoblasts exhibited single labeling either for Gp IIb-IIIa (Fig. 1) or for Gp Ib (Fig. 2) but there was never a colabeling for Gp IV. In these experiments, the membranes of macrophages were labeled serving as a positive control for Gp IV (Fig. 1). Promegakaryoblasts were small (8-10 µ), rarely showed DM or α-granules, but contained large mitochondria. The nucleus was round or indented and frequently exhibited a large nucleolus. Some cells were in mitosis or endomitosis (Fig. 1).The PPO reaction was inconsistently detected in liquid culture. For unknown reasons, PPO appears in MK in some cultures but not others. A few MK were present. They were large and fully mature exhibiting numerous DM and α-granules. They probably arose from the bone marrow promegakaryoblasts that had been put into culture on day 0 and not from CFU-MK since such large MK were absent from cultures initially depleted of Gp IIb-IIIa-positive cells (data not shown).

On day 11, there was no difference between the size, the morphology, and the labeling of MK cultured with AP alone, or AP supplemented with rh-GM-CSF or rhEpo. The size of MK varied from 10 µ to 30 µ and the majority of them were fully mature, containing DM, α-granules, small mitochondria and aggregates of glycogen particles. PPO was present in some cultures and absent from others without any relationship with the growth factors added. In large MK, the nucleus was polylobulated while it was round or indented in small MK. A minority of promegakaryoblats were found.`

There was no difference in the intensity of labeling between large and small mature MK.

About 55% of MK exhibited a labeling for only Gp IIb-IIIa while 60% exhibited labeling only for Gp Ib (Fig. 3). This labeling was present both on the cell membrane and on DM which were localized at the cell periphery; these studies were performed by the pre-embedding method (Fig. 3). As previously shown (Debili et al., 1990), antibodies cannot penetrate to the inner cytoplasm of living cells; however, when the labeling was performed by the post-embedding method on thin sections, all DM showed a labeling.

In 45% of MK, Gp IV was co-localized with Gp IIb-IIIa while 55 % of MK expressed only Gp IIb-IIIa. In 40% of MK there was a co-localization of Gp Ib and Gp IV (Fig. 4, 5) while 60 % of MK exhibited a labeling only for Gp Ib. The intensity of the labeling for Gp IV was always weak even in the fully mature MK and exhibited peripheral microfilaments (Fig. 5).

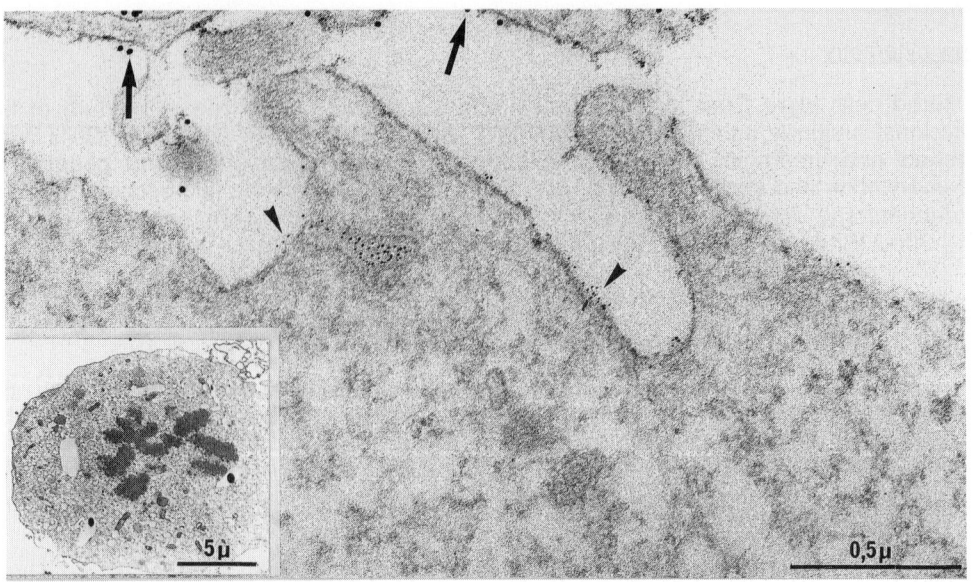

Fig. 1 A promegakaryoblast cultured for 7 days with AP + rhGM-CSF, immunolabeled for Gp IIb-IIIa and Gp IV. This cell viewed in inset is in mitosis or endomitosis. The enlargement shows no platelet organelles. The plasma membrane is labeled by small gold particles (arrow heads), indicating the presence of only Gp IIb - IIIa. A macrophage located above exhibits labeling by large gold particles (arrows) which corresponds to the presence of Gp IV.

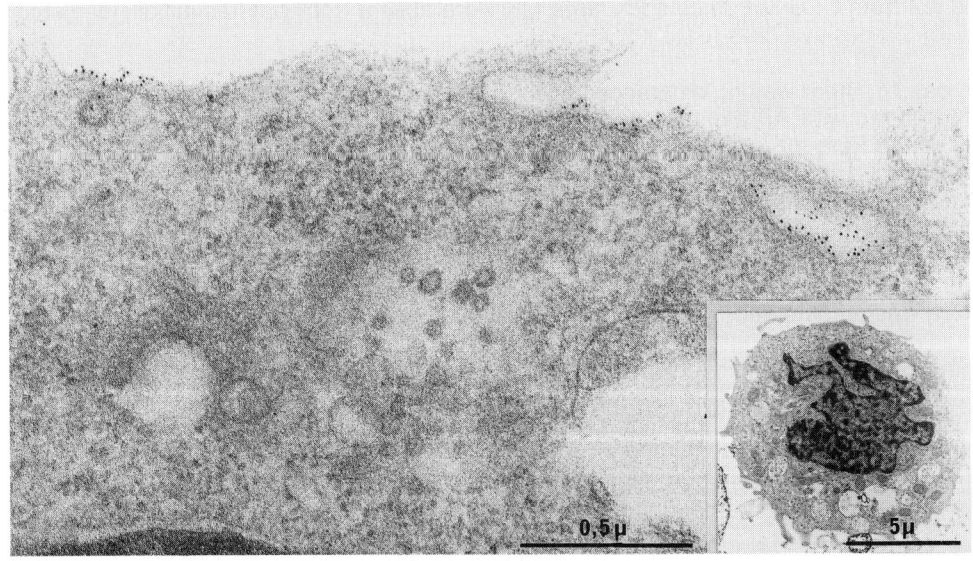

Fig. 2 A promegakaryoblast cultured for 7 days with AP + rhEpo, immunolabeled for Gp Ib and Gp IV. The cell seen in inset shows an indented nucleus. The cell surface is only labeled by small gold particles, corresponding to the binding of anti-glycocalin antibody. The lack of large gold particles indicates the absence of Gp IV.

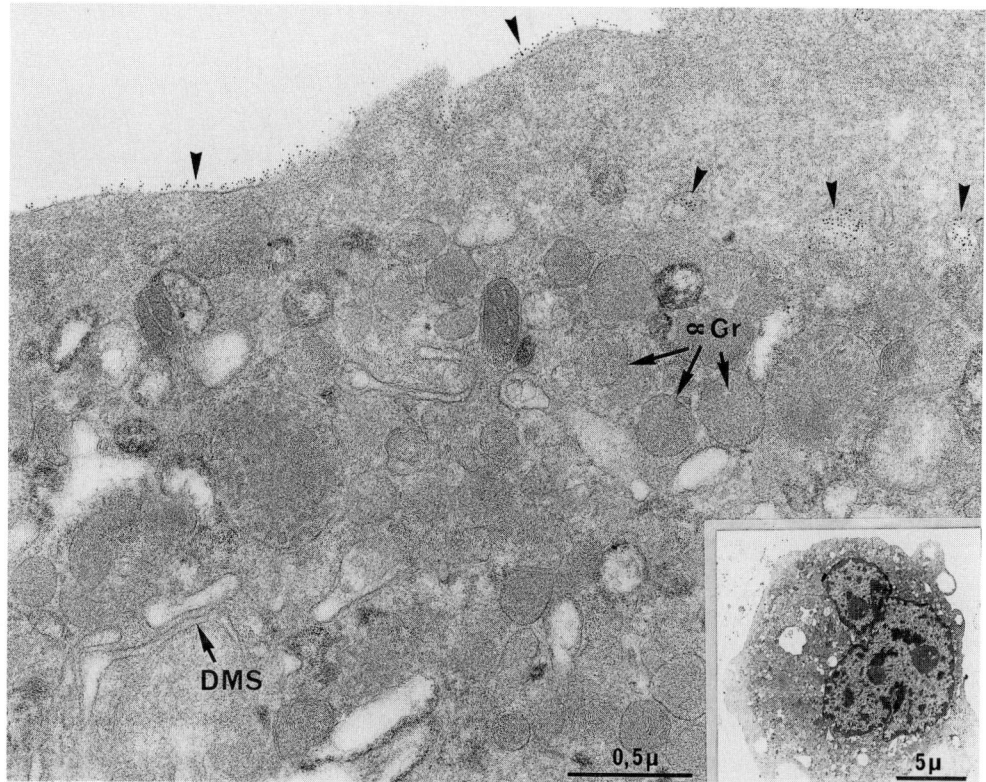

Fig. 3 A mature MK cultured for 11 days with AP, immunolabeled for Gp Ib and Gp IV. This large cell has a polylobulated nucleus. The enlargement shows numerous α-granules (α-gr), small mitochondria, multivesicular bodies and the demarcation membrane system (DMS).
Platelet peroxidase reactivity is seen by the dense reaction product in the endoplasmic reticulum. The cell membrane and DMS located close to the periphery are labeled exclusively for Gp Ib (arrow heads).

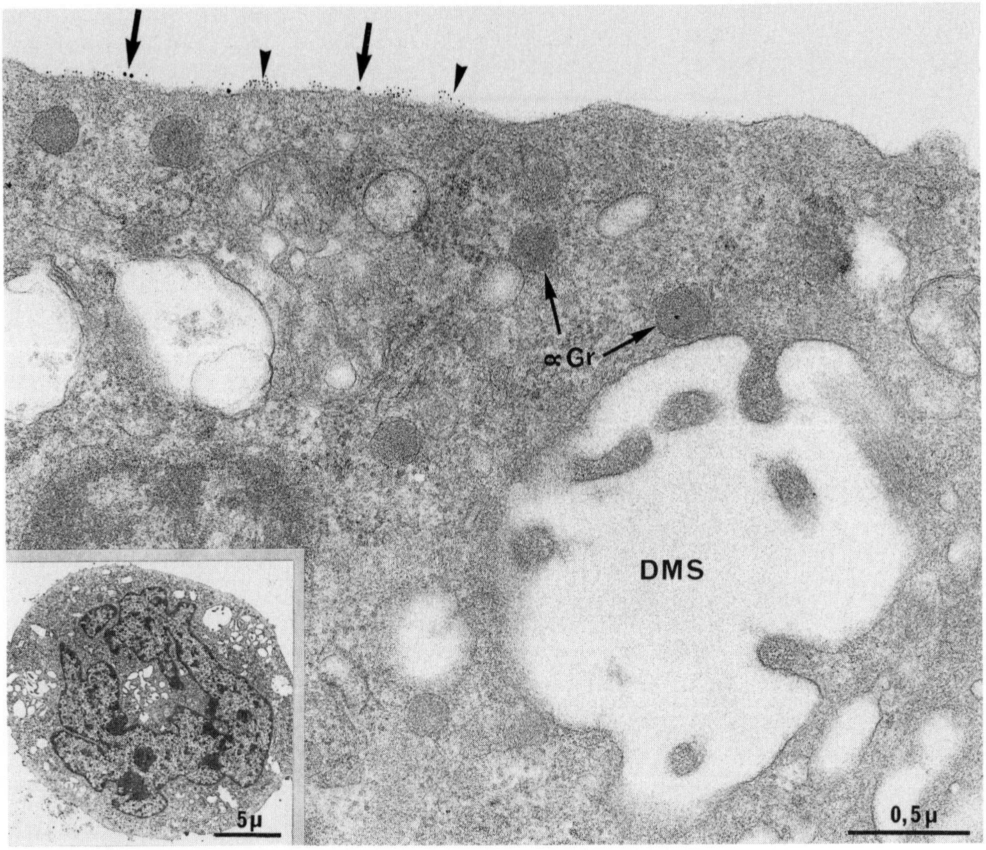

Fig. 4 A megakaryocyte cultured for 11 days with AP and, immunolabelled for Gp Ib and Gp IV. MK, viewed in inset, possesses a highly polylobulated nucleus and exhibits several groups of demarcation membrane system. An enlargement shows α-granules (α-gr) and the demarcation membrane system (DMS). Small gold particles (arrow heads) which visualized Gp Ib antigen are more numerous than large particles (arrows) which represent the Gp IV sites.

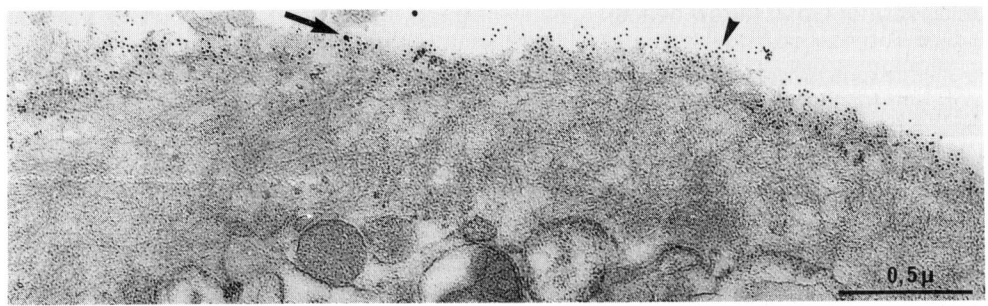

Fig 5 Enlarged portion of a mature MK treated as in Fig. 4.
This fully mature MK shows in the cell periphery numerous microfilaments. The numerous small gold particles (arrow head) indicate a strong labeling for Gp Ib while very few large gold particles represent a minimum of sites for Gp IV (arrow).

Ultrastructural immunolabeling of MK growing in the presence of AP supplemented with rhIL3.

On day 7, 80% of promegakaryoblasts exhibited only Gp IIb-IIIa; however, in contrast to cells cultured with AP alone or with AP + rhGM-CSF, or rhEpo, 20% of them expressed both Gp IIb-IIIa and Gp IV. All promegakaryoblasts were labeled both for Gp Ib and Gp IV (Fig. 6). The ultrastructure of double stained cells did not differ from that growing with AP alone.

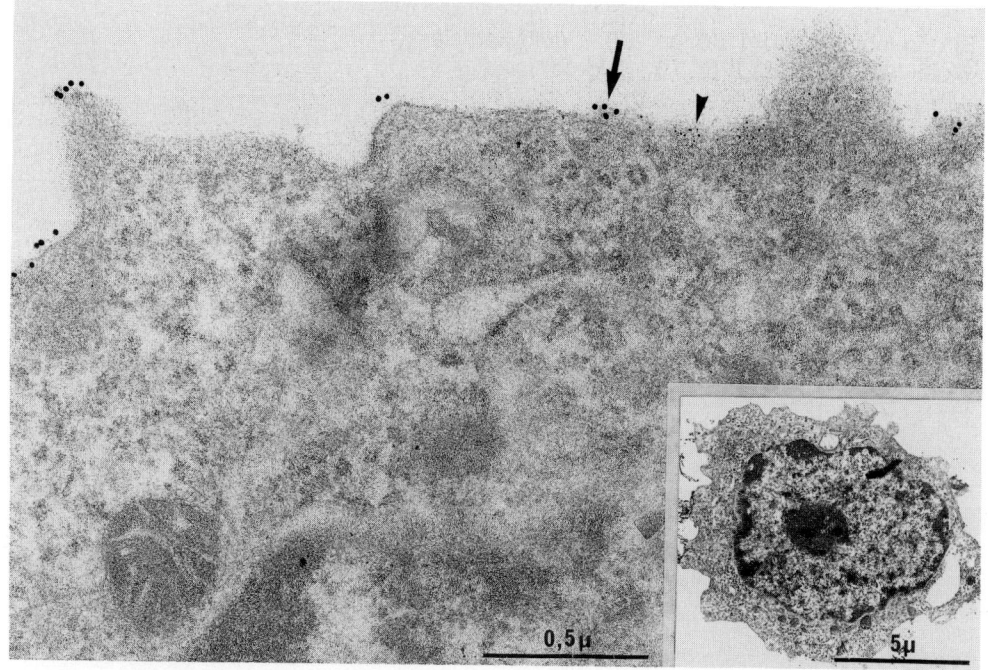

Fig. 6 A promegakaryoblast cultured 7 days with AP + rhIL3, immunolabeled for Gp Ib and Gp IV.
Note the presence of a round nucleolus with a large nucleolus in the insert.
On the enlargement, one can see a labeling for Gp Ib (small gold particles, arrow head) and for Gp IV (large gold particles, arrow).

On day 11, the majority of mature MK were small (from 8 to 18 μ). Only an exceptional MK was 30 μ. This is consistant with their ploidy value. In a separate study (Hegyi et al., 1990), it has been shown that MK grown under these conditions are 2 or 4N with only rare 8 N MK. On the other hand with AP alone, AP + rhGM-CSF or AP + rhEpo, there are frequent 8N MK and also some 16N and 32N MK.

rhIL3 had a drastic effect on the intensity of labeling by FA6-152 MoAb as seen in Figs 7 and 8. Table 2 summarizes the results.

Table 2: Summary of results

	PMKB without platelet organelles (%) Day 7 of culture with		Fully mature MK (%) Day 11 of culture with	
	AP	AP + IL-3	AP	AP + IL-3
Gp IIb-IIIa + Gp IV	0	20	§45	*100
Only Gp IIb-IIIa	100	80	55	0
Gp Ib + Gp IV	0	100	§40	*100
Only Gp Ib	100	0	60	0

*: Strong labeling (from 60 to 90 gold particles/μ)
§: Weak labeling (from 2 to 5 gold particles/μ)

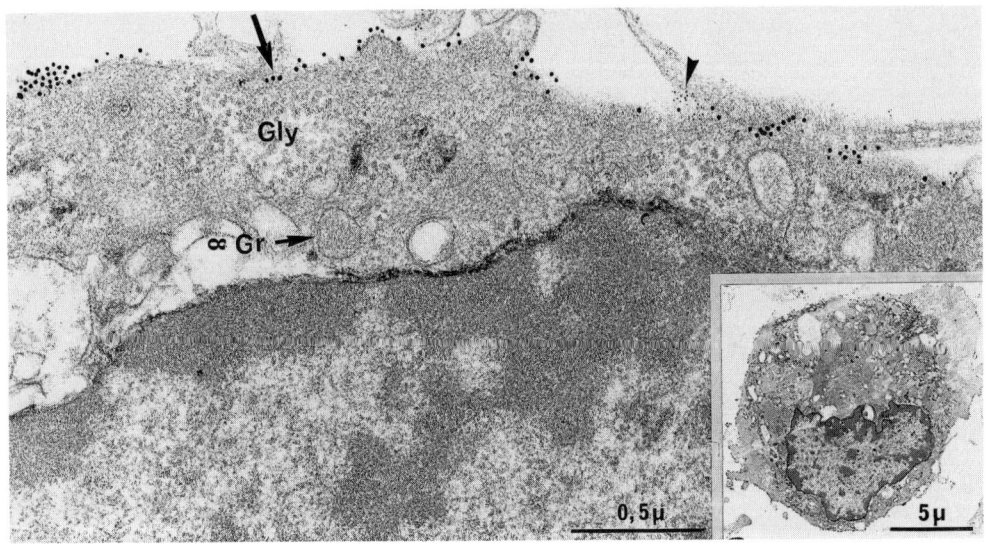

Fig. 7 A megakaryocyte cultured 11 days with AP and IL 3, immunolabeled for Gp Ib and Gp IV.
This small MK has 15 μ in diameter, the nucleus is irregular. Platelet peroxidase is present in the nuclear envelope and in the endoplasmic reticulum.

At higher magnification, an alpha granule (α-Gr) is seen and some clumps of glycogen particles (Gly); The plasma membrane exhibits labeling for both Gp Ib (arrow head) and Gp IV (arrow).

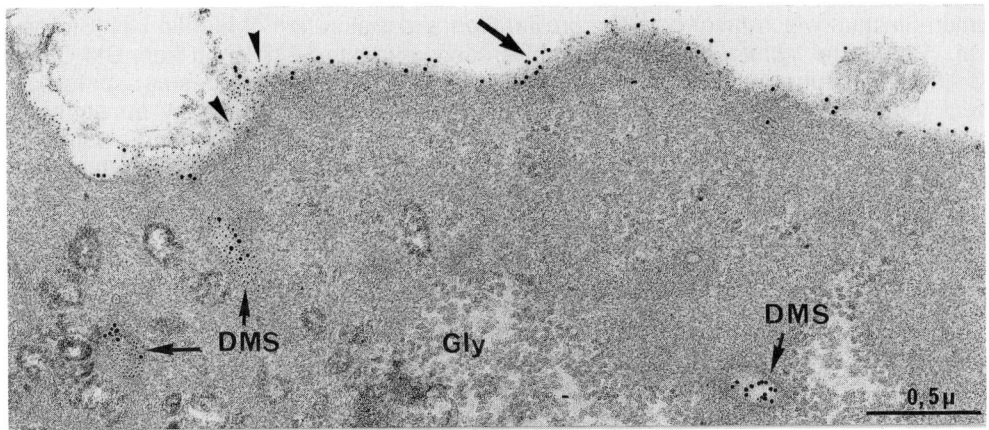

Fig. 8 A megakaryocyte cultured 11 days with AP and IL 3, immunolabeled for Gp IIb-IIIa and Gp IV.
Note the deposit of glycogen (Gly); the plasma membrane and demarcating membrane system (DMS) are strongly labeled for both Gp IIb-IIIa (arrow heads) and Gp IV (arrow).

Flow cytometry

Marrow cells were cutured in the presence of AP or AP plus IL3 for 11 days. They were double stained with a polyclonal antibody against Gp IIb-IIIa and the FA6-152 MoAb directed against Gp IV.

The expression of Gp IV was studied on the Gp IIb-IIIa positive cells i.e., MK. 50 000 MKs were analyzed in both conditions of culture.

MKs expressing GpIIb-IIIa was about twice more frequent in culture containing IL3. Whereas no clear correlation between the expression of Gp IV and the volume of MKs was observed in cultures containing IL3, a direct correlation between these two parameters was found with AP alone i.e., the large MK express more Gp IV than the small ones.

GpIIb-IIIa negative cells, mainly macrophages also express low amounts of Gp IV

DISCUSSION

In the present study, we compared the effects of different growth factors on the expression of Gp IV by double immunolabeling with either anti-Gp Ib or Gp IIb-IIIa antibodies. In this purpose we used a simple technique of culture in liquid medium (Debili et al., 1990) which allows the recovery of a sufficient number of MKs for ultrastructural immunogold localization and measurement of ploidy and quantitation of Gps by flow cytometry.

The first stimulus used was AP. It is well known that AP or aplastic serum contains several humoral factors which favor both the proliferation and maturation of human MK (Straneva et al., 1989). The factor which triggers proliferation seems to be different from GM-CSF or IL3 since the neutralization of these cytokines by specific antibodies does not abrogate its effect (Mazur et al., 1988a). However this activity can be abolished by an antiserum against *"MK colony-stimulating factor"*, a glycoprotein isolated from human plasma and partially purified (Hoffman , 1989). The fact that AP adsorbed with this antiserum retained the ability to promote cytoplasmic maturation indicates the presence of a distinct activity which has been named thrombocytopoiesis-stimulating factor (Straneva, 1989).

GM-CSF and IL3 support MK colony formation as well as AP, the activity of GM-CSF being lower that of IL3 (Teramura et al., 1989; Mazur et al., 1987). The role of Epo on megakaryocytopoiesis remains controversial (Burstein and Ishibashi, 1989; Dukes et al., 1986; Berridge et al., 1988; Dessypris et al., 1987; McDonald et al., 1987; Rossi et al., 1989; Tsukada et al., 1987; Hill and Levin, 1989; Kuter et al., 1989).

It has been previously shown that the addition of IL3 to AP increases the proliferation of MK but greatly diminishes their ploidy level (Hegyi et al 1990). The mechanism responsible for the inhibitory effect that the addition of IL3 to AP has on ploidization remains to be clarified. One possibility is that IL3 triggers the production of TGF-β since a factor present in serum which inhibits ploidization (Kuter et al 1989) was then characterized as being TGF-β (Kuter et al 1990).

If IL3 diminishes the ploidy level of MK, it does not significantly modify the quality of the maturation in these small MK.

In the present study using several hematopoietic growth factors and double immunolabeling of Gps, it was confirmed that Gp IIb-IIIa was expressed on the cell membranes of promegakaryoblasts earlier in the differentiation than Gp IV (Edelman et al., 1985) at day 7 since 80% of them cultured with AP + IL3 and 100% of them cultured with AP alone, only exhibited Gp IIb-IIIa. At this time, Gp IV expression was increased by the addition of IL3 and this effect was even more pronounced on day 11(see Table 2). In contrast addition of rhGM-CSF or rhEPO to AP did not modulate Gp IV expression.

The virtual absence of Gp IV in cultures with AP alone could be due to a weak expression of the antigen identified by FA6-152 MoAb or to a defect in final maturation related to this system of culture. In contrast, with AP + rhIL3, not only did all MK co-express Gp IIb-IIIa and Gp IV and Gp Ib and Gp IV but the labeling was considerably stronger than with AP alone. This was confirmed by flow cytometry.

There is no clear relationship between the low ploidy level and the intensity of the labeling for Gp IV, since the rare big MK cultured with AP + rIL3 also exhibited strong immunolabeling.

In conclusion, this is the first report in which the expression of one Gp on MK can be modulated by IL3 . Addition of other factors such as GM-CSF or Epo did not have this effect. In other cell systems, it has been reported that culture conditions and some cytokines, especially TGF-β can modulate the expression of integrins (Ignotz et al. 1987). Gp IV is apparently a receptor for several ligands (Oquendo et al. 1987). Several reports suggest that it is the receptor for thrombospondin (Asch et al., 1987; Kieffer et al., 1989; McGregor et al., 1989; Silverstein et al., 1989). Further studies will be required to understand the role of this modulation of Gp IV by IL3 in megakaryocytopoiesis and in platelet function.

REFERENCES

Asch, A.S., Barnwell, J., Silverstein, R.L., and Nachman, R.L. (1987): Isolation of the thrombospondin membrane receptor. J. Clin. Invest. 79: 1054-1061.

Berridge, M.V., Fraser, J.K., Carter, J.M., and Lin, F.K. (1988): Effects of recombinant human erythropoietin on megakaryocytes and on platelet production in the rat. Blood 72: 970-977.

Bray, P.F., Rosa, J.P., Johnston, G.I., Shiu, D.T., Cook, R.G., Lau, C., Kan, Y.W., McEver, R.P., and Shuman, M.A. (1987): Glycoprotein IIb chromosomal localization and tissue expression. J. Clin. Invest. 80: 1812-1817.

Breton-Gorius, J., Vanhaeke, D., Pryzwansky, K.B., Guichard, J., Tabilio, A., Vainchenker, W., and Carmel, R. (1984): Simultaneous detection of membrane markers with monoclonal antibodies and peroxidatic activities in leukemia : ultrastructural analysis using a new method of fixation preserving the platelet peroxidase. Br. J. Haematol. 58: 447-458.

Burstein, S.A., and Ishibashi, T. (1989): Erythropoietin and megakaryocytopoiesis. Blood cells 15: 193-201.

Cramer, E.M., Savidge, G.F., Vainchenker, W., Berndt, M.C., Pidard, D., Caen J.P., Masse, J.M., and Breton-Gorius, J. (1990): Alpha-granule pool of glycoprotein IIb-IIIa in normal and pathological platelets and megakaryocytes. Blood in press.

Debili, N., Kieffer, N., Nakazawa, M., Guichard, J., Titeux, M., Cramer, E., Breton-Gorius, J., and Vainchenker, W. (1990): Expression of platelet glycoprotein Ib by cultured human megakaryocytes. Ultrastructural localization and biosynthesis. Blood in press.

Dessypris, E.N., Gleaton, J.H., and Armstrong, O.L. (1987): Effect of human recombinant erythropoietin on human marrow megakaryocyte colony formation in vitro. Br. J. Haematol. 65: 265-269.

Dukes, P.P., Egrie, J.C., Strickland, T.W., Browne, J.K., and Lin, F.K. (1986): Megakaryocyte colony stimulating activity of recombinant human and monkey erythropoietin. In: Megakaryocyte development and function, eds, R.F. Levine, N. Williams, J. Levin, and B.L. Evatt, pp. 105-109. New York, Alan R. Liss.

Duperray, A., Berthier, R., Chagnon, E., Ryckewaert, J.J., Ginsberg, M., Plow, E., and Marguerie, G. (1987): Biosynthesis and processing of platelet Gp IIb-IIIa in human megakaryocytes. J. Cell Biol. 104: 1665-1673.

Edelman, P., Vinci, G., Villeval, J.L., Vainchenker, W., Henri, A., Miglierina, R., Rouger, P., Reviron J., Breton-Gorius, J., Sureau, C., and Edelman, L. (1986): A monoclonal antibody against an erythrocyte ontogenic antigen identifies fetal and adult erythroid progenitors. Blood 67: 56-63.

Hegyi, E., Nakazawa, M., Debili, N., Navarro, S., Katz, A., Breton-Gorius, J., and Vainchenker, W. (1990): Developmental changes in human megakaryocyte ploidy. Exp. Hematol. submitted.

Hickey, M.J., Williams, S.A., and Roth, G.J. (1989): Human platelet glycoprotein IX : an adhesive prototype of leucine-rich glycoproteins with flank-center structure. Proc. Natl. Acad. Sci. USA 86: 6773-6777.

Hill, R.J., and Levin, J. (1989): Regulators of thrombopoiesis : their biochemistry and physiology. Blood cells 15: 141-166.

Hoffman, R. (1989): Regulation of megakaryocytopoiesis. Blood 74: 1196-1212.

Ignotz, R.A., and Massagné, J. (1987): Cell adhesion protein receptors as targets for transforming growth factor -ß action. Cell 51: 189-197.

Jenkis, R.B., Nichols, W.L., Mann, K.G., and Solberg, L.A. (1986): CFU-M-derived human megakaryocytes synthesize glycoproteins IIb-IIIa. Blood 67: 682-688.

Kieffer, N., Bettaieb, A., Legrand, C., Coulombel, L., Vainchenker, W., Edelman, L., and Breton-Gorius, J. (1989): Developmentally regulated expression of a 78 KDa erythroblast membrane glycoprotein immunologically related to the platelet thrombospondin receptor. Biochem. J. 262: 835-842.

Knapp, W., Dörken, B., Rieber, P., Schmidt, R.E., and von dem Borne, A.E.G. Kr. (1989): CD antigens 1989. Blood 74: 1448-1450.

Kuter, D.J., Gminski, D., and Rosenberg, G.D. (1990): Platelets contain several inhibitors of megakaryocyte growth and ploidization. In press in Molecular Biology and Differentiation of megakaryocytes, eds, J. Breton-Gorius, J. Levin, A.T. Nurden, and N. Williams, New York, Alan R. Liss.

Kuter, D.J., Greenberg, S.M., and Rosenberg, R.D. (1989): Analysis of megakaryocyte ploidy in rat bone marrow cultures. Blood 74: 1952-1962.

Lopez, S.A., Chung, D.W., Fujikawa, K., Hagen, F.S., Papayannopoulou, T., and Roth, G.J. (1987): Cloning of the α chain of human platelet glycoprotein Ib : a transmembrane protein with homology to leucine-rich α 2 glycoprotein. Proc. Natl. Acad. Sci. U.S.A. 84: 5615-5619.

Lopez, S.A., Chung, D.W., Fujikawa, K., Hagen, F.S., Davie, E.W., and Roth, G.J. (1988): The α and ß chains of human platelet glycoprotein Ib are both transmembrane proteins containing a leucine- rich amino sequence. Proc. Natl. Acad. Sci. U.S.A. 85: 2135-2139.

Mazur, E.M., Cohen, J.L., Wong, G.G., and Clark, S.C. (1987): Modest stimulatory effect of recombinant human GM-CSF on colony growth from peripheral blood human megakaryocyte progenitor cells. Exp. Hematol. 15: 1128-1133.

Mazur, E.M., Cohen, J.L., Newton, J., Gesner, T.G., and Mufson, R.A. (1988a): Human serum megakaryocyte colony stimulating activity (Meg-CSA) is distinct from interleukin 3 (IL-3), granulocyte macrophage colony stimulating factor (GM-CSF) and phytohemagglutinin stimulated lymphocyte conditioned medium. Blood 72: 331a.

Mazur, E.M., Cohen, J.L., Bogart, L., Mufson, R.A., Gesner, T.G., Yang, Y.C., and Clark, S.C. (1988b): Recombinant gibbon interleukin-3 stimulates megakaryocyte colony growth in vitro from human peripheral blood progenitor cells. J. Cell. Physiol. 136: 439-446.

McDonald, T.P., Cottrell, M.B., Clift, R.E., Cullen, W.C., and Lin, K.F. (1987): High doses of recombinant erythropoietin stimulate platelet production in mice. Exp. Hematol. 15: 719-721.

McGregor, J.L., Catimel, B., Parmentier, S., Clezardin, P., Dechavanne, M., and L. L. K. Leung (1989): Rapid purification and partial characterization of human platelet glycoprotein IIIb. J. Biol.Chem. 264: 501-506.

Oquendo, R., Hundt, E., Lawler, J., and Seed, E. (1989): CD36 directly mediates cytoadherence of plasmodium falciparum parasitized erythrocytes. Cell 58: 95-101.

Rosa, J.P., Bray, P.F., Gayet, O., Johnston, G.I., Cook, J.R., Jackson, K.W., Shuman, M.A., and McEver, R.P. (1988): Cloning of glycoprotein IIIa cDNA from human erythroleukemia cells and localization of the gene to chromosome 17. Blood 72: 593-600.

Rossi, A., Vannuchi, A.M., Rafanelli, D., and Ferrini, P.R. (1989): Recombinant human erythropoietin has little influence on megakaryocytopoiesis in mice. Br. J. Haematol. 71: 463-468.

Silver, S.N., McDonough, M.M., Vilaire, G., and Bennett, J.S. (1987): The in vitro synthesis of polypeptides for the platelet membrane glycoproteins IIb and IIIa. Blood 69: 1031-1037.

Silverstein, L., Asch, S., and Nachman, L. (1989): Glycoprotein IV mediates thrombospondin-dependent platelet-monocyte and platelet-U937 adhesion. J. Clin. Invest. 84: 546-552.

Straneva, J.E., Briddell, R.A., McDonald, T.P., Yang, H.H., and Hoffman, R. (1989): Effects of thrombopoiesis stimulating factor on terminal cytoplasmic maturation of human megakaryocytes. Exp. Hematol. 17: 1122-1127.

Teramura, M., Katahira, J., Hoshino, S., Motoji, T., Oshimi, K., and Mizoguchi, H. (1989): Effect of recombinant hemopoietic growth factors on human megakaryocyte colony formation in serum free cultures. Exp. Hematol. 17: 1011-1016.

Tsukara, J., Misago, M., Sato, T., Kikuchi, M., Oda S., Chiba, S., and Eto, S. (1987): The effect of recombinant erythropoietin on murine megakaryocyte colony formation. Int. J. Cell Cloning 5: 401-411.

Vinci, G., Tabilio, A., Deschamps, J.F., Vanhaeke, D., Henri, A., Guichard, J., Tettero, P., Lansdorp, P.M., Hercend, T., Vainchenker, W., and Breton-Gorius, J. (1984): Immunological study of in vitro maturation of human megakaryocytes. Br. J. Haematol. 56: 589-605.

Wicki, A.N., and Clemetson K.J. (1985): Structure and function of platelet membrane glycoprotein Ib and V. Effects of leucocyte elastase and proteases on platelet response to von Willebrand factor and thrombin. Europ. J. Biochem. 153: 1-11.

ABSTRACT

The ultrastructural immunolocalization of platelet glycoproteins (Gp) Ib, IIb-IIIa and IV was studied on megakaryocytes (MK) maturing in liquid culture from normal bone marrow cells, in the presence of several growth factors. The results confirmed that Gp IIb-IIIa and Gp Ib were expressed on promegakaryoblasts (PMKB) earlier in the differentiation than Gp IV : on day 7, all of them cultured with plasma from aplastic patients alone or additioned with rhGM-CSF or rhEpo only exhibited Gp IIb-IIIa or Gp Ib. At this time, Gp IV expression was induced by the addition of IL3 since 20 % of PMKB co-expressed Gp IIb-IIIa and Gp IV and all of them co-expressed Gp Ib and Gp IV. This effect of IL3 was even more pronounced on day 11 and was confirmed by flow cytometry. In conclusion, the expression of Gp IV on MK can be modulated in culture by IL3.

Résumé

La localisation immuno-ultrastructurale des glycoprotéines (Gp) Ib, IIb-IIIa et IV a été étudiée durant la maturation des mégacaryocytes (Meg) cultivés en milieu liquide à partir de cellules médullaires en faisant varier les facteurs de croissance. Les résultats confirment que la Gp IIb-IIIa et la Gp Ib apparaissent plus précocément que la Gp IV : au 7ème jour de culture, en présence de plasma de sujets aplasiques, seul ou additionné de rhGM-CSF ou de rhEpo, tous les promégacaryoblastes (PMCB) expriment exclusivement la Gp IIb-IIIa ou la Gp Ib. Par contre, après addition de rhIL3, 20 % des PMCB co-expriment la GP IIb-IIIa et la Gp IV. Cet effet de l'IL3 est encore plus évident sur les Meg mûrs au 11ème jour de culture et est confirmé par cytométrie de flux. Il apparaît donc que l'expression de la Gp IV des Meg peut être modulée en culture par l'IL3.

Coexpression in the same cell in marrow culture of antigens from erythroid and megakaryocytic lineage

Z. Han, S. Bellucci, D. Pidard and J.P. Caen

INSERM U 150 – CNRS UA 334 – IVS, Hôpital Lariboisière, 75475 Paris cedex 10, France

The process of human megakaryocyte development includes hematopoietic stem cell commitment followed by megakaryocyte proliferation and maturation to give rise to platelets. Several investigators have reported that some neoplastic human cell lines express both glycophorin A and glycoprotein IIb/IIIa (GPIIb, IIIa), the specific markers for the erythroid and megakaryocytic lineages, respectively. In this study, using a double immunofluorescent staining, we have identified a population of hemopoietic cells coexpressing glycophorin A and GPIIIa, for the first time, in several (but not in all) normal human bone marrow cultures. The cells coexpressing GPIIIa and markers of myeloid lineages were not found, either using My9 which detects an antigen present on the myeloid/monocytic lineage, or MO1 which detects an antigen present on the monocytic/macrophagic lineage. The cells coexpressing GPIIIa and glycophorin A have the size of lymphocytes and appear at early time (day 1 to day 6) of culture. We have also detected a type of mixed colonies containing this phenotype on day 3 or 4 in most normal marrow samples. Such cell phenotype was not detected after 6 days of culture. These cells may represent hematopoietic cells common to megakaryocytic and erythroid lineages, at a very early stage of differenciation.

La mégacaryocytopoïèse humaine requiert plusieurs étapes : l'engagement des cellules souches hématopoiétiques vers la lignée mégacaryocytaire, la prolifération des mégacyoblastes puis la maturation des mégacaryocytes afin de donner naissance aux plaquette.Plusieurs équipes ont rapporté que certaines lignées tumorales expriment à la fois la glycophorine A et le complexe des glycoprotéines IIb/IIIa (GP IIb/IIIa) marqueurs spécifiques respectivement des lignées érythrocytaire et mégacaryocytaire. Au cours de cette étude, à l'aide d'une technique de double marquage par immunofluorescence indirecte, nous avons identifié une population des cellules hématopoïétiques coexprimant la glycophorine A et les glycoprotéines IIb/IIIa, pour la première fois, au niveau de la moëlle osseuse normale mise en culture. Il n'a pas été retrouvé de cellules coexprimant la glycoprotéine IIIa et les marqueurs de la lignée myéloïde (soit l'antigène myélomonocytaire reconnu par My9, soit l'antigène monocytique macrophagique reconnu par MO1). Les cellules coexprimant la glycoprotéine IIIa et la glycophorine A ont la taille de lymphocytes et apparaissent aux jours précoces de culture (jour 1 au jour 6. Nous avons également détecté la présence de telles cellules au sein de colonies mixtes aux jours 3-4 de culture dans la plupart des échantillons médullaires examinés. Ce phénotype cellulaire n'est plus détecté après le 8ème jour de culture. Ces cellules peuvent représenter des cellules hématopoiétiques, précurseurs des lignées érythrocytaire et mégacaryotaire, à un stade très précoce de différenciation.

Biochemistry and molecular biology of the platelet membrane glycoprotein Ib complex and the Bernard-Soulier syndrome

K.J. Clemetson, R.H. Wenger, J.M. Clemetson and J. Drouin*

Theodor Kocher Institute, University of Bern, Freiestr 1, CH-3012 Bern, Switzerland
*Ottawa General Hospital, Ontario, Canada

ABSTRACT

Glycoprotein Ib complex contains the major sialoglycoprotain on the platelet membrane surface. It is composed of two chains α and β, linked by a disulphide bond and a further chain, GPIX, which is non-covalently associated. All these components plus GPV, another single chain, are missing or deficient in Bernard-Soulier syndrome. GPIb is also affected in other genetic disorders. The primary structures of GPIb complex molecules are characterized by leucine-rich domains. The structure of the GPIbα gene and flanking regions has been determined and putative nuclear factor binding sites identified. The GPIbα gene shares an NF-E1 (GF-1, Eryf-1) site with other megakaryocyte and erythrocyte lineage genes.

INTRODUCTION

Glycoprotein (GP) Ib is the major sialoglycoprotein on the platelet membrane surface. It is a heterodimer of 160 kDa composed of a large (α-) subunit (140 kDa) and a small (β-) subunit (25 kDa) linked by a disulphide bond (Phillips and Poh-Agin, 1977). The GPIb complex also contains GPIX (20 kDa) non-covalently associated in a 1:1 ratio (Berndt et al., 1985). The general structure of the GPIb complex is shown in Fig. 1. Evidence of other glycoproteins related or possibly associated with GPIb comes from Bernard-Soulier syndrome, (BSs) a hereditary bleeding disorder, where GPIbα (Nurden and Caen, 1975), GPIbα, GPIX and also GPV (Clemetson et al., 1982) and a 210 kDa glycoprotein (Stricker et al., 1985) are missing. GPIb functions as the von Willebrand receptor on resting platelets and contains a thrombin binding site (Okumura et al., 1978) which controls the kinetic response to thrombin (Wicki and Clemetson, 1985; McGowan and Detwiler, 1986) and amplifies it by about ten-fold. The principal physiological role of GPIb is as the binding site on resting platelets for vWf on exposed subendothelium in the first stage of haemostasis. This is particularly important under conditions of high shear where other adhesion mechanisms such as that involving fibronectin cannot function. Because the GPIb-vWf axis provides adhesion under such extreme conditions the mechanism of binding is of great interest.

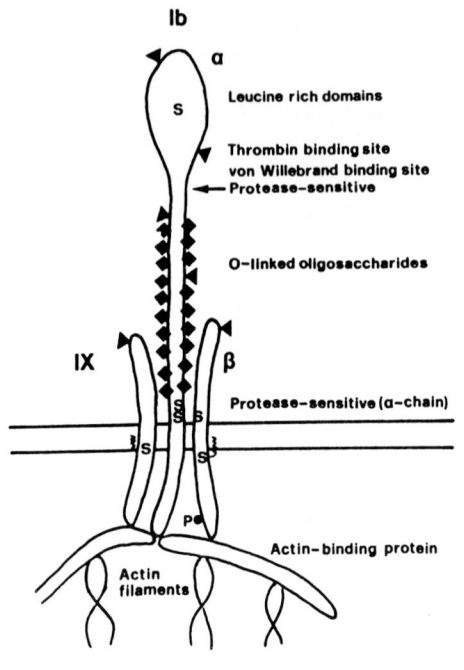

Fig. 1 Schematic model of the GPIb-IX complex showing major sequence and functional features.

A wide variety of genetic disorders including BSs are known which affect GPIb. In pseudo von Willebrand disease (Miller et al., 1983) the GPIb molecule has a higher avidity for vWf than normal leading to platelet aggregation and thus to thrombocytopenia and depletion of the higher molecular weight, more active, forms of vWf in the plasma. Bolin-Jamieson disease (Bolin et al., 1977) is a mild bleeding disorder involving polymorphism of GPIb where the thrombin binding site on GPIb may be affected. A defect in GPIb has been reported giving rise to an α-chain 20 kDa heavier than normal (Meyer, 1988). Polymorphism in GPIbα leading to four molecular weight variants has also been described in normal Japanese (Moroi et al., 1984) and Americans (Jung et al., 1986). So far there is littleevidence for alloantibodies against GPIb which would be expected if this polymorphism gave rise to antigenic differences. Since GPIbα is highly O-glycosylated, this could therefore reflect O-glycosylation differences. A major problem concerning GPIb and other platelet proteins is how tissue-specific expression is controlled during megakaryocyte differentiation. Most of the questions listed above require a detailed knowledge of the sequence and structure of the GPIb gene and the availability of cloned segments as the starting point for further investigation. With these now available a start can be made to resolve these problems.

PRINCIPAL FEATURES OF THE GPIB COMPLEX

Leucine-rich glycoprotein domains

An interesting and so far unexplained feature of all the components of the GPIb complex (apparently including GPV) is the presence of leucine-rich domains with a high degree of homology to those found in other proteins including the prototype, leucine-rich α_2-glycoprotein. Many proteins from a wide variety of sources containing such sequences are now known and a list of these are shown in Table 1. The function of this type of structure remains a puzzle but various proposals have been made including a role in the association of subunits. In the GPIb complex components the LRG sequences lie towards the N-terminal end.

TABLE 1

Consensus sequences in proteins with leucine-rich sequences
LRG is leucine rich α2-glycoprotein, PG is proteoglycan, LH is luteinizing hormone, CG is choriogonadotrophin, CPN is carboxypeptidase N 83 kDa subunit, Ad cycl is adenylate cyclase, X is any amino acid, α is leucine, isoleucine or valine.

GPIbα	Human platelet	PXGLLXXLPXLXXF-LHGNPWLCNC
GPIbβ	Human platelet	PPGLLDALPALRTAHLGANPWRCDC
GPIX	Human platelet	PPGAFDHLPQLQTLDVTQNPWHCDC
LRG	Human plasma	PPGLLQGLXQLRXFDISGNPWICDG
PGI	Human bone	PXXXFXXLXXLXXLXLXXNXIXXV
PGII	Human fibroblasts	XXGXhXXXXXLXXLXLXXNXISXV
LH-CG rec	Rat ovary	PSXαFXXLXXαXXXLXLXXXXLXXα
Ad cycl	Yeast	PXXL-XXLXXLXXLXLXXNXLXXα
CPN 83	Human plasma	PXXαFXXLXXLXXLXLXXNXLXXL
RNaseInh	Human placenta	XXXLXXPXCXLEXLXLXXCXLTXXCXXL
	Porcine liver	XXALXXXXXLXE-LXLXXNXLGDXGXXXL
Toll	Drosophila	PXXLFXHXXNLXXLXLXXNXLXXα
Chaoptin	Drosophila	PXXLFXXLXXLXXLXLXXNXLXXα
YopM	Yersina pestis	IRSLCDLPPSLEELNVSNNKLIELPA

Thrombin-binding site

The structure of the GPIb complex and its principal features is shown in Fig. 2. It has long been known that GPIbα contains a high-affinity thrombin-binding site. It is clearly established that this site affects the platelet response to thrombin but is not the receptor essential for activation. Experiments with peptides and with proteolytic cleavage indicate that at least part of the binding site lies in the area of the sequence 215-240 just after the LRG sequences in the C-terminal direction (Katagiri et al. 1990). Since heparin competes with GPIb for thrombin binding and is highly positively charged it is reasonable to think that the thrombin binding domain on GPIb must also be positively charged. This is not particularly the case for the 215-240 sequence but is definitely so for 269-287. If cysteines 248 and 264 are linked (see below) these sequences could very easily be next one another. The role of this binding site remains obscure; α-thrombin inhibited at the proteolytic site can still bind to GPIb whereas active γ-thrombin cannot. Cleavage of the thrombin binding region of GPIbα or its absence (as in Bernard-Soulier syndrome) gives platelets that show a response to α-thrombin very similar to that of intact platelets to γ-thrombin. Treatment of platelets with inactivated α-thrombin before adding active α-thrombin does not inhibit the response but rather amplifies it. These observations would tend to indicate that the binding site on GPIb modulates either the interaction of thrombin with the effective receptor or the signal transmission resulting from this interaction. There is no hard evidence yet for a detectable signal resulting from the binding of thrombin to GPIb.

Von Willebrand factor binding site

The principal physiological role for GPIb is to act as the platelet receptor for vWf during platelet adhesion to subendothelium. It was soon established that the binding site lay in the outer 45 kDa region of the GPIbα chain. More recently, experiments with peptides point to the 235-275 region in the molecule as important for interaction with vWf (Katagiri et al. 1990; Vicente et al., 1990). Since this is in close proximity to the thrombin site it may explain why certain monoclonal antibodies affect both activities. It is also of some interest to note that there are two cysteines in this sequence which are suspected to form a loop. The GPIb binding region of vWf has been shown to lie on a disulphide bridge linked loop also so that the interaction might be mostly via these two loop structures. Clearly, other parts of the GPIb complex may also play a role in maintaining the conformation of this region. A major problem in these studies is the fact that normally vWf does not interact directly with GPIb on platelets but must be associated with collagen or possibly proteoglycan which induces the necessary conformational changes. Since binding experiments under heterogeneous conditions are difficult, nearly all studies have been done using binding induced by ristocetin which may differ from the physiological situation. More recent studies have used either asialo vWf, which interacts directly with GPIb on platelets, or botrocetin (Andrews et al.,1989) which seems to induce vWf binding to GPIb in a manner closer to physiological. Another approach is to use bovine or porcine vWf which also bind human GPIb directly but again it is not clear if exactly the same domains in GPIb are involved.

Another controversial area is whether vWf binding to platelets transmits a signal i.e. causes platelet activation. The primary interaction certainly does not require such activation and fixed platelets are agglutinated under the same conditions as untreated platelets. Some authors did not see any signs of activation in the first 5 min after agglutination and could recover discoid platelets (Wicki and Clemetson, 1985) whereas others (De Marco et al., 1985) found typical indications that activation had occured. In the reverse direction the question has been asked; what happens to GPIb when platelets are activated via other receptors? Following activation with thrombin platelets bound less vWf (Michelson and Barnard, 1987)which may be due to sequestration of GPIb in the surface connected canalicular system. (Nurden et al., 1989)

Glycosylation sites and GPIb complex structure

GPIbα is probably the most heavily glycosylated protein on the platelet surface. The bulk of this is O-glycosylation which is concentrated on serine and threonine residues in repetitive sequences lying between amino-acids 363-414 and probably on flanking regions covering the region from about 300-440 in total (Lopez et al., 1987). The principal O-linked oligosaccharide found was a biantennary hexasaccharide but some biantennary tetrasaccharide was also present and the structures of both have been determined (Tsuji et al., 1983 ,Korrel et al., 1984). A rough calculation based on the molecular weight of the protein backbone, the 4 putative N-linked glycosylation sites and the average molecular weight of the O-linked oligosaccharides indicate that there must be approximately 40 O-linked chains. There are 56 serine and threonine residues between 300-440 implying a high rate of occupation with one oligosaccharide per 3-4 amino acids, giving rise to a densely packed, stiff, rod-like structure for this domain with a high degree of intramolecular hydrogen bonding. Similar structures exist at least partially in other molecules such as glycophorin. What are such structures for? An explanation could be that they are simply there to hold the receptor sites out above the other glycoproteins of the plasma membrane to enable them to interact quickly with the vWf on the subendothelium. However, the problem of a possible signal transmission to the platelet interior still remains with the difficulty of sending conformational changes through a structure of this type.

Cytoplasmic domains

All of the GPIb complex components for which the primary structure is known contain a segment traversing the membrane and a cytoplasmic region varying between 96 amino acids for GPIbα, 34 for GPIbβ and 6 for GPIX. It is known that these regions are involved in binding to actin binding protein and hence to the cytoskeleton. GPIbβ contains a phosphorylation site (Wyler et al., 1986) on serine residue 166 which is affected by cyclic AMP levels and appears to regulate actin polymerization in response to collagen (Fox et al., 1989) but not to other agonists. An active thiol group was detected just under the membrane in GPIbβ (Kalomiris and Coller, 1985) and both GPIbβ and GPIX were shown to be palmitylated on cysteine residues (Muszbek and Laposata, 1989). In the case of GPIbβ this is obviously the same cysteine as it is in an appropriate position and in GPIX there is a cysteine just inside the membrane (Hickey et al., 1989) which is the only reasonable possibility. These sites may regulate the interaction of GPIb with the membrane and could also be involved in the interaction between GPIX and GPIb. It is not clear if or how this palmitylation is regulated. In Bernard-Soulier syndrome platelets where the GPIb complex is absent the membranes are more easily deformed than normal which has been ascribed to the lack of binding to actin binding protein and hence to the cytoskeleton but the membrane segments of the complex and the associated palmitate might also be involved.

Cysteine bridges

The positions of the disulphide bridges in the GPIb complex is not yet well established and there remain a number of problems. GPIbα contains 9 cysteine residues, 2 just above the membrane crossing segment. One of these is most likely involved in the interchain bond to GPIbβ, but what of the second? This cannot be involved in an intrachain disulphide bridge to another cysteine in GPIbα as this would prevent release of glycocalicin, the water-soluble fragment of GPIbα, which is cleaved off just above the membrane, by a variety of proteases. It might form a second disulphide bond to the β-chain as there is a cysteine only 6 amino acids higher up which would be sterically favourable. However, that would leave an odd number (7) of cysteines in this subunit. Thus, it is unlikely that the second cysteine, just above the membrane in the α-chain, is involved in a disulphide bond and since it was not detectable as an active thiol group it is either inaccessible i.e. imbedded in the membrane, or acylated in some way. The remaining 7 cysteines in the α-chain probably form 3 disulphide bonds, leaving one free. This is either embedded in a globular domain such as might be formed by the leucine rich domains or again may be modified. The only candidate within the LR region is cysteine 65. GPIbβ contains 10 cysteines, one just below the membrane which is partly palmitylated, one forming the bond to the α-subunit and the other 8 which are assumed to form 4 disulphide bonds. GPIX contains 9 cysteines, one of which is just inside the membrane on the cytoplasmic face and is either completely palmitylated or also protected from thiol reagents. The other 8 are presumably in 4 disulphide bonds.

Polymorphism and immunology

Four variants of GPIbα with slightly different molecular weights have been described first in normal Japanese (Moroi et al., 1984) and then in American populations (Jung et al., 1986). Since alloantigens on GPIb are not common and because of its high degree of O-glycosylation it seems likely that these polymorphic variants are due to differences in O-glycosylation sites due either to changes in specific glycosyl transferases or to changes in the primary sequence which is not seen as immunologically different because it is inaccessible. Alloantigenic differences in GPIb have been described as the Ko system but they are so far limited to one case.

The structure of the GPIb complex and the role of GPV

Two of the major problems still unsolved are the signal transmission problem within GPIb (mentioned above) and the putative role of GPV. So far the only hard evidence for the involvement of GPV with GPIb is the fact that it is also missing in Bernard-Soulier syndrome. Preliminary studies indicate that GPV also contains leucine-rich glycoprotein type domains, another common feature. GPV has not been shown to coprecipitate with GPIb in immunological studies or vice-versa. It is clear that a molecular biology explanation for the coordinated lack of the α-, β- and IX chains could be based on a requirement for expression of all these components in order that the complex be processed. Thus, there are two major alternatives, GPV also forms part of the complex but is more weakly associated and can be removed by non-ionic detergents or GPV is not part of the complex but shares an important processing step with the other components.

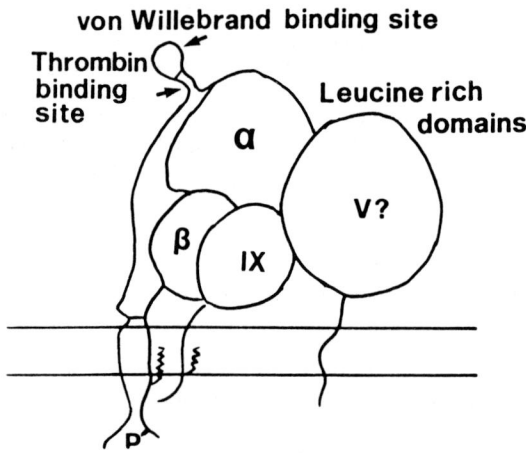

Fig. 2 A schematic model of a postulated GPIb-IX-V complex with interactions of LR domains

Such a step could be glycosylation, or could involve a not yet established function of the LRG type domains. An alternative model for the GPIb complex to accommodate a possible role for the LRG domains in subunit association also with GPV is shown in Fig. 2. GPV is known to be the major substrate for thrombin but nevertheless not the essential receptor for platelet activation. The thrombin remains bound to the cleaved off GPV fragment which might have a role elsewhere in the circulation. Electron microscopy studies of GPIb/IX complexes indicate a structure supporting earlier models with the LRG domains forming a globular region at one end of a dumbbell and the other globular region formed by the cytoplasmic domains plus the β- and IX chains (Fox et al., 1988). The major problems with this model are the signal transmission mechanism and the changes in conformation of glycocalicin compared to the intact molecule noted by several investigators (Andrews et al., 1989). Both these imply that the β- and IX chains stabilise the conformation of the outer domain of the α-subunit. Fig. 2 shows one possible way this might occur. Such structures might be less stable in the presence of detergent accounting for their rarity (but not absence!) in rotary shadowing pictures. The ease with which both glycocalicin and GPV are lost from the platelet surface after cleavage also argues against a strong interaction.

CLONING AND SEQUENCING OF THE GPIbα GENE

Cloning genes for platelet specific proteins has till recently given special problems not usually encountered with other cells since platelets have no nucleus and megakaryocytes are difficult to obtain in adequate amounts. These problems have been solved in various ways by different investigators. Several platelet proteins including GPIbα and β have been cloned by screening expression libraries derived from the human erythroleukaemic (HEL) cell-line which shows both megakaryocytic and erythroid characteristics (Lopez et al., 1987). Others have used megakaryocytes of neoplastic origin as source (Uzan et al., 1988). Where sufficient sequence data is available direct screening of genomic libraries can be used (Kobilka et al., (1987). However, evidence exists going back over twenty years that platelets still have a biosynthetic capability and therefore contain intact mRNA. Based on this extracted mRNA from platelets and used this for the preparation of a cDNA expression library in λgt11. Screening this library with monospecific polyclonal antibodies allowed the isolation of cDNA clones coding for three platelet-specific proteins, GPIbα (Wicki et al., 1989), connective tissue activating peptide-III and platelet factor 4 (Wenger et al., 1989a) demonstrating the validity of this approach. The partial GPIba clone (783 bp) was used as probe to screen a human pCV 105 cosmid library and four positive clones were isolated. These clones contained a 6.5 EcoRI fragment which hybridized to the same probe on Southern blots. One of the clones was completely sequenced (Wenger et al., 1988; Wenger et al., 1989b) and the structure is shown in Fig. 3. The exon-intron structure of the GPIbα gene is rare in eukaryotic genes and the whole precursor of GPIbα (626 amino acids is expressed by a single, exceptionally large 2.4 kb exon. In the whole gene there is a single 233 bp intron 6 bp upstream of the initiation site. Downsteam of the polyadenylation site at the 3' end 646 bp were sequenced to the EcoRI cleavage site and at the 5' end

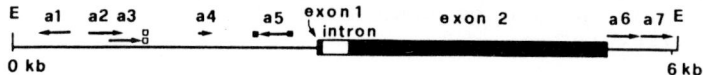

Figure 3. Structure of the GPIbα gene and its 5' and 3' flanking regions. The exon-intron structure is shown by filled and open bars. Arrows indicate the location of Alu ("a") repeats 1 to 7. Solid boxes associated with Alu 5 indicate the 14 bp direct repeat. The 55 bp pur.pyr stretch is indicated by two open boxes.

2794 bp from the EcoRI cleavage site to the putative site for start of transcription.

CANDIDATE CIS-REGULATORY ELEMENTS WITHIN THE GPIBα GENE

The sequence upstream of the transcription initiation site was searched for homologies to consensus sequences specific for transcription regulating factors. Such identifications are difficult by comparative analysis alone since there are many such sequences which are only a few bases long and they have a high degeneracy in their flanking regions. The effect of enhancer elements is also not dependent on orientation or location which means that they may be located in either the 5' or 3' directions and possibly far from the transcription start site. Thus, there is a high probability of finding matches but demonstration of authenticity requires expression experiments. Some sequences which may function as cis-regulatory elements in the GPIbα gene are listed in Table 2. No typical CCAAT or TATA elements were detected but interesting sequences were found in the regions where these normally occur, a GGCCTGCAT stretch, which contains the TGCAT sequence of the octamer motif of immunoglobulin promotors and the direct repeat CTAGAAGA begining at 2755 and 2788. Another TATA-like sequence was found just after the first Alu sequence upstream of the transcription initiation site. A sequence similar to an Sp1 binding site was found at position 2641.

Comparison with the promoter regions of other genes expressed exclusively in megakaryocytes should provide information on the significance of regulatory elements in megakaryocyte differentiation. However, only one other human platelet-specific gene, GPIIb, has been cloned so far (Prandini et al., 1988). Comparison of the 5' flanking region of the genes for GPIbα and GPIIb yields some data. An Sp1 binding site and a binding site for an erythroid-specific nuclear protein are found in both genes. Since megakaryocytes and reticulocytes are derived from the same stem cell in the bone marrow, this erythroid-specific site could be involved in tissue-specific activation of both genes. Pur.pyr sequence motifs of about 20 bp around positions -15, -518 and -575 in GPIIb are also elements common to both. In contrast, no Alu repeats were found in the published sequences flanking the the GPIIb gene and no inverted repeats longer than 10 bp nor a CP2 binding site were detected in the GPIbα gene. Undoubtedly, sequences of the promoter regions of genes for further platelet-specific proteins and functional assays with these sequences will be necessary in order to establish megakaryocyte-specific regulatory elements. Investigations in other systems indicate that a large number of factors both positive and negative are probably involved in the control of a eukaryotic gene via binding to both promotor and enhancer elements and only a few of these are actually specific for a particular gene, perhaps even different combinations can be used when the same gene is expressed in different cells.

WHAT IS THE GENETIC DEFECT IN BERNARD-SOULIER SYNDROME?

The peculiarity of BSs as a genetic disorder is the large number of proteins (4 or 5) involved. Examination of DNA from patients with BSs by Southern blotting using DNA probes directed against both GPIbα and GPIbβ gave identical results to those obtained with DNA from normal controls (Fig. 2) These patients included

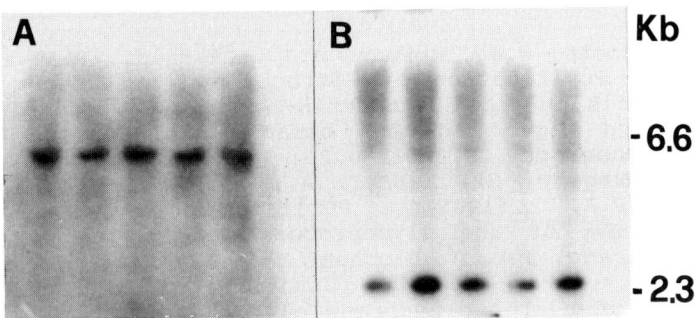

Figure 4 Genomic Southern blots of representative Bernard Soulier patients using cDNA probes for GPIbα (A) and GPIbβ (B). DNA samples were digested with BamH1. From left to right, gels show DNA from a normal control, two heterozygotes and two homozygote Bernard-Soulier patients. Additional patients gave similar results. Digestion with other restriction nucleases showed no differences between patients and normals

3 Swiss with no detectable GPIb complex glycoproteins and 2 Canadians with varying amounts. This result indicates that major deletions or rearrangements in the GPIbα or GPIbβ genes are unlikely to be the cause of BSs but does not exclude critical point mutations in the transcribed or promoter regions. A defect in the genes of other GPIb complex proteins such as GPV or GPIX which might prevent expression of the complex also cannot be excluded. Clearly, BSs may have a heterogeneous origin and further research is necessary to clarify this problem. Studies with all of the components of the GPIb complex will be needed to define which are essential for expression. Such studies should also indicate whether all the chains are necessary for biological activity and how GPV is involved. With the characterization of the GPIbα gene and its sequence and the likelihood that similar detailed information will soon exist on the GPIbβ, GPV and GPIX genes the basic tools to approach this problem should soon be available.

ABSTRACT

Le complexe de la glycoproteine Ib renferme la sialoglycoprotein la plus importante de la surface plaquettaire et joue un rôle primordial dans l'adhésion à la paroi du vaisseau lésé. Il se compose de 2 chaines a et β unie par une liason disulfure et d'une chaine supplémentaire GPIX associée de manière non covalente. Tous ces composés ainsi que GPV, font defaut ou sont défectueux dans le syndrôme de Bernard-Soulier. La structure primaire des molécules du complexe GPIb révèle des domaines riches en leucine. La structure du gène de GPIbα et les régions qui lui sont juxtaposées ont été élucidées et les éventuels sites de liason pour les facteurs nucléaires identifiés. Le gène de GPIbα renferme un site NF-E1, propriété partagée avec d'autres gènes de lignées megakaryocytaires et erythrocytaires.

REFERENCES

Andrews, R.K., Booth, W.J., Gorman, J.J., Castaldi, P.A. and Berndt, M.C. (1989): Purification of Botrocetin from Bothrops jararaca venom. Analysis of the Botrocetin-mediated interaction between von Willebrand factor and the human platelet membrane GPIb-IX complex. *Biochemistry* 28, 8317-8326.

Berndt, M.C., Gregory, C., Kabral, A., Zola, H., Founier, D. and Castaldi, P.A. (1985): Purification and preliminary characterization of the glycoprotein Ib complex in the human platelet membrane. *Eur. J. Biochem.* 151, 637-649.

Bolin, R.B., Okumura, T. and Jamieson, G.A. (1977): New polymorphism of platelet membrane glycoproteins. *Nature* 269, 69-70.

Bray, P.F., Barsh, G., Rosa, J.-P., Luo, X.Y., Magenis, E. and Shuman, M.A. (1988). Physical linkage of the genes for platelet membrane glycoproteins IIb and IIIa. *Proc. Natl. Acad. Sci. USA* 85, 8683-8687.

Clemetson, K.J., McGregor, J.L., James, E., Dechavanne, M. and Lüscher, E.F. (1982): Characterization of the platelet membrane glycoprotein abnormalities in Bernard-Soulier syndrome and comparison with normal by surface-labeling techniques and high-resolution two-dimensional gel electrophoresis. *J. Clin. Invest.* 70, 304-311.

De Marco, L., Girolami, A., Russell, S. and Ruggeri, Z.M. (1985): Interaction of asialo von Willebrand factor with glycoprotein Ib induces fibrinogen binding to the glycoprotein IIb/IIIa complex and mediates platelet aggregation. *J. Clin. Invest.* 75: 1198-1203.

Fox, J.E.B., Aggerbeck, L.P. and Berndt, M.C. (1988): Structure of the glycoprotein Ib-IX complex from platelet membranes. *J. Biol. Chem.* 263, 4882-4890.

Fox, J.E.B. and Berndt, M.C. (1989): Cyclic AMP-dependent phosphorylation of glycoprotein Ib inhibits collagen-induced polymerization of actin in platelets. *J. Biol. Chem.* 264, 9520-9526.

Jung, S.M., Plow, E.F. and Moroi, M. (1986): Polymorphism of platelet glycoprotein Ib in the United States. *Thromb. Res.* 42, 83-90.

Kalomiris, E.L. and Coller, B.S. (1985): Thiol-specific probes indicate that the β-chain of platelet glycoprotein Ib is a transmembrane protein with a reactive endofacial sulfhydryl group. *Biochemistry* 24, 5430-5436.

Katagiri, Y., Hayashi, Y., Yamamoto, K., Tanoue, K., Kosaki, G. and Yamazaki, H. (1990): Localization of von Willebrand and thrombin-interactive domains on human platelet glycoprotein Ib. *Thromb. Haemostas.* 63, 122-126.

Korrel, S.A., Clemetson, K.J., van Halbeek, H., Kamering, J.P., Sixma, J.J. and Vliegenthart, J.F. (1984): Structural studies on the O-linked carbohydrate chains of human platelet glycocalicin. *Eur. J. Biochem.* 140, 571-576.

Kobilka, B.K., Matsui, M., Kobilka, T.S., Yang-Feng, T.L., Francke, U., Caron, M.G., Lefkowitz, R.J. and Regan, J.W. (1987): Cloning, sequencing and expression of the gene coding for the human platelet α_2-adrenergic receptor. *Science* 238, 650-656.

Lopez, J.A., Chung, D.W., Fujikawa, K., Hagen, F.S., Papayannopoulou, T. and Roth, G.J. (1987): Cloning of the α chain of human platelet glycoprotein Ib: A transmembrane protein with

INTRODUCTION

In hematopoiesis, the commitment of the progenitor cell and the later differentiation steps depend on the establishment of specific patterns of gene expression achieved through networks of regulatory factors. While some of these factors may be expressed in a cell specific maner, they can be associated with a panel of ubiquitous factors as well. Very little is known about the factors that regulate the transcription of lineage specific genes in hematopoiesis. Most of the informations have been accumulated from the expression of the globin genes system in the erythrocytes. Factors like NFE1 have been cloned (Tsai et al, 1987), and studies on the function of this factor in the transcription of categories of genes is in progress. Until now, similar studies have not been performed and no transcription factors have been identified in megakaryocytes.

These cells represent only a small percentage of the total marrow cells. With the progress of liquid culture of human megakaryocytes however (Berthier et al, 1987) and the caracterisation of an increasing number of permanent cell lines with megakaryocytic features, analysis of megakaryocytopoiesis at the molecular level is now feasible. Nuclear factors important in cell differentiation can be identify using a marker gene, that is highly specific to the lineage, and is in expressed at an early stage of differentiation. In megakaryocytopoiesis, glycoprotein IIb (GPIIb) fulfil these criteria. The molecule is the α subunit of the platelet integrin GPIIb-IIIa. Platelet GPIIb-IIIa and the vitronectin receptor share the same β subunit, the GPIIIa (Ginsberg et al, 1988). While GPIIIa and VNRα are expressed in different cells, the GPIIb mRNA has only been found in megakaryocytes or in cell lines with megakaryocytic features.

Despite a controversy on the expression of GPIIb-IIIa as early as in the CFU-Meg (Berridge et al, 1985 ; Fraser et al, 1986 ; Kantz et al, 1988) it is now admitted that GPIIb-IIIa is an early marker of megakaryocytopoiesis and appears at least at the transitional cell level.

We have recently isolated the gene encoding GPIIb and caracterized the transcription start site (Prandini et al, 1988). A fragment of 1.9 kb containing a portion of the 5' flanking region was sequenced.

In this paper we have further analysed this sequence, and we demonstrate that this region contains promoter elements responsible for the specific expression of the gene. Multiple binding sites for nuclear proteins were identified. This study provides evidence for the existence of megakaryocyte specific DNA binding proteins.

MATERIAL AND METHODS

Cells and nuclear extracts

Nuclear extracts were prepared from three cell lines, Hela, Hel and Lama 84, and from human megakaryocytes and endothelial cells. The

Megakaryocyte specific expression of human platelet GPIIb gene

G. Uzan, M.H. Prandini, M. Prenant, F. Martin and G. Marguerie

INSERM U 217, Laboratoire d'Hématologie, Centre d'Etudes Nucléaires, BP 85X, 38041 Grenoble Cedex, France

ABSTRACT

One of the major objectives in the study of megakaryocytopoiesis is to identify the mechanisms by which the progenitor cells are committed to the megakaryocytic lineage. One approach to address this question is to idenfify a marker gene which is specific and expressed at an early stage of the differentiation. Nuclear factors that regulate the transcription of this gene in a tissue specific maner can be isolated, and there potential role in the differentiation of the megakaryocytes can be tested in functional assays. One gene of interest is the GPIIb gene. GPIIb wich is the α subunit of the platelet integrin GPIIbIIIa, is only expressed in megakaryocytes, and the molecule is detected at an early stage of the differentiation. The GPIIb gene was isolated, and a genomic subclone containing the 5' flanking region was sequenced. This region encoded the signal peptide and 31 amino acids of the mature protein. The transcription start site was localized, and the 5' flanking region was analyzed for DNA binding protein sites. A sequence, centred at position -54 was identical to the transcription factor NFE1 binding site. This factor was originaly described as an erythroid specific DNA binding protein. The potential implication of this molecule in the expression of megakaryocitic genes support the accumulating evidences regarding megakaryocyte and erythrocyte similarities. DNA binding activity for megakaryocyte nuclear factors was investigated in band shift assays. Two fragments, extending from -152 to -428 and from -428 to -588 exhibited retarded bands when nuclear extract from megakaryocytic cell lines were used. This suggests that megakaryocyte specific factors may controle the transcription of the GPIIb gene.

chromosomal localization of the human blood platelet membrane glycoprotein Ibα gene. *Gene*, 85, 519-523.

Wicki, A.N. and Clemetson, K.J. (1985): Structure and function of platelet membrane glycoproteins Ib and V. *Eur. J. Biochem.* 153, 1-11.

Wicki, A.N., Walz, A., Gerber-Huber, S.N., Wenger, R.H., Vornhagen, R. and Clemetson, K.J. (1989): Isolation and characterization of human blood platelet mRNA and construction of a cDNA library in λgt11. *Thromb. Haemostas.* 61, 448-453.

Wyler, B., Bienz, D., Clemetson, K.J. and Lüscher, E.F. (1986): Glycoprotein Ibβ is the only major phosphorylated major membrane glycoprotein in human platelets. *Biochem. J.* 234, 373-379.

homology to leucine-rich α2-glycoprotein. *Proc. Natl. Acad. Sci. USA* 84, 5615-5619.

McGowan, E.B. and Detwiler, T.C. (1986): Modified platelet responses to thrombin: Evidence for two types of receptor or coupling mechanisms. *J. Biol. Chem.* 261, 739-746.

Meyer, M., Schellenberg, I., Hofmann, B. and Vogel, G. (1988): A platelet disorder due to a structural abnormality of membrane glycoprotein Ib. *Folia Haematol.* 115, 515-518.

Michelson, A.D. and Barnard, M.R. (1987): Thrombin-induced changes in platelet membrane glycoproteins Ib, IX, and IIb-IIIa complex. *Blood* 70, 1673-1678.

Miller, J.L., Kupinski, J.M., Castella, A. and Ruggeri, Z.M. (1983): von Willebrand factor binds to platelets and induces aggregation in platelet-type but not type IIB von Willebrand disease. *J. Clin. Invest.* 72, 1532-1542.

Moroi, M., Jung, S.M. and Yoshida, N. (1984): Genetic polymorphism of platelet glycoprotein Ib. *Blood* 64, 622-629.

Muszbek, L. and Laposata, M. (1989): Glycoprotein Ib and glycoprotein IX in human platelets are acylated with palmitic acid through thioester linkages. *J. Biol. Chem.* 264, 9716-9719.

Nurden, A.T. and Caen, J.P. (1975): Specific roles for platelet surface glycoproteins in platelet function. *Nature* 255, 720-722.

Nurden, A.T., Hourdillé, P., Heilmann, E., Jallu, V., Pintigny, D., Clemetson, K.J., Chevaleyre, J. and Vezon, G. (1989): Thrombin induces a rapid redistribution of GPIb-IX complexes within the membrane systems of human platelets. *Blood* 74, 129a.

Okumura, T., Hasitz, M. and Jamieson, G.A. (1978): Platelet glycocalicin. *J. Biol. Chem.* 253, 3435-3443

Phillips, D.R. and Poh-Agin, P. (1977): Platelet plasma membrane glycoproteins. *J. Biol. Chem.* 252, 2121-2126.

Prandini, M.H., Denarier, E., Frachet, P., Uzan, G. and Marguerie, G. (1988): Isolation of the human platelet glycoprotein IIb gene and character-ization of the 5′ flanking region. *Biochem. Biophys. Res. Comm.* 156, 595-601.

Rosa, J.-P., Bray, P.F., Gayet, O., Johnston, G.I., Cook, R.G., Jackson, K.W., Shuman, M.A. and McEver, R.P. (1988): Cloning of glycoprotein IIIa cDNA from human erythroleukemia cells and localization of the gene to chromosome 17. *Blood* 72, 593-600.

Stricker, R.B., Wong, D., Saks, S.R., Corash, L. and Shuman, M.A. (1985): Acquired Bernard-Soulier syndrome. *J. Clin. Invest.* 76, 1274-1278.

Tsuji, T., Tsunehisa, S., Watanabe, Y., Yamamoto, K., Tohyama, H. and Osawa, T. (1983): The carbohydrate moiety of human platelet glycocalicin. The structure of the major ser/thr-linked sugar chain. *J. Biol. Chem.* 258, 6335-6339.

Vincente, V., Houghten, R.A. and Ruggeri, Z.M. (1990): Identification of a site in the a chain of platelet glycoprotein Ib that participates in von Willebrand factor binding. *J. Biol. Chem.* 265, 274-280

Wenger, R.H., Kieffer, N., Wicki, A.N. and Clemetson, K.J. (1988): Structure of the human blood platelet membrane glycoprotein Ibα gene. *Biochem. Biophys. Res. Comm.* 156, 389-395.

Wenger, R.H., Wicki, A.N., Walz, A., Kieffer, N. and Clemetson, K.J. (1989a): Cloning of cDNA coding for connective tissue activating peptide III from a human platelet-derived λgt11 expression library. *Blood* 73, 1498-1503.

Wenger, R.H., Wicki, A.N., Kieffer, N., Adolph, S., Hameister, H. and Clemetson, K.J. (1989b): The 5′ flanking region and

megakaryocytes are cultured as described elsewhere (Berthier et al, 1987).
The nuclear extracts were prepared according to (Ohlson, H. and Edlund, 1986).

Primer extension
Total RNA was extracted from human megakaryocytes using the thiocyanate-guanidinium method and the poly A^+ mRNA were purified by chromatograghy on oligo (dT) cellulose column. The 5' end labelled oligonucleotide (7.10^6 cpm) was hybridized to poly A^+ mRNA and elongated using the protocol and reagents of the first strand cDNA synthesis kit (Amersham England).

RNase mapping
RNase mapping with Sp6 probes was carried out essentially as previously described. The templates used for the generation of the anti-sens RNA probes were obtained by cloning a 1.4 kb Nco I-EcoR I fragment and a 1 kb Bgl I-Bgl I fragment isolated from the 1.9 kb 5'subclone, in the appropriate orientation, in the PGEM 1 plasmid. For synthesis of the Sp6 probes, the templates were linearized by Dde I and Pvu II respectively. Total RNA (50 µg) was hybridized overnight to 5.10^6 cpm of probe at 45°C and digested with RNase T1 and RNase A. The RNase resistant products were subsequently analysed on 6% acrylamide sequencing gel.

Gel retardation assay
Five overlapping fragments spaning the region between nucleotide +95 to nucleotide -853 were generated by digestion with restriction enzyme or amplified by polymerase chain reaction (PCR). These fragment were analyzed by gel retardation assays (Singh et al, 1986). For the binding reaction, 0.2 to 0.5 µg of radiolabeled DNA fragment ($\simeq$10 000 cpm) were mixed with 2 to 5 µg of nuclear extracts in a final volume of 30 µl containing : 10 mM Tris-HCL pH 7.5, 25 to 100 mM KCl, 1 mM DTT, 5% glycerol and 1 to 5 µg of poly dI-dC are used as described in individual experiments. The sample were incubated for 30 mn at room temperature and analyzed on 6% polyacrylamide gels in 0.5 xTBE buffer. The gels were preelectrophorezed twice at 180 V for 1 hour and electrophorezed at the same voltage for 2 to 3 hours at +4°C. After electrophoresis the gels were dried and autoradiographed overnight.

RESULTS

Characterization of the 5' end of the gene and localization of the transcriptionnal start site.
An 18 bases long oligonucleotide corresponding to the sequence of the 5'

end of the GPIIb cDNA was used to define more precisely the 5' region of the gene. This probe hybridized with a 1.9 Kb Eco RI Eco RI fragment from a genomic clone. This fragment was subcloned in the PGEM1 plasmid and sequenced. The complete sequence is shown in Fig 1.

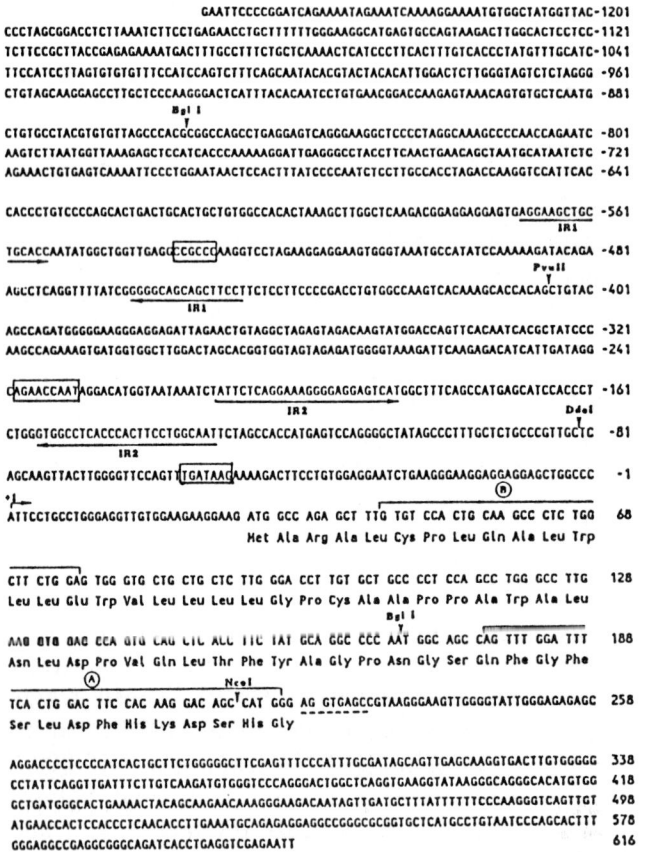

Fig 1 : DNA sequence of the first exon and 5' flanking region of GPIIb gene. The nucleotide +1, designated by an arrow corresponds to the transcription start site. Horizontal arrows indicate inverted repeats. Sequences corresponding to potential DNA binding sites are boxed. Oligonucleotides A and B were used in primer extension experiments.

Comparison with the cDNA sequence and the N-terminal domain of GPIIb indicates that this fragment contains the putative translation initiation codon ATG, the entire signal peptide and 31N-terminal amino acid residues of mature GPIIb. This exon is followed by an intron extending up to the end of this 1.9 Kb fragment. The exon-intron boundary sequence is consistent with the consensus sequence GT (A/G) AGT.

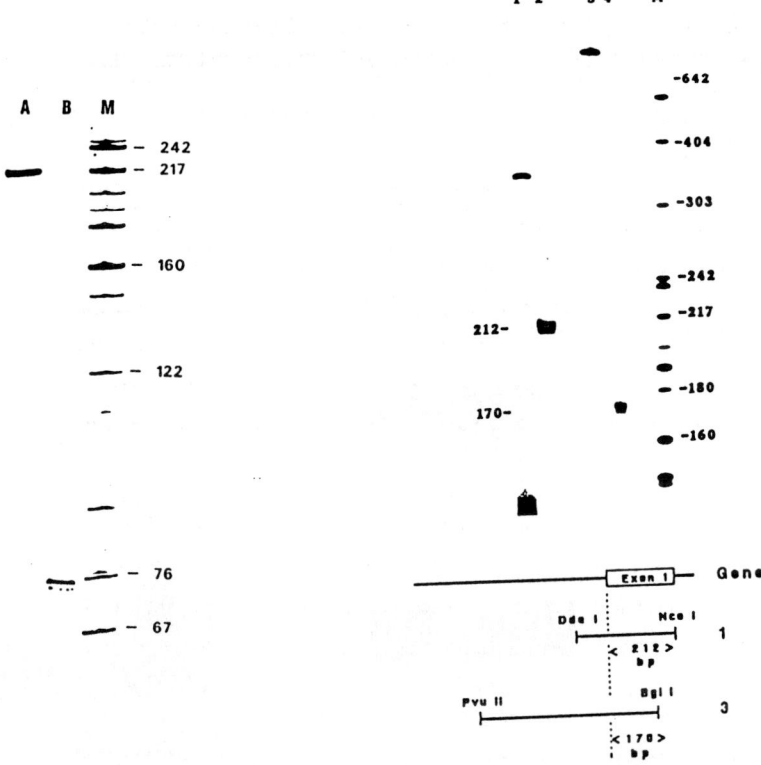

Fig. 2 : Primer extension and RNAse mapping experiments. Two oligonucleotides (Fig. 1) complementary to GPIIb mRNA were end labeled and elongated with AMV reverse transcriptase after hybridization with poly A^+ mRNA from megakaryocytes. The oligonucleotide A and B extended a 217 and a 76 based products, respectively. Two probes were used for RNAse mapping. One extended between Nco I and Dde I site (lane 1), the others extending between Bgl I and PVU II sites (lane 3). After hybridization with total magakaryocyte RNA and digestion with ribonucleases, protected fragments were detected on lane 2 and 4.

To identify the transcription initiation site for human GPIIb mRNA, a combination of primer extension and RNase mapping analysis was used. The primer extension experiments were performed with two oligonucleotides (A and B) corresponding to different positions on the exon. The extended products were resolved on a 6% denaturing polyacrylamide gel. After autoradiography, two fragments of 217 and 76 bases long respectively were visualized (Fig. 2). The RNase mapping

35

analysis were performed using two anti-sens RNA probes hybridized with total RNA from megakaryocytes. The protected fragments extend 212 bases from the Nco I site and 170 bases from the Bgl I site.

RNase mapping and primer extension analysis both indicated a similar 5' terminus, suggesting that the exon is the first one in the GPIIb gene and that its 5' end corresponds to the transcriptionnal start site indicated as +1.

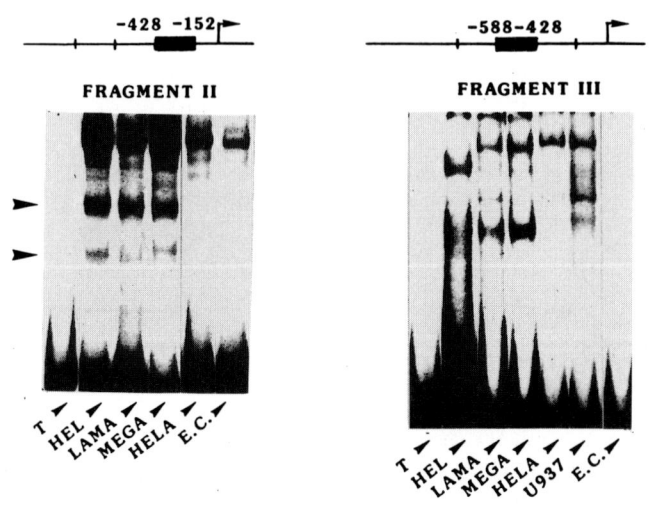

Fig 3 : Gel mobility shift of two different fragments from GPIIb gene 5' flanking region. Position of the fragments are indicated over the solid boxes. Nuclear proteins extracts from HEL, LAMA, megakaryocytes, Hela and Endothelial cells were used. The control with the probe alone is indicated by a T. Arrows indicate the position for specific DNA-protein interactions.

DNA/ protein interactions within GPIIb gene 5' flanking region

To determine if any of the protein interacting with the GPIIb gene were megakaryocyte specific, five overlapping fragment extending from nucleotide +95 to nucleotide -853 were analyzed in retardation gel assays using protein nuclear extracts prepared from different cell lines. Two of these fragments formed specific as well as ubiquitous DNA/protein complexes. A fragment of 276 bp covering the region comprised between nucleotides -152 at -428 showed retarded bands of lower electrophoretic mobility with nuclear extracts from HEL, megakaryocyte, Lama, Hela and endothelial cells. Two other bands of higher mobility are also detectable when nuclear extracts from megakaryocytic cells were used. Similar results were observed when a 160 bp fragment spanning from nucleotide -428 to -588 was used.

DISCUSSION

The gene encoding for GPIIb was isolated and the last 5' genomic fragment hybridizing with GPIIb cDNA probes was subcloned and sequenced. This fragment of 1.9 Kb in length contained the first exon, as determined by RNAse mapping and primer extension. The transcription start site was indicated as +1 in the sequence. The only ATG between nucleotide +1 and the codon corresponding to the amino terminal Leucine of mature GPIIb is at position +33. The sequence of the coding region corresponding to the signal peptide and for the 31 N-terminal amino acid of mature GPIIb is in total agreement with the sequence deduced from GPIIb cDNA (Poncz et al, 1987). This coding sequence is then interrupted by the first intron. We tried to identify in the 5' flanking region of the gene, consensus sequences corresponding to binding sites for nuclear factors. There is no consensus sequences corresponding to a TATA box between -25 to -40. It is also the case for GPIb, which is an another marker for megakaryocytopoiesis (Wenger et al, 1988). This observation suggest that for these genes, the RNA polymerase II positionning depends on other mechanisms than for TATA box containing genes. Centered at position -54, the sequence TGATAA is in total agreement with a NFE 1 (GF1) binding site A/T GAT AA/G. NFE1 was originaly described as an erythroid specific DNA binding protein. The proteins was recently cloned (Tsai et al, 1988), and the interaction of this molecule with various erythroid genes as human β and γ globin genes was demonstrated (de Boer et al, 1988 ; Martin et al, 1989 ; Mantovani et al, 1988). If NFE1 is realy implicated in GPIIb gene transcription, this will support early evidence (McLeod et al, 1980 ; Hoffman et al, 1989) concerning the similarities between megakaryocyte and erythrocyte progenitors. The sequence ACCAAT, centered at position -233 is homologous to a CAAT binding region. The other sequences which could represent DNA binding sites for nuclear factors were of less stringent homologies.

DNA binding activity for megakaryocyte specific nuclear factors was investigated within the region extending from nucleotides +95 to -853. Five different fragments were generated within this region by the polymerase chain reaction. These fragments were incubated with nuclear extracts from different cell lines and analysed in gel retardation assays. Two of these fragments, extending from nucleotides -152 to -428 and -428 to -588 showed retarded bands corresponding to specific complexes. These complexes were only detected when nuclear extracts from megakaryocytic cell lines were used indicating that the GPIIb gene contains multiple binding sites for nuclear proteins and suggesting the existence of specific megakaryocyte nuclear factors. Thus the GPIIb gene may be controlled by a specific mechanism, and may represent a good target gene for studying megakaryocyte differentiation

REFERENCES

Berridge, M.V., Ralph, S.J. and Tan, A.S. (1985) : Cell lineage antigens of the stem cell mekagaryocyte platelet lineage are associated with the platelet IIb-IIIa glycoprotein complex. Blood 66, 76-82.

Berthier, R., Marin, MP., Duperray, A., Prenant, M., Newton, I., Schweitzer, A., Hollard, D. and Marguerie, G. (1987) : Megakaryocytic development in liquid cultures of cryopreserved leukocyte stem cell concentrates from chronic myelogenous leukemia patients. Exp. Hematol. 15, 750-755.

de Boer, E., Antoniou, M., Mignotte, V., Wall, L. and Grosveld, F. (1988) : The human β-globin promoter ; nuclear protein factors and erythroid specific induction of transcription. Embo. J. 7, 4203-4212.

Fraser, J.K., Leahy, M.F. and Berridge, M.V. (1986) : Expression of antigens of the platelet glycoprotein IIbIIIa complex on human hematopoietic stem cells. Blood 68, 762-769.

Ginsberg, M.H., Loftus, J.C. and Plow, E.F. (1988) : Cytoadhesins, integrins and platelets. Thromb. Hemostas. 59, 1-6.

Kanz, L., Mielke, R. and Franzer, A.A. (1988) : Analysis of human hematopoietic progenitor cells for the expression of glycoprotein IIIa. Exp. Hematol. 16, 741-747.

Ohlson, G. and Edlund, T. (1986) : Sequence specific interactions of nuclear factors with the insulin gene enhancer. Cell 45, 35-44.

Poncz, H., Eizman, R., Heidenreich, R., Silver, S.M., Vilaire, G., Surrey, S., Schwartz, E. and Bennet, J.S. (1987) : Structure of the platelet membrane glycoprotein IIb. J. Biol. Chem. 262, 8476-8482.

Prandini, M.H., Denarier, E., Frachet, P., Uzan, G. and Marguerie, G. (1988) : Isolation of the human platelet GPIIb gene and characterization of the 5' flanking region. Biochem. Res. Com. 156, 35-54.

Singh, H., Sen, R., Baltimore, D. and Sharp, P.A. (1986) : A nuclear factor that binds to a conserved sequence motif in transcriptional control element of immunoglobulin genes. Nature 319, 154-158.

Tsai, S.F., Martin, D.I.K., Zon, L.I., D'Andrea, A.D., Wong, G.G. and Orkin, S.H. (1989) : Cloning of cDNA for the major DNA-binding protein of the erythroid lineage through expression in mammalian cells. Nature

339, 446-451.

Wenger, R.H., Kieffer, N., Wicki, A.N. and Clemetson, K.J. (1988) : Structure of the human blood platelet membrane glycoprotein Ibα gene. Biophys. Res. Com. 156, 389-395.

Résumé

L'un des principaux objectifs de l'étude de la mégacaryocytopoïèse est l'identification des facteurs qui permettent à la cellule souche de se différencier et d'acquérir le phénotype mégacaryocytaire.

L'une des approches possibles pour identifier de tels facteurs est de choisir un gène marqueur, exprimé de façon précoce et spécifique dans cette lignée. Les facteurs nucléaires qui régulent la transcription de ce gène d'une façon tissu spécifique peuvent être isolés, et leur rôle éventuel dans la différenciation des mégacaryocytes peut être testé. Le gène codant pour la GPIIb est un bon candidat. La GPIIb, qui constitue la sous unité α de l'intégrine plaquettaire GPIIb-IIIa n'est exprimée que dans les mégacaryocytes, et cette expression est détectée à des stades précoces de la différenciation. Le gène de la GPIIb a été isolé, et un sous-clone génomique contenant une partie de la région 5' flanquante a été séquencé. Ce fragment d'ADN code pour le peptide signal et pour 31 acides aminés de la protéine mature. Le site d'initiation de la transcription a été localisé, et les sites de fixation de protéines nucléaires ont été analysés.

Une séquence, centrée à -54 contient un motif identique a celui du site de liaison du facteur de transcription NFE1. Ce facteur a été décrit initialement comme étant spécifique de la lignée érythrocytaire. L'implication de ce facteur dans la régulation de gènes mégacaryocytaires confirmerait la parenté existant entre les deux lignées. Par ailleurs, deux fragments situés entre -152 et -428 et entre -428 et -588 fixent des protéines uniquement lorsque des extraits nucléaires de mégacaryocyte ou de lignée à caractère mégacaryocytaire sont utilisés. Ceci suggère que la transcription du gène de la GPIIb fait intervenir des facteurs spécifiques du mégacaryocyte.

Molecular and cellular biology of glycoprotein IIIb (GPIV, CD36)

B. Catimel*,**, S. Parmentier*, L.K.K. Leung*** and J.L. McGregor*,***

INSERM U 331, *Faculté de Médecine Alexis Carrel, **Institut Pasteur, Lyon, France
***Stanford Medical school, California, USA

SUMMARY

Membrane glycoprotein, IIIb, also known as GPIV and clustered as CD36, is a major human blood platelet glycoprotein. In contrast to the 3 other major glycoproteins (GPIb, GPIIb and GPIIIa) which are known to play a vital role in platelet adhesion and aggregation, little is known about the function of GPIIIb. This review summarizes the recent work concerning the structure, function and possible role of GPIIIb in platelets and other cells.

BIOCHEMISTRY AND STRUCTURE:

GPIIIb, also know as GPIV or CD36[1], is present in different amounts in platelets of normal donors[2] and shows a relative increase, associated with a decrease of platelet GPIb[3,4,5,6], in platelets of patients with myeloproliferative disorders. Recently, a new platelet specific alloantigen, designed Nak^a[7], has been found on GPIIIb[8]. In addition to platelets, GPIIIb has been identified on endothelial cells and certain tumor cell lines by monoclonal antiboby OKM5[9,10,11,12]. GPIIIb was previously isolated from C32 melanoma cells and platelets by immunoaffinity chromatography with monoclonal antibody OKM5[7], from Triton X-114 membrane platelet extracts that were extensively degraded with chymotrypsin[13] or by a combination of lectin affinity chromatography and preparative SDS-PAGE[14]. Recent work has allowed the purification of GPIIIb, under non-denaturing conditions, from Triton X-114 platelet extracts by tandem anion-exchange and size exclusion fast protein liquid chromatography (FPLC)[15]. Alternatively, anion-exchange followed by lectin affinity and size exclusion chromatography[16] has also been used to isolate GPIIIb. Glycoprotein IIIb is composed of a single highly glycosylated polypeptide chain, with an apparent molecular mass of 88 kDa and an apparent isoelectric point (pI) ranging between 4.4 and 6.3[17,18]. This pI heterogeneity is probably due to variable sialic acid contents[19]. GPIIIb migrates with a relatively slow anodal mobility on crossed immunoelectrophoresis[20]. Analysis of GPIIIb showed that it contains large amounts of acidic and hydroxy amino acids and 26 % (w/w) carbohydrate consisting of galactose, mannose, N-acetyl glucosamine, N-acetyl galactosamine and sialic acid as principal sugars[12,14]. GPIIIb contains both N- and O-linked sugar chains. The successful cloning of a placenta cell cDNA coding for CD36 has provided a primary structure of GPIIIb[21]. The sequence of the cDNA clone consists of 1870 residues and the resulting polypeptide would possess 471 residues with a molecular weight of 53 kDa. The high glycosylation (26%, 10 potential sites of N-glycosylation) could explain the discrepancy between the predicted polypeptide and the apparent molecular mass of GPIIIb. The transmembrane domain contains 27 hydrophylic residues preceded by a short intercellular domain (6 residues). The N-terminal region of GPIIIb also possesses a potential transmembrane domain (23 hydrophobic residues) followed by a hydrophilic hexapeptide. The molecule could also contain 2 potential associated-membrane domains. These hydrophobic regions could explain the resistance in situ of GPIIIb to proteolysis by trypsin and chymotrypsin[11,15,22].

ROLE OF GPIIIb AND THROMBOSPONDIN IN PLATELET AGGREGATION:

GPIIIb has been identified as a receptor site for thrombospondin on activated platelets[9,15]. Thrombospondin, a major multifunctional adhesive protein released by platelet upon stimulation[23,24,25], supports hemagglutination of fixed erythrocytes and acts as an endogenous platelet lectin[26,27,28]. Thrombospondin (TSP) has a broad tissue distribution[29] and may mediate a variety of cell-cell and cell-matrix interactions[24,25,26,30,31,32,33,33,34,35,36,37,38]. This adhesive protein (TSP) is thought to play an important role in platelet aggregation[39,40,41]. The plasmatic level of thrombospondin is low (20-30 ng/ml)[42] and the TSP expression on platelet surface is dependent on the release of TSP from platelet alpha-granules ($20\mu g/10^9$) following thrombin stimulation[43]. The formation of a macromolecular complex between thrombospondin, fibrinogen and GPIIb/IIIa has been proposed as a major stage in the mechanism leading to irreversible platelet aggregation[37]. Previous work by Leung & Nachman using an ELISA system indicates that TSP has the ability to interact with fibrinogen bound to GPIIb/IIIa[44]. Electron microscopy work shows the colocalization of TSP, fibrinogen and GPIIb/IIIa[45,46,47]. However, it is important to note that TSP can bind to stimulated platelets from patients with Glanzmann's thrombasthenia (platelets which lack GPIIb/IIIa)[41,48], suggesting that TSP binds to sites independent from GPIIb/IIIa and fibrinogen. Recent studies have shown that fibrinogen contains at least two unique sequences which are recognized by thrombospondin[49]. Fab fragments of polyclonal and monoclonal antibodies[37,41] directed against TSP inhibit the second wave of ADP-induced aggregation and partially inhibit thrombin and collagen-induced aggregation. Experiments with monoclonal antibodies against defined domains of thrombospondin[50] were showed to inhibit platelet aggregation or agglutination. A monoclonal antibody against the 18kDa COOH-terminal domain of TSP inhibited platelet aggregation[51]. However, antibodies directed against the 25kDa NH_2-terminal domain inhibited thrombospondin-induced agglutination of fixed platelet but did not affect, with one exception[52], platelet aggregation[53,54]. Studies have shown that platelets have two classes of TSP-binding sites[39,48,55]. One is cation-independent with low capacity (2.000-3.000 binding sites on resting platelets) and the other is cation dependent with high capacity (16.000 binding sites on thrombin-activated platelets). When the binding of exogenous thrombospondin to thrombin-stimulated platelets was examined, 36.000 TSP molecules/cell was reported[56]. Recent studies have shown that GPIIIb is responsible, in part, for the cation-dependent binding of TSP to the surface of activated platelet[7,15]. The binding of TSP to purified GPIIIb is calcium dependent and is not inhibited by the RGD peptide[7,15]. The role of GPIIIb as a functional thrombospondin receptor was recently confirmed by the specific and calcium-dependant binding of TSP to purified GPIIIb incorporated into liposomes[57]. However, it remains to be explained why the expression of a CD36 cDNA clone in COS cells did not show an increased binding of purified human thrombospondin[19]. Monospecific anti-GPIIIb antibodies interfered with the expression of endogeneous thrombospondin on thrombin-activated platelets and partially inhibited collagen- and thrombin-induced platelet aggregation[15]. Monoclonal antibody OKM5, directed against GPIIIb, inhibits endogeneous TSP binding to thrombin- and ionophore-activated platelets[7]. Another monoclonal antibody against GPIIIb (FA6-152) was recently described to inhibit platelet aggregation as well as endogeneous TSP binding to the platelet surface[58]. It is of interest that the number of binding sites of anti-GPIIIb monoclonal antibodies on platelets is in the same range (11 000 to 25 000)[57,59], as that reported for endogenous thrombospondin binding to thrombin-activated platelets. This suggests that the stoechiometry of TSP binding to GPIIIb on the platelet surface is 1:1. Thrombospondin may interact with the platelet surface by at least two different mechanisms: via the COOH-terminal domain with GPIIIb on activated platelets and via the NH_2-terminal heparin binding domain with the heparan sulfate of resting platelet membranes. In addition to fibrinogen[42,48], TSP is also known to interact with multiple ligands such as fibronectin[60,61] and plasminogen[62] which bind to platelets. Thrombospondin also contains a RGD sequence[23,63]. The RGD sequence is known to mediate the interaction of adhesive proteins such as fibrinogen, fibronectin, vitronectin, von Willebrand factor with cell surfaces[64,65]. Thrombospondin was recently reported to interact in vitro through its RGD site with the vitronectin receptor[66,67] and the platelet GPIIb/IIIa[68]. The thrombospondin RGD sequence is cryptic under normal conditions and its availability is regulated by the calcium concentration[23,62,67]. The interaction of TSP with the surface of activated-platelets is complex and may involve more than one class of binding sites. This could explain the number of binding-sites of exogenous thrombospondin to stimulated-platelet membranes.

GPIIIb IN PLATELET ADHESION TO COLLAGEN:

Platelet interaction with collagen is a crucial event in haemostasis. Fibrillar collagen is the most thrombogenic constituent of the vascular endothelium[69]. Recent studies have shown that platelet GPIIIb may act as a primary receptor for collagen and mediate platelet-collagen adhesion[14,70]. Purified GPIIIb binds to collagen type I fibrils. Fab fragment of monospecific antibody to GPIIIb inhibited platelet adhesion, shape change and secretion induced by collagen. Platelet adhesion to collagen was shown to be inhibited by Fab fragments of monospecific antibody to GPIIIb. This antibody is able to reverse adhesion that occured within the first 5-8 minutes and to inhibit adhesion occuring therafter[69]. GPIIIb may play a role in the first step of recognition and in initial attachment to collagen. A second mechanism, GPIIIb independent, may occur for the spreading of platelets. Recent studies have shown the role of platelet glycoprotein GPIa/IIa or VLA-2 in platelet-collagen adhesion[71].

ROLE OF GPIIIb IN CYTOADHESION OF *PLASMODIUM FALCIPARUM*-INFECTED ERYTHROCYTES:

The adherence of trophozoide-infected erythrocytes to vasular endothelium plays an important role in the biology of *Plasmodium falciparum*. By this mechanism, the parasites promote their survival by escaping passage through the immunologically active spleen. The sequestration of infected erythrocytes in the brain vessels is responsible for the frequently lethal syndrome of central nervous malaria. Infected erythrocytes adhere under in vivo or in vitro conditions to endothelial cells[72] via electron dense protusions called knobs[73]. Extensive evidence shows that infected erythrocytes also bind to monocytes[74] and some human melanoma cell lines[73,75,76]. Moreover, the adherence of parasitized erythrocytes is inhibited by monoclonal antibody OKM5 to these specific target cells[73]. Recent studies have demonstrated the role of GPIIIb in the cytoadherence of infected erythrocytes[9,19,77]. Thrombospondin has also been reported to mediate the cytoadherence of *Plasmodium falciparum*-infected erythrocytes[34,78]. The binding of parasitized erythrocytes to GPIIIb is unaffected by the absence of calcium and thrombospondin[9]. The expression of a CD36 cDNA clone in COS cells supports the cytoadherence of infected erythrocytes[19]. The interaction of TSP and GPIIIb with infected erythrocytes under different conditions suggests the presence of two different ligands or one with different functional domains. A third cell-adhesion molecule for parasitized erythrocytes, ICAM-1 or intercellullar adhesion molecule-1[79], which is a ligand for the leucocyte integrin LFA-1[80], has recently been identified on endothelial cells. Moreover, COS cells transfected with ICAM-1 cDNA bind parasitized erythrocytes[78].

GPIIIb AND THROMBOSPONDIN IN INFLAMMATION AND ARTERIOSCLEROSIS:

Interaction between activated platelets with mononuclear phagocytes at sites of platelet injury has been shown to be one of the first events in experimental arteriosclerosis[81,82]. Thrombospondin was shown to mediate an interaction between thrombin-stimulated platelets and both U937 cells (an histiocytic cell line that has many characteristics of human monocytes[83]) and monocytes[28]. These dependent platelet-monocyte interactions are mediated by GPIIIb[29]. The phenomenon of platelet satellitism with U937 and monocytes is inhibited by preincubating platelets or U937 cells with anti-GPIIIb monoclonal or polyclonal antibodies. Thrombospondin can cross-link platelets and monocytes via its attachment to the respective GPIIIb of both cells. Another platelet glycoprotein, GMP140 or PADGEM (platelet activation dependant granule-external protein)[84] was also shown to mediate interaction of activated platelets with neutrophils and monocytes[85].

GPIIIb AND THROMBOSPONDIN IN TUMOR CELL METASTASIS:

Metastasis is a process by which tumor cells colonize distant tissue via the circulatory system. The metastatic system is complex and includes stages by which tumor cells enter and exit the circulatory system and grow in a new site. Recent works have implicated platelets in the metastatic process[86,87]. Platelet-melanoma cell interaction was recently shown to be mediated by the platelet GPIIb/IIIa complex and by a GPIIb/IIIa-like glycoprotein present on melanoma cell lines[88,89,90]. A monoclonal antibody, directed against the blood platelet GPIIb/IIIa, inhibits human melanoma growth in vivo[91]. Thrombospondin supports adhesion and spreading of several tumor cell lines like human squamous carcinoma cells and melanoma cells[92,93,94]. Thrombospondin adhesion activity is lost following removal of the 18kDa COOH-terminal domain. The NH_2-terminal heparin-binding domain of thrombospondin does not promote adhesion but is involved in the spreading of cells. Thrombospondin also interacts with sulfated glycolipids and proteoglycans of human melanoma cells[95]. These results suggest that on some tumor cells, more than one receptor is involved in thrombospondin binding. The carboxyl-terminal domain region and perhaps other regions of the molecule bind to receptor(s) (GPIIIb) on the tumor cell surface that promote initial attachment but not cell spreading. Interaction of the heparin-binding domain with cell surface sulfated glycolipids and proteoglycans mediates spreading. The important role of thrombospondin in the metastatic process was confirmed by its role of potentiator in tumor cell metastasis[96] and by its role in the killing of monocytes by human squamous epithelial cells[97]. This monocyte killing was inhibited by monoclonal antibodies against the heparin-binding region and against the non-heparin-binding regions of the TSP molecule. TSP and TSP-receptors on both cells played a role in monocyte-mediated killing of squamous epithelial cells. A recent study has shown that C32 human melanoma cells expressed different amounts of GPIIIb[98]. Heterogeneous C32 melanoma cells, GPIIIb-rich and GPIIIb-poor cells, were identified and separated by fluorescence activated cell sorting. GPIIIb-rich melanoma cells, compared to GPIIIb-poor cells, showed a different morphology on light microscopy (dendritic appearance), had a significant growth and demonstrated an enhanced binding to TSP coated to plastic. The growth advantage of these GPIIIb-rich melanoma cells was also demonstrated in vivo in a nude mouse model. The GPIIIb expression in C32 melanoma cells may represent a marker for a more malignant phenotype

GPIIIb IS RELATED TO EPITHELIAL MEMBRANE GLYCOPROTEIN PAS-IV:

PAS-IV is a 78 kDa integral membrane protein found in lactating mammary epithelial cells and capillary endothelial cells[99]. The N-terminal sequence of PAS-IV was found to be nearly identical to that of GPIIIb[100]. GPIIIb and PAS-IV show the same reactivity with monoclonal antibodies OKM5 and OKM8[100]. PAS-IV binds to thrombospondin in a concentration-dependant and saturable manner. However, the maximum binding of thrombospondin was 50% of that of GPIIIb and was not inhibited by EDTA. GPIIIb supports *Plasmodium falciparum*-infected erythrocytes in a dose-dependent manner while no significant binding of infected-erythrocytes to PAS-IV is observed[100]. GPIIIb and PAS-IV appear to be structurally and immunologically related but show significant differences in their functional properties. It is interesting to note that thrombospondin is found in human colostrum and milk, but TSP is present in the aqueous phase and not associated with the milk fat globule membrane[37]. Using anti-PASIV monoclonal antibodies, an immunoreactive protein of 85kDa is specifically detected in the microsomal fraction of heart and lung tissues[101]. Human peripherical blood monocytes synthesize a GPIIIb-like protein of 94 kDa (unpublished observation, JL McGregor, L.K.K. Leung). Recently, a 78kDa erythroblast membrane glycoprotein has been found to be immunologically related to platelet GPIIIb[57]. Its expression is developmentally regulated during erythroid differentiation: it is present on fetal erythroblasts, fetal mature erythrocytes but is absent from adult erythrocytes. This protein is also detected in human erythroleukaemic (HEL) cells as two bands of 85 and 88kDa[57]. These results suggest the presence of multiple forms of immunoreactive GPIIIb-like proteins in different tissues. GPIIIb, PASIV and the 78 kDa erythroblast membrane protein may belong to a family of related cell adhesive protein receptor.

The broad tissue distribution of platelet membrane glycoprotein IIIb, along that of thrombospondin, raises the possibility that the TSP-IIIb interaction, in addition to its role in platelet aggregation, may be important in cell-cell and cell-matrix interaction and plays a role in the regulation of thrombosis, inflammation and pathology of arteriosclerosis. Moreover, by its role as primary receptor for collagen on human platelets and for *Plasmodium falciparum*-infected erythrocytes, GPIIIb may represent a new class of cell adhesion molecules.

REFERENCES

1 - Shaw, S., Characterization of human leucocyte differentiation antigens. (1987) Immunology Today 8: 1-3.

2 - Jamieson, G.A., Okurama, T., Fischback, B., Johnson, M.M., Egan, J.J. & Weiss, H.J. Changes in distribution of platelet membrane glycoproteins in patients with myeloproliferatives disorders.(1979) J. Lab. Clin. Med. 93: 652-660.

3 - Bolin, R.B., Okurama, T. & Jamieson, G.A. Changes in distribution of platelet membrane glycoprotein in patient with myeloproliferative disorders. (1977) Am. J. Hematol. 3: 63-67.

4 - Vainer, H. & Bussel, A. Altered platelet surface glycoproteins in chronic myeloid leukemia. (1977) Int. J. Cancer. 19: 134-150.

5. Wautier, J.L., Souchon, M., Dupuis, D., Caen, J.P. & Nurden, A.T. A platelet defect in a patient with eosinophilic leukemia: Absent ristococetin-induced platelet aggregation associated with a reduced platelet sialic acid content. (1979) Scan. J. Haematol. 26: 123-129.

6. Eche, N., Sie, P., Caranobe, C., Nouvel, C., Pris, J. & Boneu, B. Platelet in myeloproliferative disorders. III glycoprotein profile in relation to platelet function and density. (1981) Scand. J. Haematol. 26: 123-129.

7. Ikeda, H., Mitani, T., Ohnuma, M., Haga, H.,Ohtzuka, S., Sato, T., Nakase, T. & Sekiguchi, S. A new platelet specific antigen NAK[a] involved in the refractoriness of HLA-matched platelet transfusion. (1989) Vox Sang. 57:213.

8. Tomiyama, Y., Take, H., Ikeda, H., Mitani, T., Furubayashi, T., Mizutami, H., Yamamoto, N., Tandon, N.N., Sekiguchi, S., Jamieson, G.A., Kurata, Y., Yonezawa, T. & Tarui, S. Identification of the platelet-specific alloantigen, Nak[a], on platelet membrane glycoprotein IV. (1990) Blood 75: 684-687.

9. Asch, A.S., Barnwell, J., Silverstein, R.L. & Nachman, R.L. Isolation of the thrombospondin membrane receptor. (1987) J. Clin. Invest. 79: 1054-1061.

10. Knowles, D.M., Tolidjian, B., Marboe, C., D'Agati, V., Grimes, M. & Chess, L. Monoclonal anti-human monocytes OKM1 and OKM5 possess distinctive tissue distributions including differential reactivity with vascular endothelium. (1984) J. Immunol. 132: 2170-2173.

11. Barnwell, J.W., Asch, A.S., Nachman, R.L., Yamaya, M., Aikawa, M. & Ingravallo, P. A human 88-kD membrane glycoprotein (CD36) functions in vitro as a receptor for cytoadherence ligand of *Plasmodium falciparum*-infected erythrocytes. (1989) J. Clin. Invest. 84: 765-.772.

12. Ockenhouse, C.F., Magowan, C. & Chulay, J.D. Activation of monocytes and platelets by monoclonal antibodies or malaria-infected erythrocytes binding to the CD36 surface receptor in vitro. (1989) J. Clin. Invest. 84: 468-475.

13. Tandon, N.N. & Jamieson, G.A. Role of platelet membrane glycoprotein IV in platelet-collagen interaction: a microtiter assay to study platelet adherence. (1987) Throm. Haemost. abs. 1107.

14. Tsuji, T. & Osawa, T. Purification and chemical characterization of platelet membrane glycoprotein IV. (1986) J. Biochem. 100: 1077-1082.

15. McGregor, J.L., Catimel, B., Parmentier, S., Clezardin, P., Dechavanne, M. & Leung, L.K.K. Rapid purification and partial characterization of human platelet IIIb. (1989) J. Biol. Chem. 264: 501-506.

16. Tandon, N.N., Lipski, R.H., Burges, W.H. & Jamieson, G.A. Isolation and Characterization of platelet GPIV. (1989) J. Biol. Chem. 264: 7570-7575.

17. Mc Gregor, J.L., CLemetson, K.J., James, E., Luscher, E.F. & Dechavanne, M. Characterization of human blood platelet membrane glycoproteins by their isoelectric point and apparent molecular weight using 2D-electrophoresis and surface labelling. (1980) Biochim. Biophys. Acta. 599: 473-483.

18. Clemetson, K.J. & Mc Gregor, J.L. Characterization of platelet glycoproteins. (1987) in Platelets in Biology and Pathology III. (Macintyre, E.E. & Gordon, J.L., eds.) pp160-220, Academic press, New York.

19. Mc Gregor, J.L., Clemetson, K.J., James, E., Capitano, A., Greenland, T. , Luscher, E.F. & Dechavanne, M. (1981) Eur. J. Biochem.116: 379-388.

20. Yamamoto, N., De Romeuf, C., Tandom, N.N. Jamieson, G.A. A resolution in reported discrepancies in the characteristics of platelet glycoproteins IV (GPIV) and IIIb (GPIIIb). (1990) Thromb. Haemostasis. 63: 97-102.

21. Ockendo, P., Hundt, E., Lawler, J. & Seeds, B. CD36 directly mediates cytoadherence of Plasmodium falciparum-parasitized erythrocytes. (1989) Cell. 58: 95-101.

22. Poldolsack, B. Effect of thrombin, chymotrypsin and aggregate gamma-globulins on the human platelet membrane. (1977) Thromb. Haemostasis. 37: 396-406.

23. Lawler, J. The structural and functional properties of thrombospondin. (1986) Blood. 67: 1197-1209.

24. Silverstein, R.L., Leung, L.K.K. & Nachman, R.L. Thrombospondin, a versatile multifunctional platelet glycoprotein. (1986) Artheriosclerosis. 6: 245-248.

25. Lawler, J. & Hynes, R.O. Structural organization of the thrombospondin molecule. (1987) Seminars in Thrombosis and Hemostasis. vol 13 n°3: 245-253.

26. Jaffe, E.A., Leung, L.K.K., Nachman, R.L., Levin, R.I. & Moscher, D.F. Thrombospondin is the endogenous lectin of human platelets. (1982) Nature. 295: 246-248.

27. Haverstick, D.M., Dixit, V.M., Grant, G.A., Frazier, W.A. & Santoro, S.A. Localization of the hemagglutinating activity of platelet thrombospondin to a 140 000-dalton thermolytic fragment. (1984) Biochemistry. 23: 5597-5603.

28. Gartner, T.K., Doyle, M.J. & Moscher, D.F. Effect on anti-thrombospondin antibodies on the hemagglutination activity of the endogenous platelet lectin and thrombospondin. (1984) Thromb. Haemostasis. 52: 354-357.

29. Wight, T.N., Raugi, G.J., Mumbi, S.M. & Bornstein, P. Light microscopic immunolocalization of thrombospondin in human tissues. (1985) J. Histochem. Cytochem. 33: 295-302

30. Silverstein, R.L. & Nachman, R.L. Thrombospondin binds to monocytes, macrophages and mediates platelet-monocytes adhesion. (1987) J. Clin. Invest. 79: 867-874.

31. Silverstein, R.L., Asch, A.S. & Nachman, R.L. GPIV mediates thrombospondin dependant platelet-monocytes adhesion. (1989) J. Clin. invest. 84: 546-552.

32. Murphy-Ullrich, J.E. & Moscher, D.F. Interaction of thrombospondin with endothelial cells: receptor-mediated binding and degradation. (1987) J. Cell. Biol. 105: 1603-1611.

33. Dawes, J., Clezardin, P. & Pratt, D.A. Thrombospondin in milk, other breast secretions and breast tissue. (1987) Seminars in Thrombosis and Hemostasis. vol 13, n° 3 : 378-384.

33. Wilkner, N.E., Dixit, V.N., Frazier, W.A. & Clark, R.A. Human keratinocytes synthetyse and secrete the extracellular matrix protein, thrombospondin. (1987) J. Invest. Dermatol. 88: 207-211.

34. Majack, R.A., Goodman, L.V. & Dixit, V.M. Cell surface thrombospondin is functionally essential for vascular smooth muscle cell proliferation. (1988) J. Cell. Biol. 106: 415-422.

35. O'Sea, K.S. & Dixit, V.N. Unique distribution of the extracellular componant thrombospondin in the developing mouse embryo. (1988) J. Cell. Biol. 107: 2737-2748.

36. Roberts, D.D., Sherwood, J.A., Spitalnik, S., Panton, L.J., Howard, R.J., Dixit, V.M., Frazier, W.A.,

Miller, L.H. & Ginsberg, V. Thrombospondin binds falciparum malaria parasitized erythrocytes and may mediate cythoadherence. (1985) Nature. 318: 64-66.

37. Jaffe, E.A., Ruggiero, J.T., Leung, L.K.K., Doyle, P.J., McKeown-Longo, P.J. & Moscher, D.F. Cultured fibroblast synthetyse and secrete thrombospondin and incorporate into cellular matrix.(1983) Pro. Natl. Acad. Sci. USA. 80: 999-1002.

38. Robey, P.G., Young, M.F., Fischer, L.W.& McClain, T.D. Thrombospondin is an osteobast-derived componant of mineralized extracellular matrix. (1989) J. Cell. Biol. 108: 719-727.

39. Leung, L.K.K. Role of thrombospondin in platelet agregation. (1984) J. Clin. Invest. 74: 1764-1777.

40. Dixit, V.M., Haverwick, D.M., O'Rourke, K.M., Hennessy, W.M., Grant, G.A. & Frazier, W.A. A monoclonal antibody against human thrombospondin inhibits platelet agregation. (1985) Proc. Natl. Acad. Sci. USA. 82: 3472-3476.

41. Boukerche, H. & Mc Gregor, J.L. Characterization of a anti-thrombospondin monoclonal antibody P8 that inhibits human blood platelet functions. (1987) Eur. J. Biochem. 171: 383-392.

42. Saglio, S.D. & Slayter, H.S. Use of a radioimmunoassay to quantify thrombospondin. (1982) Blood. 59: 162-166..

43. Phillips, .R., Jennings, L.K. & Prasanna, H.R. Calcium-mediated association of protein G (Thrombin-sensitive protein, thrombospondin). (1980) J. Biol. Chem. 255: 11629-11632.

44. Leung, L.K.K. & Nachman, R.L. Complex formation of platelet thrombospondin with fibrinogen. (1984) J. Clin. Invest. 70: 742-749.

45. Asch, A.S., Leung, L.K.K., Polley, M.J. & Nachman, R.L. Colocalization of thrombospondin and fibrinogen with the glycoprotein IIb/IIIa complex. (1985) Blood. 66: 926-933.

46. Hourdille, P., Hasitz, M., Belloc, F. & Nurden, A.T. Immunocytochemical study of the binding of fibrinogen and thrombospondin to ADP and thrombin-stimulated platelets. (1985) Blood. 65: 912-920.

47. Isenberg, W.M., McEver, R.P., Phillips, D.R., Schuman, M.A. & Benton, D.F. The platelet fibrinogen receptor: an immunogold-surface replica study of agonist-induced ligand binding and receptor clustering. (1987) J. Cell. Biol. 104: 1655-1663.

48. Aiken, M.L., Ginsberg, M.H. & Plow, E.F. Identification of a new class of inducible receptors on platelets. Thrombospondin interacts with platelets via a GPIIb/IIIa independant mechanism. (1986) J. Clin. Invest. 78: 1713-1716.

49. Bacon-Baguley, T., Ogilvie, M.L., Gartner, T.K. & Waltz, D.A. Thrombospondin binding to specific sequences within the Aα-and Bβ-chains of fibrinogen. (1990) J. Biol. Chem. 265: 32317-2323.

50. Galvin, N.J., Dixit, V.M., O'Rourke, K.M., Santoro, S.A., Grant, G.A. & Frazier, W.A. Mapping of epitopes for monoclonal antibodies against human platelet thrombospondin with electron microscopy and high sensitivity amino acid sequencing. (1985) J. Cell Biol. 101: 1434-1444.

51. Dixit, V.M.,Haverwick, D.M., O'Rourke, K.M., Hennessy, V.M., Grant, V.A., Santoro, S.A. & Frazier, W.A. A monoclonal antibody against human thrombospondin inhibits platelet aggregation. (1985) Proc. Natl. Acad. Sci. USA. 82: 3472-3476.

52. Gartner, T.K., Walz, D.A., Aiken, M., Starrspires, L. & Ogilvie, M.L. Antibodies against a 23 kDa heparin binding fragment of thrombospondin inhibit platelet aggregation. (1984) Biochem. Biophys.

Res. Comm. 124: 290-295.

53. Dixit, V.M., Haverstick, V.M., O'Rourke, K.M., Hennessy, S.W., Grant, G.A. & Frazier, W.A. Effect of anti-thrombospondin monoclonal antibodies on the aggluntnation of erythrocytes and fixed, activated platelets by purified thrombospondin. (1985) Biochemistry. 24: 4270-4275.

54. Clezardin, P., McGregor, J.L., Lyon, M., Clemetson, K.J. & Huppert, J. Characterization of two murine monoclonal antibodies (P10,P12) directed against different determinants on human blood platelet thrombospondin. (1986) Eur. J. Biochem. 154: 95-102.

55. Aiken, M.L., Ginsberg, M.H. & Plow, E.F. (1987) Divalent cation-dependant and independant surface expression of thrombospondin on thrombin-stimulated human platelets. (1987) Blood. 69:58-64.

56. Wolff, R., Plow, E.F. & Ginsberg, M.H. Interaction of thrombospondin with resting and stimulated human platelets. (1986) J. Biol. Chem. 261: 6840-6846.

57. Berk, G.I., Asch, A.S., Scotto, A.W., Silverstein, R.L. & Nachman, R.L. Glycoprotein IIIb incorporated into liposomes binds thrombospondin. (1989) Blood. 74 (suppl.1) 645 (Abstract).

58. Kieffer, N., Bettaieb, A., Legrand, C., Coulombel, L., Vainchenker, W., Edelman, L. & Breton-Gorius, J. Developmentally regulated expression of a 78 kDa erythroblast membrane glycoprotein immunologically related to the platelet thrombospondin receptor. (1989) Biochem. J. 262: 835-842.

59. Aiken, M.L., Ginsberg, M.H., Byers-Ward, V. & Plow, E.F. A monoclonal antibody to glycoprotein IV induces platelet activation. (1987) Blood. 70 (suppl.1) 346a.(Abstract).

60. Lahav, J., Lawler, J. & Gimbrone, M.A. Thrombospondin interactions with fibronectin and fibrinogen: mutual inhibition in binding. (1984) Eur. J. Biochem. 145: 151-156.

61. Lahav, J., Schwartz, M.A. & Hynes, R.O. Analysis of platelet adhesion with a radioactive chemical crosslinking reagent: Interaction of thrombospondin with fibronectin and collagen. (1982) Cell. 31: 253-262.

62. Silverstein, R.L., Leung, L.K.K., Harpel, P.C. & Nachman, R.L. Complex formation of platelet thrombospondin with plasminogen: Modulation of activation by tissue activator. (1984) J. Clin. Invest. 74: 1625-1633.

63. Frazier, W.A., Dixit, V.A., Galvin, N.J. & Rotwein, P.R. Complete aminoacid sequence derived from cDNA. (1987) Seminars in Thrombosis and haemostasis. vol 13 n°3 255-266.

64. Hynes, R.O. Integrines: a family of cell surface receptor. (1987) Cell. 238: 549-544.

65. Ruoslahi, E. & Pierschbacher, M.D. New perspective in cell adhesion: RGD and integrins. (1987) Science. 238491-497.

66. Lawler, J., Weinstein, R. & Hynes, R.O. Cell attachment to thrombospondin: The role of Arg-Gly-Asp, calcium and integrin receptors. (1988) J. Cell. Biol. 107: 2352-2361.

67. Lawler, J. & Hynes, R.O. An integrin receptor on normal and thrombasthenic platelets that binds thrombospondin. (1989) Blood. 74 2022-2027.

68. Karczewski, J., Knudsen, K.A., Smith, L., Murphy, A., Rothman, V.L. & Tuszynski, G.P. The interaction of thrombospondin with platelet glycoproteins GPIIb/IIIa. (1989) J. Biol. Chem. 264: 21322-21326.

69. Baumgartner, H.R. Platelet interaction with collagen fibrills in flowing blood. Reaction of human platelets with a chymotrypsin-digested endothelium. (1977) Thrombos. Haemostasis. 37: 1-16.

70. Tandon, N.N., Kralisz, U. & Jamieson, G.A. Identification of glycoprotein IV (CD36) as a primary receptor for platelet collagen adhesion. (1989) J. Biol. Chem. 264: 7576-7583.

71. Staatz, W.D., Radjpara, S.M., Wayner, E.A., Carter, W.G. & Santoro, S.A. The platelet membrane glycoprotein Ia-IIa complex mediates the magnesium-dependant adhesion of platelet to collagen. (1988) J. Cell. Biol. 108: 1917-1924.

72. Udeinya,, I.J., Schmidt, J.A., Aikawa, M., Miller, M. & Green, I. Plasmodium malaria infected erythrocytes bind to cultured human endothelial cells. (1981) Science. 213: 555-557.

73. Trager, W., Rudzinska, M.A. & Bradbury, P.C. The fine structure of *Plasmodium falciparum* and its host erythrocytes in natural infection in man. (1966) Bull WHO. 35: 883-889.

74. Barnwell, J.W., Ockenhouse, C.F. & Knowles, D.M. Monoclonal antibody OKM5 inhibits the in vitro binding of *plasmodium falciparum*-infected erythrocytes to monocytes, endothelial and C32 melanoma cells. (1985) J. Immuno. 135: 3494-3497.

75. Schmidt, J.A., Udeinya, I.J., Leech, J.H., Hay, R.J., Aikawa, M., Barnwell, J., Green, I. & Miller, L.H. *Plasmodium falciparum* malaria. An amelanotic melanoma cell line bears receptor for the knob ligand on infected-erythrocytes. (1982) J. Clin. Invest. 70: 379-386.

76. Planton, L.J., Leech,J.H., Miller, L.H. & Howard, R.J. Cytoadherence of *Plasmodium falciparum*-infected erythroctes to human melanoma cell lines correlates with OKM5 antigen. (1987) Infect. Imm. 55: 2754-2758.

77. Ockenhouse, C.F., Magowan, C. & Chulay J.D. Activation of monocytes and platelets by monoclonal antibodies or malaria-infected erythrocytes binding to the CD36 surface receptor in vitro. (1989) J. Clin. Invest. 84: 468-475.

78. Rock, E.P., Roth, T.H., Rojas-Corona, R.D., Sherwood, J.A., Nagel, R.L., Howard, R.J. & Kaul, D.K. Thrombospondin mediates the cytoadherence of *Plasmodium falciparum*-infected red cells to vascular endothelium in shear flow conditions. (1988) Blood. 71: 71-75.

79. Berendt, A.R., Simmons, D.L., Tansey, J., Newbold, C.I. & Marsh, K. Intercellular adhesion molecule-1 is an endothelial cell adhesion receptor for *Plasmodium falciparum*. (1989) Nature. 341: 57-59.

80. Marlin, S.D. & Springer, T.A. Purified intercellullar adhesion molecule-1 (ICAM) is a ligand for lymphocyte function-associated antigen-1. (1989) Cell. 51: 813-819.

81. Faggiotto, A., Ross, R. & Harker, L. Studies of hypercholesterolemia in the non-human primate. (1984) Arteriosclerosis. 4: 323-356.

82. Gerrity, R.G. The role of monocytes in atherosclerosis.(1981) Am. J. Path. 103: 181-200.

83. Sundstrom, C. & Nilsson, K. Establishment and characterization of a human histiolitic cell line (U937). (1976) Int. J. Cancer.17: 565-577.

84. Hsu-lin, S.C., Berman, C.L., Furie, B.C., August, D. & Furie, B. A platelet membrane protein expressed during platelet activation. (1984) J. Biol. Chem. 259: 9121-9126.

85. Larsen, E., Celi, A., Gilbert, G.E., Furie, B.C., Erban, J.K., Bonfanti, R., Wagner, D.D. & Furie, B. Padgem protein: A receptor that mediates the interaction of activated platelets with neutrophils and monocytes. (1989) Cell. 59: 305-312.

86- Gasic, G.P., Tuszynski, G.P. & Gorelik, E. Interaction of the hemostatic system and immune system in the metastatic spread of tumor cells. (1986) Int. Rev. Exp. Path.29: 173-208.

87- Metha, P. Potential role of platelets in the pathogenesis of tumor metastasis. (1988) Blood. 63: 55-63.

88- Knudsen, A.K., Smith, L., Smith, S., Karczewksi, & Tuszynski, G.P. Role of GPIIb/IIIa-like glycoprotein in cell-substratum adhesion of human melanoma cells (1988) J. Cell. Path. 136: 471-478.

89- Grossi, I.M., Hatfield, J.S., Fitzgerald, L.A., Newcombe, M., Taylor, J.D. & Honn, K.V. Role of cell glycoproteins immunologically related to glycoproteins Ib andIIb/IIIa in tumor cell platelets and tumor cell-matrix interactions. (1988) Faseb. J. 2: 2385-2395.

90- Boukerche, H., Berthier-Vergnes, O., Dore, J.F., Leung, L.K.K. & McGregor, J.L. Platelet-melanoma cell interaction is medietad by the glycoprotein IIb/IIIa complex. (1989) Blood. 74: 658-653.

91- Boukerche, H., Berthier-Vergnes, O., Tabone, E., Dore, J.F., Leung, L.K.K. & McGregor, J.L. A monoclonal antibody (LYP18) directed against the blood platelet glycoprotein GPIIb/IIIa complex inhibits human melanoma growth in vivo (1989) Blood. 74: 909-912.

92- Varani, J., Dixit, V.M., Fliegel, S.E., McKeever, P.E. & Carey, T.M. Thrombospondin induced attachment and spreading of human squamous carcinoma cells. (1986) Exp. Cell. Res. 167: 376-390.

93- Riser, B.L., Varani, J., O'Rourke, K. & Dixit, V.A. Thrombospondin binding by human squamous carcinoma and melanoma cells: Relationship to activity. (1988) Exp. Cell. Res. 174: 319-329.

94- Roberts, D.D., Sherwood, J.A. & Ginsburg, V. Platelet thrombospondin mediates attachment and spreading of human melanoma cells. (1988) J. Cell. Biol. 104: 131-139.

95- Robets, D.D. Interaction of thrombospondin with sulfated glycolipids and proteoglycans of human melanoma cells. (1988) Cancer Reseach. 48:6785-6793.

96- Tuszynski, G.P., Gasic, T.B., Rothman, V.L., Knudsen, K.A. & Gasic, G.J. Thrombospondin, a potentiator cell metastasis. (1989) Cancer Research. 47: 4130-4137.

97- Riser, B.L., Mitra, R., Perry, P., Dixit, V. & Varani, J. Monocytes killing of human squamous epithelial cells: Role of thrombospondin. Cancer Research. 49: 6123-6129.

98- Wong, J.E.L., ASch, A.S., Silverstein, R.L. & Nachman, R.L. Glycoprotein IV expression in C32 human melanoma cell culture is marker for a more malignant phenotype. (1989) Blood 74. Suppl. 1 638 (Abstract).

99- Greenwalt, D.E. & Mather, H.I. Characterization of an appically derived epithelial glycoprotein from bovin milk, which is expressed in capillary endothelia in diverse tissues. (1985) J. Cell. Biol. 100: 6123-6129.

100- Catimel, B., McGregor, J.L., Hasler, T., Greenwalt, D.E., Howard, R.J. & Leung, L.K.K. Epithelial membrane PAS-IV is related to glycoprotein IIIb: Binding to TSP and malaria erythrocytes. (1989) Blood74. Suppl. 1 (Abstract).

101- Greenwalt, D.E., Johnson, V.G. & Mather, I.H. Specific antibodies to PAS-IV, a glycoprotein of bovine milk-fat-globule-membrane, binds to a similar protein in cardiac endothelial cells and leung bronchioles. (1985) Biochem. J. 228: 233-240.

Résumé

La glycoproteine IIIb (GPIIIb) ou GPIV est une protéine majeure de la membrane plaquettaire. La GPIIIb est homologue ou identique à l'antigène CD36 identifié sur les cellules endothéliales, monocytes et certaines lignées cellulaires tumorales. En tant que récepteur de la thrombospondine, la GPIIIb joue un rôle important dans l'agrégation plaquettaire, l'interaction plaquettes-monocytes et le processus métastatique. Elle intervient aussi dans l'adhésion plaquette-collagène et joue un rôle majeur dans la cytoadhérence des érythrocytes infectés par le *Plasmodium falciparum* à l'endothélium vasculaire.

Cette revue récapitule les récent travaux concernant la structure et les différentes fonctions de la glycoprotéine IIIb dans les interactions cellule-cellule et cellule-matrice.

GMP-140, an inducible receptor for leukocytes on platelets and endothelium

R.P. McEver

St. Francis Medical Research Institute and Department of Medicine, University of Oklahoma Health Sciences Center, and Cardiovascular Biology Research Program, Oklahoma Medical Research Foundation, Oklahoma City, OK 73104, USA

Cellular activation is required for platelets and endothelial cells to mediate many functions related to hemostasis and inflammation. Activation-dependent processes include generation of lipid products, release of stored molecules from secretory granules, and rearrangement of membrane glycoproteins at the cell surface (Phillips & Shuman, 1986; Simionescu & Simionescu, 1988). We have focused our studies on a membrane protein, termed GMP-140, that is expressed on the surface of platelets and endothelium only after these cells are activated.

SUBCELLULAR LOCATION OF PLATELET GMP-140

GMP-140 was initially identified following the characterization of a monoclonal antibody, S12, prepared by immunizing mice with thrombin-activated platelets (McEver & Martin, 1984). When incubated with unstimulated platelets, radiolabeled S12 IgG or Fab fragments bound to less than 1000 sites per cell. However, when platelets were activated with thrombin, about 10,000 S12 molecules bound to each cell. The thrombin-induced increase in binding suggested that S12 identified either an activation-induced conformational change in a plasma membrane molecule or an internal membrane antigen that is redistributed to the cell surface following platelet stimulation.

The S12-binding protein was isolated by immunoaffinity chromatography of Lubrol-PX platelet lysates on S12-agarose (McEver & Martin, 1984). When analyzed by SDS-PAGE, the protein migrated with an apparent Mr of 140,000 under reducing conditions. To determine its subcellular location, we used an immunogold procedure on frozen thin sections of human platelets (Stenberg et al., 1985). Immunogold label was concentrated along membranes of α-granules in unstimulated cells. We therefore named the protein GMP-140, to indicate that it is a granule membrane protein of apparent Mr 140,000. Following platelet activation, immunogold label for GMP-140 was redistributed to the surface-connected canalicular system and plasma membrane as a result of membrane fusion. The redistribution occurs within seconds and results in a uniform dispersal of GMP-140 along the plane of the plasma membrane (Isenberg et al., 1986). Similar observations were made independently by Furie and coworkers, who called the protein PADGEM protein (platelet activation dependent-granule external membrane protein) (Hsu-Lin et al., 1984; Berman et al., 1986). Recently GMP-140 has been given the cluster designation CD62 (Knapp et al., 1989).

IDENTIFICATION OF GMP-140 IN ENDOTHELIAL CELLS

To determine whether GMP-140 was expressed only in platelets, an immunoperoxidase procedure was used to examine the distribution of GMP-140 in a variety of human tissues (McEver et al., 1989). In addition to its presence in platelets and their progenitor cells, megakaryocytes, GMP-140 antigen was detected in vascular endothelial cells of all organs examined. The endothelial cell protein was concentrated in postcapillary venules; only patchy distribution was noted in arteries, arterioles, and capillaries. Immunogold labeling of unstimulated endothelial cells indicated that GMP-140 was concentrated along the membranes of electron-dense granules but not along the plasma membrane. These granules resembled Weibel-Palade bodies, the organelles in which are stored high molecular weight multimers of von Willebrand factor (vWF) (Weibel & Palade, 1964; Sporn et al., 1986). Double-label studies with antibodies to both GMP-140 and vWF colocalized both proteins to the same granules, confirming the location of GMP-140 in Weibel-Palade bodies (McEver et al., 1989; Bonfanti et al., 1989).

Immunocytochemistry and binding studies with radiolabeled S12 indicated that activation of endothelium with agonists such as thrombin and histamine induced rapid redistribution of GMP-140 to the cell surface, presumably by fusion of Weibel-Palade membranes with the plasma membrane (McEver et al., 1989; Hattori et al., 1989a). The dose-dependent agonist effect on GMP-140 expression paralleled the dose-dependent secretion of vWF into the medium. In contrast to activated platelets, where GMP-140 remains on the plasma membrane for at least an hour following in vitro activation (George et al., 1986), the expression of GMP-140 on the surface of stimulated endothelium is transient, peaking at 3 min and declining to basal levels by 20-30 min (Hattori et al., 1989a). The transient appearance of surface GMP-140 appears to be due to sequential degranulation and endocytosis (Hattori et al., 1989a).

USE OF MONOCLONAL ANTIBODIES TO GMP-140

The data summarized above indicate that GMP-140 is found in secretory granule membrane of two vascular cell types, platelets and endothelium. Following stimulation with agonists such as thrombin, both cell types rapidly fuse their granules with the plasma membrane, release granular contents, and express GMP-140 on the cell surface. Therefore, monoclonal antibodies to GMP-140 are useful markers of secretion-associated platelet and endothelial activation. Flow cytometry is a particularly sensitive approach for identifying a small population of activated platelets in anticoagulated whole blood or in a sample of isolated platelets (Shattil et al., 1987; Johnston et al., 1987). This approach has been used in a limited number of studies of patients with disorders involving platelet activation (George et al., 1986; Abrams et al., 1990) as well as in studies of platelet storage (George et al., 1988). One report has also documented the use of radiolabeled S12 to identify endothelial cells activated by deposition of the terminal complement proteins C5b-9 (Hattori et al., 1989b).

Antibodies to GMP-140 may also prove useful as noninvasive markers of thrombi in vivo. Because activated platelets should be concentrated at sites of thrombi, infusion of radiolabeled antibodies to GMP-140 may result in rapid visualization of thrombi without accompanying blood pool activity due to labeling of unstimulated platelets. Two groups have reported promising results in imaging experimental thrombi in baboons (Palabrica et al., 1989) and rabbits (Miller et al., 1989).

STRUCTURE OF GMP-140

The rapid expression of GMP-140 on the surface of activated platelets and endothelium suggested that the protein might serve an important role as an inducible receptor at sites of vascular inflammation or injury, where these cells would be activated. To provide insight into potential function, the structure of GMP-140 was studied. Purified platelet GMP-140 contains 30% carbohydrate organized into complex N-linked oligosaccharides (Johnston et al., 1989a). Pulse-chase studies of [^{35}S]cysteine-labeled HEL cells (a human cell line with features of megakaryocytes) or human umbilical vein endothelial cells indicated that core high mannose oligosaccharides are first added to the GMP-140 precursor; these are then processed into complex forms in the Golgi apparatus (Johnston et al., 1989a; McEver et al., 1989). Prior to carbohydrate addition, three or four precursors of GMP-140 of slightly different Mr were noted, suggesting heterogeneity of GMP-140 at the protein level (Johnston et al., 1989a).

To determine the primary structure of GMP-140, we cloned and sequenced cDNAs from a human endothelial cell cDNA library (Johnston et al., 1989b). The deduced amino acid sequence of the clones matched extensive protein sequence obtained directly from peptides of purified platelet GMP-140. The sequence predicts a large protein with multiple independently folded domains. Twelve potential sites for addition of N-linked carbohydrate are present, all of which are likely to be filled based on the carbohydrate compositional analysis. Following a 41-residue signal peptide, the mature protein contains 789 amino acids. Beginning at the N terminus, there is a 119-residue region homologous to Ca^{2+}-dependent lectins, a 36-residue epidermal growth factor (EGF)-like domain, nine tandem consensus repeats similar to those in complement-binding proteins, a transmembrane domain, and a short cytoplasmic tail. Two different types of in-frame deletions were noted in some of the cDNA clones. One type predicts a deletion of 62 amino acids encoding the seventh consensus repeat; this variant predicts a protein containing eight instead of nine repeats. The other variant predicts a deletion of 40 amino acids encompassing the transmembrane domain; these clones predict a soluble form of GMP-140. Preliminary analysis of genomic clones indicates that each of the regions deleted in the cDNAs corresponds precisely to an exon (G.I. Johnston and R.P. McEver, unpublished observations). This suggests that the different forms of GMP-140 are derived from alternative splicing of messenger RNA. Such variable splicing could explain the apparent heterogeneity of the GMP-140 precursors previously noted in metabolically labeled HEL cells (Johnston et al., 1989a). The unexpected prediction of a soluble form of GMP-140 is of particular interest and is the subject of current investigation.

GMP-140 BELONGS TO A NEW GENE FAMILY OF RECEPTORS

The domain organization of GMP-140 is remarkably similar to those of two other vascular cell surface molecules that were recently cloned. The first is endothelial leukocyte adhesion molecule-1 (Bevilacqua et al., 1989). The second is the Mel 14 antigen, a structure found on murine neutrophils, monocytes, and a majority of lymphocytes, best known for its role in "homing" lymphocytes to high endothelial venules of peripheral lymph nodes (Lasky et al., 1989; Siegelman et al., 1989). The human equivalent of the Mel 14 antigen has also been cloned (Tedder et al., 1989; Camerini et al., 1989; Bowen et al., 1989; Siegelman & Weissman, 1989); this molecule has been termed LAM-1 or the Leu 8/TQ1 antigen. Like GMP-140, ELAM-1 and LAM-1 contain an N-terminal lectin-like domain, followed by an EGF-like domain, a variable number of consensus repeats (six in ELAM-1 and two in LAM-1), a transmembrane domain, and a short cytoplasmic tail. The lectin and EGF domains of the three molecules share over 60% amino acid identity and the consensus repeats also demonstrate sequence similarity. The genes for GMP-140 and LAM-1 have been mapped by in situ hybridization to the long arm of human chromosome chromosome 1 at bands q21-24 (Tedder et al., 1989; Johnston et al., 1988). Pulsed field electrophoresis of genomic DNA in conjunction with Southern blotting indicate that the genes for GMP-140, LAM-1, and ELAM-1 are all tightly clustered on chromosome 1 in a region spanning no more than 200 kb; this clustering has been conserved in both the mouse and human genomes (Watson et al., 1990). The name "selectins" has been given to this new family of related cell surface molecules.

LEUKOCYTE ADHESIVE FUNCTION OF GMP-140

Both ELAM-1 and the Mel 14 antigen (LAM-1) have defined roles in mediating interactions of leukocytes with vascular endothelium, suggesting that GMP-140 might share a related function. One possibility was that GMP-140 could be a rapidly inducible receptor for neutrophils and monocytes when expressed on the surface of activated platelets and endothelium. Previous studies demonstrated that activated platelets interact with neutrophils and monocytes in a Ca^{2+}-dependent manner (Jungi et al., 1986). In addition, endothelium stimulated with thrombin becomes adhesive for neutrophils within minutes (Zimmerman et al., 1985); these kinetics are different than the cytokine-induced endothelial adhesiveness for neutrophils that requires several hours and parallels the surface expression of ELAM-1 (Bevilacqua et al., 1987). Endothelial GMP-140 (McEver et al., 1989), like ELAM-1 (Cotran et al., 1986), is concentrated in postcapillary venules, the sites where leukocytes migrate across endothelium in inflammatory foci.

Several lines of evidence indicate that GMP-140 does indeed interact with neutrophils and monocytes. COS cells transfected with cDNAs encoding GMP-140 become adhesive for neutrophils and HL-60 cells, as assayed by formation of neutrophil rosettes over the transfected cells; rosette formation is inhibited by polyclonal antibodies to GMP-140 and by some, but not all, monoclonal antibodies to GMP-140 (Geng et al., 1990). Neutrophils and HL-60 cells bind to GMP-140 immobilized on plastic microtiter wells but not to other immobilized proteins; this binding is inhibited by monoclonal antibodies to GMP-140 and by fluid-phase GMP-140 (Geng et al., 1990). Fixed neutrophils bind to GMP-140-coated wells, indicating that active neutrophil metabolism is not required for adhesion (Geng et al., 1990). Cell binding requires extracellular Ca^{2+}. However, lower concentrations of Ca^{2+} will support maximal adhesion if Mg^{2+} is also present; this suggests that at least two binding sites for divalent cations participate in the adhesive interaction (Geng et al., 1990). Activated, but not unactivated, platelets form rosettes around neutrophils and monocytes but not around lymphocytes; the binding requires Ca^{2+} and is inhibited by monoclonal and polyclonal antibodies to GMP-140 and by fluid-phase GMP-140 (Larsen et al., 1989; Hamburger & McEver, 1990). Human endothelial cells stimulated with rapid activators such as histamine become adhesive for neutrophils within minutes (Geng et al., 1990); the adhesiveness is transient and declines to basal levels within 20-30 min, a pattern similar to the transient expression of GMP-140 on the surface of activated endothelium (Hattori et al., 1989a). Furthermore, binding of neutrophils to rapidly activated endothelium is inhibited by monoclonal antibodies to GMP-140 (Geng et al., 1990).

These studies indicate that GMP-140 promotes rapid binding of neutrophils and monocytes to the surface of activated platelets and endothelium. Therefore, GMP-140 shares functional as well as structural similarity with the other known selectins, ELAM-1 and LAM-1. These molecules, along with the $\beta2$ leukocyte integrins (Kishimoto et al., 1989) and several receptors which belong to the immunoglobulin gene superfamily (Marlin & Springer, 1987; Staunton et al., 1989; Rice & Bevilacqua, 1989; Osborn et al., 1989), mediate a variety of leukocyte adhesive interactions critical to the inflammatory response. The other major protective reponse to tissue injury is the hemostatic pathway, in which platelets play a major role. Because GMP-140 mediates interactions of leukocytes with both activated platelets and endothelium, it may provide an important link between the hemostatic and inflammatory responses. The multidomain organization of GMP-140 suggests that it may also have functions other than leukocyte recognition that remain to be defined.

REFERENCES

Abrams, C.S., Ellison, N., Budzynski, A.Z. & Shattil, S.J. (1990) Blood 75, 128-138.

Berman, C.L., Yeo, E.L., Wencel-Drake, J.D., Furie, B.C., Ginsberg, M.H. & Furie, B. (1986) J. Clin. Invest. 78, 130-137.

Bevilacqua, M.P., Pober, J.S., Mendrick, D.L., Cotran, R.S. & Gimbrone, M.A., Jr. (1987) Proc. Natl. Acad. Sci. USA 84, 9238-9242.

Bevilacqua, M.P., Stengelin, S., Gimbrone, M.A., Jr. & Seed, B. (1989) Science 243, 1160-1165.

Bonfanti, R., Furie, B.C., Furie, B. & Wagner, D.D. (1989) Blood 73, 1109-1112.

Bowen, B.R., Nguyen, T. & Lasky, L.A. (1989) J. Cell Biol. 109, 421-427.

Camerini, D., James, S.P., Stamenkovic, I. & Seed, B. (1989) Nature 342, 78-82.

Cotran, R.S., Gimbrone, M.A., Jr., Bevilacqua, M.P., Mendrick, D.L. & Pober, J.S. (1986) J. Exp. Med. 164, 661-666.

Geng, J.-G., Bevilacqua, M.P., Moore, K.L., McIntyre, T.M., Prescott, S.M., Kim, J.M., Bliss, G.A., Zimmerman, G.A. & McEver, R.P. (1990) Nature 343, 757-760.

George, J.N., Pickett, E.B., Saucerman, S., McEver, R.P., Kunicki, T.J., Kieffer, N. & Newman, P.J. (1986) J. Clin. Invest. 78, 340-348.

George, J.N., Pickett, E.B. & Heinz, R. (1988) Transfusion 28, 123-126.

Hamburger, S.A. & McEver, R.P. (1990) Blood 75, 550-554.

Hattori, R., Hamilton, K.K., Fugate, R.D., McEver, R.P. & Sims, P.J. (1989a) J. Biol. Chem. 264, 7768-7771.

Hattori, R., Hamilton, K.K., McEver, R.P. & Sims, P.J. (1989b) J. Biol. Chem. 264, 9053-9060.

Hsu-Lin, S.-C., Berman, C.L., Furie, B.C., August, D. & Furie, B. (1984) J. Biol. Chem. 259, 9121-9126.

Isenberg, W.M., McEver, R.P., Shuman, M.A. & Bainton, D.F. (1986) Blood Cells 12, 191-204.

Johnston, G.I., Pickett, E.B., McEver, R.P. & George, J.N. (1987) Blood 69, 1401-1403.

Johnston, G.I., Le Beau, M.M., Lemons, R.S. & McEver, R.P. (1988) Blood 72 (Suppl), 327-327.

Johnston, G.I., Kurosky, A. & McEver, R.P. (1989a) J. Biol. Chem. 264, 1816-1823.

Johnston, G.I., Cook, R.G. & McEver, R.P. (1989b) Cell 56, 1033-1044.

Jungi, T.W., Spycher, M.O., Nydegger, U.E. & Barandun, S. (1986) Blood 67, 629-636.

Kishimoto, T.K., Larson, R.S., Corbi, A.L., Dustin, M.L., Staunton, D.E. & Springer, T.A. (1989) in Advances in Immunology, Vol. 46

(Dixon, F.J., Ed.) pp 149-182, Academic Press, New York.

Knapp, W., Dorken, B., Rieber, P., Schmidt, R.E., Stein, H. & von dem Borne, A.E.G.Kr. (1989) Blood 74, 1448-1450.

Larsen, E., Celi, A., Gilbert, G.E., Furie, B.C., Erban, J.K., Bonfanti, R., Wagner, D.D. & Furie, B. (1989) Cell 59, 305-312.

Lasky, L.A., Singer, M.S., Yednock, T.A., Dowbenko, D., Fennie, C., Rodriguez, H., Nguyen, T., Stachel, S. & Rosen, S.D. (1989) Cell 56, 1045-1055.

Marlin, S.D. & Springer, T.A. (1987) Cell 51, 813-819.

McEver, R.P. & Martin, M.N. (1984) J. Biol. Chem. 259, 9799-9804.

McEver, R.P., Beckstead, J.H., Moore, K.L., Marshall-Carlson, L. & Bainton, D.F. (1989) J. Clin. Invest. 84, 92-99.

Miller, D.D., Boulet, A., Garcia, O., Heyl, B., Palmaz, J., Perez, J., Pak, K.Y., Neblock, D., Berger, H. & Daddona, P. (1989) Circulation II-516 (Abstract)

Osborn, L., Hession, C., Tizard, R., Vassallo, C., Luhowskyj, S., Chi-Rosso, G. & Lobb, R. (1989) Cell 59, 1203-1211.

Palabrica, T.M., Furie, B.C., Konstam, M.A., Aronovitz, M.J., Connolly, R., Brockway, B.A., Ramberg, K.L. & Furie, B. (1989) Proc. Natl. Acad. Sci. USA 86, 1036-1040.

Phillips, D.R. & Shuman, M.A. (1986) Biochemistry of platelets. Academic Press, Orlando, Florida.

Rice, G.E. & Bevilacqua, M.P. (1989) Science 246, 1303-1306.

Shattil, S.J., Cunningham, M. & Hoxie, J.A. (1987) Blood 70, 307-315.

Siegelman, M.H. & Weissman, I.L. (1989) Proc. Natl. Acad. Sci. U. S. A. 86, 5562-5566.

Siegelman, M.H., van de Rijn, M. & Weissman, I.L. (1989) Science 243, 1165-1172.

Simionescu, N. & Simionescu, M. (1988) Endothelial cell biology in health and disease. Plenum Press, New York.

Sporn, L.A., Marder, V.J. & Wagner, D.D. (1986) Cell 46, 185-190.

Staunton, D.E., Dustin, M.L. & Springer, T.A. (1989) Nature 339, 61-64.

Stenberg, P.E., McEver, R.P., Shuman, M.A., Jacques, Y.V. & Bainton, D.F. (1985) J. Cell Biol. 101, 880-886.

Tedder, T.F., Isaacs, C.M., Ernst, T.J., Demetri, G.D., Adler, D.A. & Distèche, C.M. (1989) J. Exp. Med. 170, 123-133.

Watson, M.L., Kingsmore, S.F., Johnston, G.I., Siegelman, M.H., Le Beau, M.M., Lemons, R.S., Bora, N.S., Howard, T.A., Weissman, I.L., McEver, R.P. & Seldin, M.F. (1990) <u>Clin. Res.</u>, in press (Abstract)

Weibel, E.R. & Palade, G.E. (1964) <u>J. Cell Biol. 23</u>, 101-112.

Zimmerman, G.A., McIntyre, T.M. & Prescott, S.M. (1985) <u>J. Clin. Invest. 76</u>, 2235-2246.

ABSTRACT

GMP-140 is a membrane glycoprotein located in secretory granules of human platelets and endothelial cells. When these cells are stimulated, the protein is rapidly redistributed to the plasma membrane; therefore, monoclonal antibodies to GMP-140 are useful markers of activated platelets and endothelium. The cDNA-derived amino acid sequence indicates that GMP-140 contains an N-terminal lectin-like domain, followed by an EGF-like domain, nine tandem consensus repeats similar to those in complement-binding proteins, a transmembrane domain, and a cytoplasmic tail. Some cDNAs also predict variant forms of GMP-140, including a putative soluble form of GMP-140 lacking the transmembrane domain. GMP-140 is structurally related to two other vascular cell surface molecules: ELAM-1, a cytokine-inducible endothelial cell receptor for neutrophils, and a lymphocyte homing receptor that mediates adherence of lymphocytes to high endothelial venules of peripheral lymph nodes. The genes for these three molecules, which have been termed selectins, are clustered on the long arm of human chromosome 1. GMP-140 mediates adhesion of neutrophils and monocytes to the surface of activated platelets and endothelium. Therefore, GMP-140 and the other selectins constitute a new family of receptors that mediate leukocyte adhesive interactions fundamental to the inflammatory response.

Résumé

La GMP-140 est une glycoprotéine membranaire localisée dans les granules secrétoires des plaquettes et des cellules endothéliales. Quand ces cellules sont stimulées la protéine est rapidement redistribuée sur la surface de la membrane plasmique, et peut être rapidement détectée par des anticorps monoclonaux (MAb) anti GMP-140. La séquence en acides aminés de la GMP-140, dérivée du séquençage de son ADNc, indique une homologie significative de cette protéine avec deux autres glycoprotéines de surface du système vasculaire le ELAM-1 et la gp^{90Mel}. Les gènes de ces 3 molécules se situent sur le chromosome 1. La GMP-140 joue le rôle de médiateur de l'adhésion des neutrophiles et des monocytes à la surface des plaquettes et des cellules endothéliales activées. En conclusion, la GMP-140 ainsi que ELAM-1 et la gp^{90Mel}, font partie d'une nouvelle famille de récepteurs, les sélectines, qui jouent un rôle fondamental dans la réponse inflammatoire.

A new family of cell-cell adhesion molecules : ELAM-1, GP90^{MEL-14} and GMP-140

S. Parmentier, L. McGregor and J.L. McGregor

INSERM U 331, Faculté de Médecine Alexis Carrel, 8, rue Guillaume Paradin, 69372 Lyon Cedex 08, France

SUMMARY

Cells interact with the extracellular matrix and other cells through families of receptors such as integrins (composed of an α and β subunits) and the immunoglobulin superfamily. Recently, a new family of adhesion molecules, the LEC-CAMs (Lectin cell adhesion molecule) (Stoolman et al., 1989) family, was reported to be involved in cell-cell interactions. Three LEC-CAMs have been discovered: (1) Endothelial Leukocyte Adhesion Molecule 1 (**ELAM-1**), which is expressed by cytokine-stimulated endothelial cells; (2) the homing receptor **gp90^{MEL-14}**, which is expressed by lymphocytes that recirculate into lymph nodes; (3) Granule Membrane Protein (**GMP-140**), which is expressed by activated platelets and endothelial cells. LEC-CAMs share common structural features: they are transmembrane, highly glycosylated proteins, with a major extracellular portion. The N-terminal extracellular segment is a lectin-like domain, followed by an Epidermal Growth Factor (EGF) region, and by repeats of complement regulatory protein motifs. LEC-CAMs are functionally involved in cell-cell contacts, such as the adhesion of neutrophils to endothelial cells (ELAM-1), the binding of homing lymphocytes to high endothelial venules (gp90^{MEL-14}) and the rosetting of activated platelets with monocytes (GMP-140).

INTRODUCTION

Several families of adhesion molecules have been shown to play a vital role in cell-matrix and cell-cell interactions (Menko et al., 1987; Springer et al., 1982; Wilcox et al., 1985). These interactions are essential in the body defense processes, such as movement of lymphocytes into peripheral lymph nodes, migration of leukocytes into inflammatory sites by extravasation (Marx, 1989) and specific attachment of blood platelets to injured platelets to injured endothelium in hemostasis and thrombosis (George, 1985). A common feature of these complex processes is the non random recruitment of circulating cells at specific sites, where the vascular endothelium has been altered. For example, resting platelets adhere to immobilized subendothelial components such as collagen, fibronectin and laminin through respective integrins GPIa-IIa or VLA-2 (Kunicki et al., 1988), GPIc-IIa or VLA-5 (Piotrowicz et al., 1988) and GPIc'-IIa or VLA-6 (Sonnenberg et al., 1988). The GPIIb-IIIa complex, the fibrinogen receptor on stimulated platelets (Bennett et al., 1983) and GPVr-IIIa, the vitronectin receptor on endothelial cells (Chen et al., 1987), are members of the integrin family. The adhesion of resting platelets to subendothelial von Willebrand factor is mediated by a complex, GPIb-IX (Sakariassen et al., 1986), not related to the integrin family. Leukocytes can adhere to altered endothelial cells through LFA-1, a member of the integrin family (Hynes, 1987), interacting with ICAM-1, a member of the immunoglobulin superfamily (Staunton et al., 1989) present on endothelial cells. Another group of membrane receptors, Hermes/CD44 (Goldstein et al., 1989), found in a large number of tissues, is involved in the adhesion of lymphocytes to endothelial cells.

Some lymphocytes can recirculate in lymph nodes, by selective recognition of high endothelial venules (Lasky et al., 1989). This specific interaction is mediated by a homing receptor (Lasky et al., 1989). This homing receptor, **gp90^{MEL-14}** in mouse, does not resemble to any previously described adhesion molecule, except the Endothelial Leukocyte Adhesion Molecule 1 (**ELAM-1**) (Bevilacqua et al., 1989) and the platelet Granule Membrane Protein (**GMP-140**) (Johnston etal., 1989), also known as Protein Activation Dependent Granule External Membrane (PADGEM). The aim of this review is to give a summary of the structural and functional features recently reported on this new family of adhesion proteins, the **LEC-CAMs** (Stoolman et al., 1989).

ENDOTHELIAL LEUKOCYTE ADHESION MOLECULE 1 (ELAM-1).

Endothelial Leukocyte Adhesion Molecule (ELAM-1) is expressed on endothelial cells stimulated by Interleukin-1 (Il-1) or Tumor Necrosis Factor (TNF) (Pober et al., 1986; Bevilacqua et al., 1987). The expression of ELAM-1 reaches a maximum within 4 hours and decreases over 24 hours. Monoclonal antibody H18/7, directed against ELAM-1, blocks the adhesion of human neutrophils and HL-60 cells to stimulated endothelial cells (Bevilacqua et al., 1987). ELAM-1 was shown to support the adhesion of tumor cells to endothelium (Bevilacqua et al., 1987; Rice et al., 1989). It is conceivable that the interaction between tumor and endothelial cells is mediated through the carbohydrates of tumor cells and the lectin-like domain of ELAM-1 (Rice, 1989). These studies show that ELAM-1 is involved in adhesive interactions between endothelium and leukocytes or tumor cells leading to extravasation (Rice, 1989).

ELAM-1 shows an apparent molecular weight of 115kD, under reducing conditions, in SDS-polyacrylamide gel electrophoresis (SDS-PAGE). The protein sequence (Bevilacqua et al., 1989), consisting of 589 amino acids, predicts a transmembrane protein. There are 32 amino acids in the C-terminal cytoplasmic segment, 21 in the transmembrane region and 536 in the extracellular domain (Bevilacqua et al., 1989). The major portion of the molecule is extracytoplasmic and bears 11 potential sites of N-linked glycosylation.

THE HOMING RECEPTOR GP90^{MEL-14}.

Recirculating mouse lymphocytes express a homing receptor, gp90^{MEL-14}, recognized by the monoclonal antibody MEL-14 (Gallatin et al., 1983). This homing receptor gp90^{MEL-14} is expressed only by lymphocytes that attach to high endothelial venules (HEV) of peripheral lymph nodes (Gallatin et al., 1983). Monoclonal antibody MEL-14 blocks the binding of normal or neoplastic lymphocytes to HEV (Sher et al., 1988), and their accumulation within peripheral lymph nodes in vivo (Mountz et al., 1988). Recent studies support that gp90^{MEL-14}, through its lectin domain (Yednock et al., 1987-1,2; Lasky et al., 1989), mediates the binding of lymphocytes to a carbohydrate ligand on high endothelium venules (Bowen et al., 1990). A homologue of gp90^{MEL-14} is found on mouse neutrophils, and defined as gp100^{MEL-14} (Kishimoto, 1989). This adhesion protein is involved in neutrophil extravasation (Lewinsohn et al., 1987) during inflammation. Once neutrophils have been activated, they lose gp100^{MEL-14} from their surface. Moreover, the neutrophils that have passed accross endothelium are free of any gp100p^{MEL-14}, suggesting that gp100^{MEL-14}-mediated adhesion to injured endothelium is a key step preceding neutrophil extravasation (Kishimoto et al., 1989).

gp90^{MEL-14}, with an apparent molecular weight of 90kD, in SDS-PAGE (Gallatin et al., 1983) is a highly glycosylated and ubiquitinated (Siegelman et al., 1986) transmembrane protein, consisting of 334 amino acids, with 18 amino acids in the cytoplasmic region, 12 in the transmembrane segment and 304 in the extracellular portion (Siegelman et al., 1989). Ten potential N-linked glycosylation sites are present on the extracellular portion, but no O-linked glycosylation was detected. The human pan-leukocyte antigen Leu-8 was recently found to be homologous to gp90^{MEL-14} (Camerini et al., 1989).

PLATELET GRANULE MEMBRANE PROTEIN (GMP-140/PADGEM).

Granule membrane protein (GMP-140) (McEver et al., 1984), also known as platelet activation-dependent granule-external membrane (PADGEM) (Hsu-Lin et al., 1984), is an integral membrane glycoprotein (Berman et al., 1986) that is expressed on the platelet surface following degranulation (Stenberg et al., 1986). Moreover, a recent study in the baboon shows that the expression of GMP-140 on young platelets is decreased as compared to controls (Savage et al., 1989). GMP-140 is also found in vascular endothelial cells, colocated with von Willebrand Factor in Weibel-Palade bodies (McEver et al., 1989). Rapid expression of GMP-140 to the endothelial surface occurs following stimulation with histamine, thrombin, PMA, calcium ionophore A23187 (Hattori et al., 1989-1) and complement protein C5b-9 (Hattori et al., 1989-2). Endothelial surface GMP-140 is maximal 3 minutes after stimulation, and disappears by 20 minutes. The rapid expression of GMP-140 on endothelial surface suggests that GMP-140 could play an important role in the migration of leukocytes accross altered endothelium (McEver et al., 1989), as ELAM-1, in response to inflammatory stimuli. Consistently, GMP-140, as ELAM-1, is mostly expressed in small veins and venules, where leukocyte migration occurs first upon inflammation (Cotran et al., 1986). Recently, platelet GMP-140 or PADGEM has been shown to mediate the interaction of activated platelets with neutrophils and monocytes (Larsen et al., 1989). It is conceivable that GMP-140, as expressed by activated platelets, plays a role in the clearance of such platelets from circulation by monocytes-macrophages (Larsen et al., 1989). There is no data available on the role of GMP-140 in the binding of stimulated platelets to endothelial cells. In addition, the role of GMP-140 in platelet aggregation has not been yet demonstrated. However, recent observations show that, 15 minutes after thrombin stimulation, GMP-140 is the only membrane glycoprotein found in areas of contact between platelets that have irreversibly aggregated (Johnston et al., 1989-1). Despite these valuable studies on GMP-140, its role in platelet functions remains unknown.

GMP-140, recognized by monoclonal antibodies S12 (McEver et al., 1984) and KC4 (Hsu-Lin et al., 1984), shows an apparent molecular weight of 140kD in SDS-PAGE. Its cDNA-derived primary structure was obtained from endothelial cells and predicts a transmembrane protein of 789 amino acids (Johnston et al., 1989-1). There are 35 residues in the C-terminal cytoplasmic tail, 24 in the transmembrane domain and 730 in the extracellular portion. GMP-140 is highly glycosylated (Johnston et al., 1989-2) and the extracellular chain bears 12 N-linked glycosylation sites. These structural homologies with ELAM-1 and gp90^{MEL-14} may help investigators to understand the functions of platelet and endothelial GMP-140.

ELAM-1, GP90^{MEL-14} AND GMP-140 SHARE A COMMON STRUCTURAL ORGANIZATION.

LEC-CAMs share a number of common structural features: all of them are transmembrane single-chain polypeptides, bearing internal disulfide bridges and being highly glycosylated (Bevilacqua et al., 1989; Siegelman et al.,1989; Johnston et al., 1989). In addition, the extracellular portions of ELAM-1, gp90^{MEL-14} and GMP-140 show a similar organization: a lectin domain is present at the N-terminal site, followed by a the epidermal growth factor (EGF) region, and by a series of repeats similar to those found in complement regulatory proteins (Bevilacqua et al., 1989; Siegelman et al., 1989; Johnston et al., 1989).

The lectin domain

Located on the N-terminal region of LEC-CAMs, this portion of 120 amino acids is related to the lectin-like protein family (Bevilacqua et al., 1989). ELAM-1 and gp90^{MEL-14} lectin domain shows homologies with the previously described CD23 (IgE receptor), with the asialoglycoprotein receptor and with mannose-binding protein (Bevilacqua et al., 1989). In the case of gp90^{MEL-14}, the role of the lectin domain was well studied. The monoclonal antibody MEL-14 inhibits the binding of lymphocytes to peripheral lymph node high endothelial venules (Gallatin et al.,1983; Mountz et al.,1988). In addition, monoclonal antibody MEL-14 inhibits the binding of lymphocytes to immobilized phosphomonoester mannan (Yednock, 1987-2). Recent studies show that MEL-14 recognizes a site located in part on the lectin domain, and this binding is abolished when the EGF domain is removed (Bowen, 1990). These data suggest that 1) the lectin domain of gp90^{MEL-14} plays a key role in adhesion of lymphocytes to postcapillary venule endothelium in lymph nodes; 2) the conformation of the lectin domain depends on the presence of the EGF domain. It is conceivable that ELAM-1 and GMP-140 show similar structural properties. However, further studies are necessary to support this hypothesis.

The EGF region

Following the lectin domain, there is a segment of about 40 residues, containing 6 Cysteines (Bevilacqua et al.; Siegelman et al.; Johnston et al., 1989), related to EGF motif (Cooke, 1987). This sequence is similar to that found in growth factors, cell surface receptors, extracellular matrix proteins, blood clotting factors, plasminogen activators and complement (Lasky et al., 1989). The role of the EGF region is unknown. However, it is conceivable that the EGF region contributes to maintain the lectin domain in an appropriate conformation, as it was demonstrated for gp90^{MEL-14} (Bowen et al., 1990).

The complement regulatory protein repeats

This domain consists of repeats of 60-62 amino acids. There are 9 repeats on GMP-140 (Johnston et al., 1989-1) 6 on ELAM-1 (Bevilacqua et al., 1989) and 2 in gp90^{MEL-14} (Siegelman et al., 1989). These repeats are homologous to those found in complement regulatory membrane proteins such as complement receptors 1 and 2 (CR1 and CR2), decay accelerating factor (DAF), membrane cofactor protein (MCP), and plasmas proteins such as C3-and C4-binding proteins. Very likely LEC-CAMs may bind the complement proteins C3b or C4b so as to regulate the amplification of the complement cascade, as DAF (Lasky et al., 1989).

CONCLUSION

The LEC-CAM family is involved in cell-cell interactions, especially in the selective captation of circulating blood cells by endothelial cells, on sites of injury. Neutrophils are attracted by inflamed endothelial cells through ELAM-1, prior to diapedesis, migration and 'cleaning' of the inflamed area. Through gp100^{MEL-14}, neutrophils can select inflamed endothelial cells prior to pass accross the endothelium. Lymphocytes that bear gp90^{MEL-14} are able to select high endothelial venules in lymph nodes prior to migration and close contact with the processed antigen. We do not know yet the ligand of ELAM-1 on neutrophils and the ligand of gp100^{MEL-14} on endothelial cells. A very attractive and simple hypothesis is that ELAM-1 and gp90/100^{MEL-14} and/or GMP-140 and gp90/100^{MEL-14} specifically bind to each other. Alternatively, it is conceivable that LEC-CAMs interact with other cell adhesion molecules. However, there is no data available concerning the identity of the membrane ligands specific for LEC-CAMs. The expression of LEC-CAMs on the cell surface is very quick and transient (except in platelets, where GMP-140 was detected in aggregates 15 minutes after thrombin activation (Johnston et al., 1989-2)), suggesting that LEC-CAMs initialize an early cell-cell contact, before disappearing from the surface while migrating accross the endothelium, as demonstrated for neutrophil gp100^{MEL-14} (Kishimoto et al., 1989). In acute inflammatory reactions, neutrophils cause severe damages not only to invaders, but to normal tissues. Therefore the understanding of the mechanism of action of LEC-CAMs will be useful in clinical applications, especially in looking whether LEC-CAMs can be neutralized to prevent excessive injury. LEC-CAMs may also participate in the interaction of tumor cells with microvascular endothelium. ELAM-1 was shown to support the adhesion of a colon carcinoma cell line (Rice et al., 1989) This observation indicated that tumor cell extravasation that occurs during metastatic process is partly mediated by ELAM-1. However, the membrane antigen expressed by tumor cells and recognized by ELAM-1 remains to be identified. The homing receptor gp90^{MEL-14} is expresed by a large proportion of lymph node metastases (Sher et al., 1988). The role of LEC-CAMs in mediating metastatic invasion needs to be further investigated and may provide valuable tools for diagnosis and treatment of metastatic diseases.

ACKNOWLEDGMENTS

This work was supported by Association pour la Recherche sur le Cancer (ARC subvention 6586), by the British Council, the Department of Biologie Humaine, Université de Lyon, and by the Ligue Nationale Française contre le Cancer.

REFERENCES

Bennett, J.S., Hoxie, J.A., Leitmen, S.F., Vilaire, G. and Cines, D.B. (1983) Inhibition of the fibrinogen receptor on human platelets by a monoclonal antibody. *Proc.Natl.Acad.Sci.USA* 80, 2417-2431.

Berman, C.L., Yeo, E.L., Wencel-Drake, J.D., Furie, B.C., Ginsberg, M.H. and Furie, B. (1986).A platelet alpha granule membrane protein that is associated with the plasma membrane after activation. *J. Clin. Invest.* 78, 130-137.

Bevilacqua, M.P., Pober, J.S., Mendrick, D.L., Cotran, R.S. and Gimbrone, M.A.Jr.(1987). Identification of an inducible endothelial-leukocyte adhesion molecule, ELAM-1. *Proc.Natl.Acad.Sci.USA* 84, 9238-9242.

Bevilacqua, M.P., Stengelin, S., Gimbrone, M.A.Jr and Seed, B. (1989). Endothelial Leukocyte Adhesion Molecule 1: an inducible receptor for neutrophils related to complement regulatory proteins and lectins. *Science* 243, 1160-1165.

Bowen, B.R., Fennie, C. and Lasky, L.A. (1990) The Mel14 antibody binds to the lectin domain of the murine peripheral lymph node homing receptor. *J.Cell Biol.*110, 147-153.

Camerini, D., James, S.P., Stamenkocic, I. and Seed, B. (1989) Leu-8/TQ1 is the human equivalent of the Mel-14 lymph node homing receptor. *Nature* 342, 78-82.

Chen, C.S., Thiagarajan, P., Schwartz, S.M., Harlan, J.M. and Heimark, R.L. (1987). The platelet glycoprotein IIb/IIIa-like protein in human endothelial cells promotes adhesion but not initial attachment to extracellular matrix. *J.Cell Biol.* 105, 1885-1892.

Cooke, R.M., Wilkinson, A.J., Baron, M., Pastore, A., Tappin, M.J., Campbell, I.D., Gregory, H. and Sheard, B. (1987). The solution structure of human epiderma growth factor. *Nature* 327, 339-341.

Cotran, R.S., Gimbrone, M.A. Jr, Bevilacqua, M.P., Mendrick, D.L. and Pober, J.S. (1986). Induction and detection of a human endothelial activation antigen in vivo. *J.Exp.Med.*164, 661-666.

Gallatin, W.M., Weissman, I. and Butcher E.C. (1983). Cell-surface molecule involved in organ-specific homing of lymphocytes. *Nature* 304, 30-34.

George, J.N. (1985). The role of membrane glycoproteins in platelet formation, circulation and senescence. Review and hypotheses. *In* Platelet membrane glycoproteins, J.N. George, A.T. Nurden and D.R. Phillips , Editors. Plenum, New York, pp 395-412.

Goldstein, L.A., Zhou, D.F.H., Picker, L.J., Minty, C.N., Bargatze, R.F., Ding, J.F. and Butcher, E.C. (1989). A human lymphocyte homing receptor, the Hermes antigen, is related to cartilage proteoglycan core and link proteins. *Cell* 56, 1063-1072.

Hattori, R., Hamilton, K.K., Fugates, R.D., McEver, R.P. and Sims, P.J. (1989-1).Stimulated secretion of endothelial von Willebrand Factor is accompanied by rapid redistribution to the cell surface of the intracellular granule membrane protein GMP-140. *J. Biol. Chem.* 264, 7768-7771.

Hattori, R., Hamilton, K.K., McEver, R.P. and Sims, P.J. (1989-2).Complement proteins C5b9 induce secretion of high molecular weight multimers of endothelial von Willebrand Factor and translocation of granule membrane protein GMP-140 to the cell surface. *J. Biol. Chem.* 264, 9053-9060

Hsu-Lin, S.C., Berman, C.L., Furie, B.C., August, D. and Furie, B. (1984). A platelet membrane protein expressed during platelet activation and secretion. *J. Biol. Chem.* 259, 9121-9126.

Hynes, R.O. (1987) Integrins: a family of cell surface receptors. *Cell* 48, 549-554.

Johnston, G.I., Cook, R.G. and McEver, R.P.(1989-2). Cloning of GMP-140, a granule membrane protein found in platelets and endothelial cells. *Cell* 56, 1033-1044

Johnston, G.I., Kurosky, A. and McEver, R.P.(1989-1).Structural and biosynthetic studies of the granule membrane protein GMP-140, from human platelets and endothelial cells. *J. Biol. Chem* 264: 1816-1823.

Kishimoto, T.K., Jutila, M.A., Berg, E.L. and Butcher, E.C. (1989) Neutrophil Mac-1 and MEL-14 adhesion proteins inversely regulated by chemotactic factors. *Science* 245, 1238-1241.

Kunicki, T.J., Nugent, D.J., Staats, S.J., Orchekowski, R.P., Wayner, E.A., and Carter, W.G. (1988). The human fibroblast class II extracellular matrix receptor mediates platelet adhesion to collagen and is identical to the platelet membrane glycoprotein Ia-IIa complex. *J. Biol. Chem.* 263, 4516-4519.

Larsen, E., Celi, A., Gilbert, G.E., Furie, B.C., Erban, J.K., Bonfanti, R., Wagner, D.D. and Furie, B. (1989). PADGEM protein: a receptor that mediates the interaction of activated platelets with neutrophils and monocytes. *Cell* 59, 305-312.

Lasky LA, Singer MS, Yednock TA, Dowbenko D, Fennie C, Rodriguez H, Nguyen T, Stachel S and Rosen SD: Cloning of a lymphocyte homing receptor reveals a lectin domain. *Cell* 56, 1045- 1989.

Lewinsohn, D.M., Bargatze, R.F. and Butcher, E.C. (1987). Leukocyte-endothelial cell recognition: evidence of a common molecular mechanism shared by neutrophil, lymphocytes, and other leukocytes. *J.Immunol.* 138, 4313-4321.

Marx, J.L. (1989). New family of adhesion proteins discovered. *Science* 243, 1144.

McEver, R.P .and Martin, M.N. (1984). A monoclonal antibody to a membrane glycoprotein binds only to activated platelets. *J. Biol. Chem.* 259, 9799-9804.

McEver, R.P., Beckstead, J.H., Moore, K.L., Marshall-Carlson, L. and Bainton, D.F. (1989).GMP-140, a platelet alpha-granule membrane protein, is also synthetized by vascular endothelial cells and is localized in Weibel-Palade bodies. *J. Clin. Invest* 84, 92-99.

Menko, S.A. and Boettiger, D. (1987). Occupation of the extracellular matrix receptor, integrin, is a control point for myogenic differentiation. *Cell* 51, 51-58.

Mountz, J.D., Gause, W.C., Finkelman, F.D. and Steinberg, A.D.(1988) Prevention of lymphadenopathy in MRL-lpr/lpr mice by blocking peripheral node homing with MEL-14 in vivo. *J.Immunol.* 140, 2943-2949.

Piotrowicz, R.S., Orchewski, R.P., Nugent, D.J., Yamada, K.Y., and Kunicki, T.J. (1988) Glycoprotein Ic-IIa functions as an activation-independent fibronectin receptor on human platelets. *J. Cell. Biol.* 106, 1359-1364.

Pober, J.S., Bevilacqua, M.P., Mendrick, D.I., Lapierre, L.A., Riers, W. and Gimbrone, M.A. Jr. (1986). Two distinct monokines, interleukin 1 and tumor necrosis factor, each independently induce biosynthesis and transient expression of the same antigen on the surface of cultured huamn vascular endothelial cells. *J.Immunol.*136, 1680-1687.

Rice, G.E. and Bevilacqua, M.P. (1989) An inducible endothelial cell surface glycoprotein mediates melanoma adhesion. *Science* 246, 1303-1306.

Sakariassen, K.S., Nievelstein, P.F., Coller, B.S. and Sixma, J.J. (1986). The role of platelet membrane glycoproteins Ib and IIb-IIIa in platelet adherence to human artery subendothelium. *Br.J.Haematol.* 63, 681-691.

Savage, B., Hunter, C.S., Harker, L.A., Woods, V.L. Jr and Hanson, S.R. (1989) Thrombin-induced increase in surface expression of epitopes on platelet membrane glycoprotein IIb/IIIa complex and GMP-140 is a function of platelet age. *Blood* 74, 1007-1014.

Sher, B.T., Bargatze, R., Holzmann, B., Gallatin, W.M., Matthews, D., Wu, N., Picker, L., Butcher, E.C. and Weissman, I.L. (1988). Homing receptors and metastasis. *Adv.Canc.Res.*51, 361-390.

Siegelman, M., Bond, M.W., Galltin, W.M., St.John, T., Smith, H.T., Fried, V.A. and Weissman, I.L. (1986). Cell surface molecule associated with lymphocyte homing is a ubiquitinated branched-chain glycoprotein. *Science* 231, 823-829.

Siegelman, M.H., van de Rijn, M. and Weissman, I.L. (1989) Mouse lymph node homing receptor cDNA clone encodes a glycoprotein revealing tandem interaction domains. *Science* 243, 1165-1172.

Sonnenberg, A., Modderman, P.W. and Hogervorst, F. (1988). Laminin receptor on platelets is the integrin VLA-6. *Nature* 336, 487-489.

Springer, T.A., Davignon, D., Ho, M.K., Kurzinger, K., Martz, E. and Sanchez-Madrid, F. (1982). LFA-1 and Lyt-2,3, molecules associated with T lymphocyte-mediated killing; and Mac-1 and LFA-1 homologue associated with complement receptor function. *Immunol.Rev.* 68, 171-195.

Staunton, D.E., Dustin, M.L. and Springer, T.A. (1989). Functional cloning of ICAM-2, a cell adhesion ligand for LFA-1 homologous to ICAM-1. *Nature* 339, 61-64.

Stenberg, P.E., McEver, R.P., Shuman, M.A., Jacques, Y.V. and Bainton, D.F. (1986).A platelet alpha-granule membrane protein (GMP-140) is expressed on the plasma membrane after activation. *J. Cell Biol.* 101, 880-886.

Stoolman, L.M.(1989). Adhesion molecules controlling lymphocyte migration. *Cell* 56, 907-910.

Wilcox, M. and Leptin, M. (1985). Tissue-specific modulation of a set of related cell surface antigens in Drosophila. *Nature* 316, 351-354.

Yednock, T., Butcher, E.C., Stoolman, L. and Rosen, S. (1987-1) Receptors involved in lymphocyte homing: relationship between a carbohydrate-binding receptor and the Mel-14 antigen. *J.Cell Biol.*104, 725-731.

Yednock, T., Stoolman, L. and Rosen, S. (1987-2) Phosphomannosyl-derivatized beads detect a receptor involved in lymphocyte homing. *J.Cell Biol.*104, 713-723.

Résumé

Les cellules interagissent avec la matrice extracellulaire et les autres cellules grâce à des familles de récepteurs comme les intégrines (formés de deux sous-unités, α et β) et comme la superfamille des immunoglobulines. Récemment, on a découvert une nouvelle famille de molécules d'adhésion, les LEC-CAMs (Lectine cell adhesion molecules) impliquées dans les interactions cellule-cellule. On connaît trois LEC-CAMs: (1) "Endothelial Leukocyte adhesion Molecule 1" (**ELAM-1**), exprimée à la surface des cellules endothéliales stimulées par des cytokines; (2) le "homing recepteur" gp90^{MEL-14}, exprimé par les lymphocytes recirculants dans les ganglions lymphatiques et la "Granule Membrane Protein de 140kD" (**GMP-140**), exprimée à la surface des plaquettes et des cellules endothéliales activées. Les LEC-CAMs ont en commun des particularités structurales: ce sont des protéines transmembranaires, monomériques, fortement glycosylées, et dont la majeure partie est extracellulaire. L'extrémité N-terminale, extracellulaire, porte un domaine caractéristique des lectines, suivi d'une région homologue au facteur de croissance épidermique (EGF), et d'une zone constituée de plusieurs répétitions de motifs caractéristiques des protéines régulatrices du complément. Les LEC-CAMs sont impliquées dans les contacts cellule-cellule, tels que l'adhésion des neutrophiles aux cellules endothéliales (ELAM-1), l'attachement des lymphocytes aux veinules postcapillaires des ganglions (gp90MEL-14) et la formations de rosettes entre les plaquettes activées et les monocytes (GMP-140).

Structure and function of platelet glycoprotein IC-IIA (VLA-6)

A. Sonnenberg*, P.W. Modderman*, P. van der Geer**, M. Aumailley*** and R. Timpl***

*Department of Immunohematology, Central Laboratory of the Netherlands Red Cross Blood Transfusion Service and Laboratory for Experimental and Clinical Immunology, University of Amsterdam, The Netherlands
**The Salk Institute, La Jolla, California 92037, USA
***Max-Planck-Institut für Biochemie, D-8033 Martinsried, Allemagne

Abstract

A glycoprotein Ic-IIa complex found on human platelets is specifically recognized by a rat monoclonal antibody GoH3 against glycoprotein Ic. This structure is identified as VLA-6 of the VLA protein family because it is detected by the monoclonal antibody, mAb A-1A5, against the common VLA-β^1 subunit, but not by antibodies against the α1-5 subunits of the VLA protein family. Platelets express four forms of VLA-6, in which the α^6 subunits are different. Two of these forms arise by different glycosylation and the two others possibly by alternative proteolytic processing of the α^6 subunit. VLA-6 ($\alpha^6\beta^1$) functions as a specific receptor for laminin and recognizes a site on the terminal half of the long arm of laminin. In addition to VLA-6, platelets express VLA-2 ($\alpha^2\beta^1$) and VLA-5 ($\alpha^5\beta^1$). There is no evidence for additional VLA structures on platelets. VLA-2 and VLA-5 serve as receptors for collagen and fibronectin, respectively. These two adhesion receptors together with VLA-6 are likely to initiate adhesion to exposed subendothelial matrix.

Introduction

Adhesion of platelets to exposed subendothelial matrix components is an initial event in hemostasis. The adhesion of platelets to damaged blood vessels results in platelet activation which is accompanied by changes in cell shape, degranulation and platelet aggregation. These platelet responses to matrix components depend on the function of specific receptors on the platelet plasma membranes.

The family of cell surface receptors known as integrins includes multiple receptors for extracellular matrix proteins (1,2). Integrins are heterodimeric integral membrane proteins, comprised of an α subunit noncovalently associated with a β subunit. Eleven different α subunits and six different β subunits have thus far been identified. The $β^1$, $β^2$ and $β^3$ subunits associate with multiple distinct α subunits and define three integrin subfamilies; VLA-proteins (3), Leu-Cam proteins (4) and cytoadhesins (5). The VLA protein family has at least seven members (3,6,7) and includes receptors for laminin, fibronectin and collagen; the Leu-Cam family has three leukocyte-specific receptors involved in cell-cell interactions and the cytoadhesins consist of the platelet glycoprotein IIb-IIa complex and the vitronectin receptor. Three additional β subunits ($β^4$, $β^5$ and $β^p$) form heterodimeric complexes with α subunits previously reported to be associated with one of the three original β subunits. For example, the $α^6$ subunit associates on platelets with $β^1$, whereas on epithelial cells this subunit is complexed with the $β^4$ subunit (8-10).

The primary structure of many α and β subunits has been determined from nucleotide sequencing of the corresponding cDNAs. The α subunits all have large extracellular domains containing 3-4 divalent cation binding domains, a single transmembrane domain and a short cytoplasmic domain. Some α subunits ($α^1$, $α^2$, $α^L$, $α^M$ and $α^X$) have an inserted "I-domain" that is homologous with a domain in a number of collagen binding proteins. Five α subunits ($α^3$, $α^5$, $α^6$, $α^{IIb}$ and $α^V$), are composed of a heavy and a light chain. The β subunits have large extracellular domains with 48-56 cysteine residues, most of which are clustered in four repeated motifs. This high cysteine content may account for the increase in electrophoretic mobility of the β subunit on SDS-PAGE when reducing agents are present. The cytoplasmic domains of the β subunits are relatively small (28-41 amino acids). Only the $β^4$ subunit has an exceptionally long cytoplasmic domain of around 1000 amino acids (11,12).

The cytoplasmic domains of integrins are thought to interact with components of the cytoskeleton. In this regard CSAT, a mixture of chicken integrins, has been shown to bind to talin (13). Binding has also been demonstrated between talin and vinculin (14) and it is suggested that these two proteins together with α-actinin (collectively named linker proteins) anchor the actin filaments to the cell surface membrane (15). Thus, integrins may provide a link between the extracellular matrix and the cytoskeleton.

In this chapter, we summarize findings on the identification, characterization and function of the antigen complex defined by the monoclonal antibody GoH3. We show that this antibody recognizes the glycoprotein Ic-IIa complex, that this complex is identical to VLA-6 and functions as a specific receptor for the E8 fragment of laminin.

Results

Identification of the human platelet antigen recognized by mAb GoH3.

Two different kinds of analyses can be employed to define the major platelet glycoproteins; two-dimensional nonreduced-reduced gel analysis (16,17) and two-dimensional isoelectric focussing/SDS-polyacrylamide gel electrophoresis (18-20). The first method was used to define the antigen complex recognized by GoH3 as platelet glycoproteins Ic-IIa (21). This analysis, however, is no longer satisfactory to define platelet antigens, as other molecules with the same nonreduced/reduced properties as the antigen complex defined by GoH3 were identified (see Table 1). Therefore, we also have applied two-dimensional isoelectric focussing/SDS-polyacrylamide gel electrophoresis to further define the antigen complex recognized by GoH3. As shown in Fig.1 analysis of the GoH3 antigens by this procedure showed that Ic resolved as a series of spots with pI of 5.0-5.4 and that IIa has a pI of 4.6-4.8. These pI values correspond to those of the authentic glycoproteins Ic and IIa and therefore we like to conclude that the GoH3-defined antigen complex actually represents the Ic-IIa complex.

Platelet glycoprotein Ic-IIa is a VLA protein.

VLA proteins are heterodimeric complexes that share a common β^1 subunit but have distinct α subunits (3). The relationship between Ic-IIa and VLA proteins was established by preclearing experiments with mAb A-1A5, directed against the common β^1 subunit of the VLA protein family (3) and with mAb GoH3, directed against the Ic subunit of the Ic-IIa complex (21). When all the Ic-IIa complexes were removed from lysates of ^{125}I-labeled platelets by three cycles of preclearing with mAb GoH3, a substantial amount of total VLA was removed (Fig. 2). The VLA proteins that remained detectable probably represent VLA-2 and VLA-5 (see below). In the reciprocal experiment, preclearing three times with mAb A-1A5 removed all VLA proteins and Ic molecules that were associated

Table 1

Platelet names	Other names	CD nomenclature	References
GP1c	VLA α^5-subunit	CDw49e	22
	VLA α^6-subunit	CDw49f	21
	VNR α^V-subunit	CD51	23
GPIIa	VLA β^1-subunit	CD29	24
	GPIIa'	CD31	25
	GMP140	CD62	26

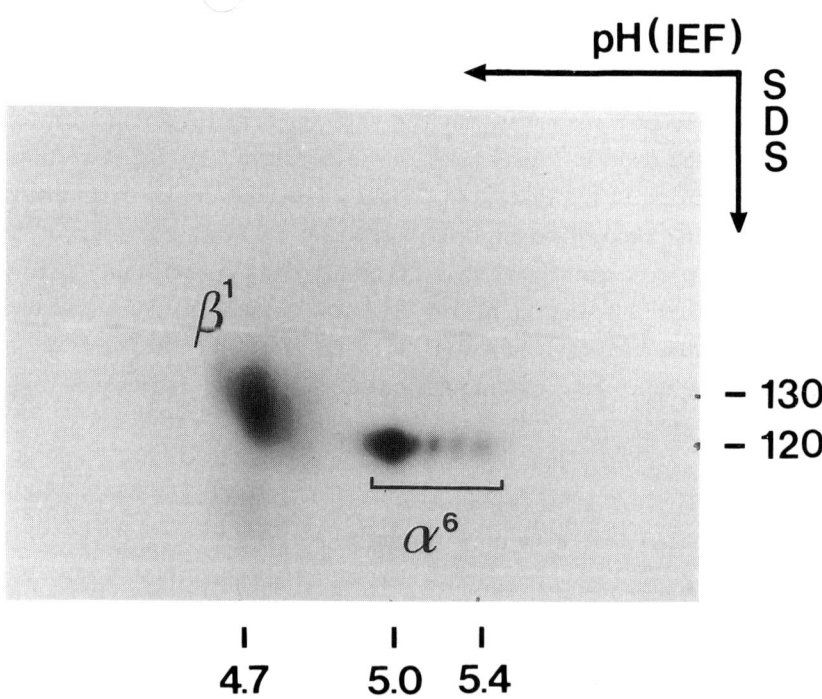

Fig. 1. Isoelectric focussing/SDS-PAGE two dimensional gel analysis of VLA-6 subunits. Lysates from ^{125}I-labeled platelets were immunoprecipitated using mAb GoH3. After isoelectric focussing of nonreduced samples in tube gels, a second dimension on a SDS-5% polyacrylamide gel was carried out under reducing conditions.

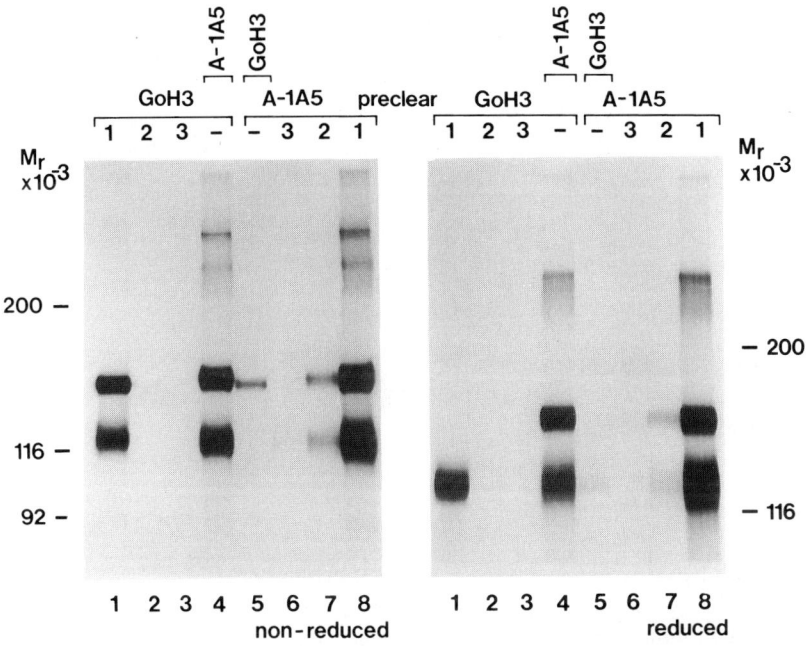

Fig. 2. Analysis of antigens recognized by mAbs GoH3 and A-1A5 in precleared lysates. Lysates of ^{125}I-labeled platelets were precleared three succesive times with either mAb GoH3 (lanes 1-3) or mAb A-1A5 (lanes 8-6). Lysate precleared of GoH3-immunoreactive material was then immunoprecipitated with A-1A5 (lane 4) and lysate precleared of A-1A5-immunoreactive material with GoH3 (lane 5).

with IIa but not free Ic molecules. These results indicate that the Ic-IIa complex is a VLA protein. Furthermore, the experiments suggest that in addition to complexes of Ic-IIa, also free Ic is present on platelets.

Platelet glycoprotein Ic-IIa complex is VLA-6.

Immunoprecipitation analysis with VLA-α subunit-specific antibodies revealed that VLA proteins present on platelets included VLA-2, VLA-5 and the antigen

79

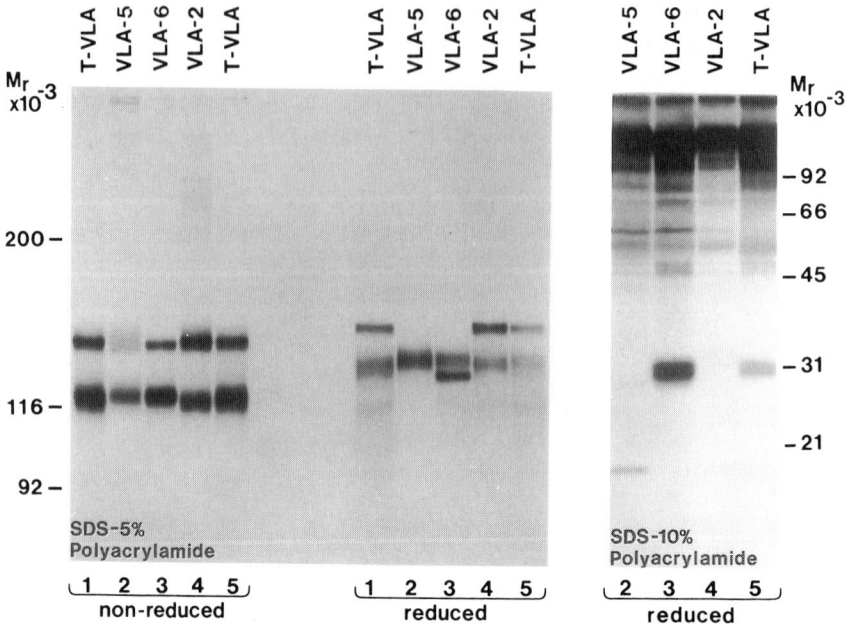

Fig. 3. Electrophoretic analysis of VLA proteins on platelets. Total VLA (lanes 1 and 5), VLA-2 (lane 2), VLA-5 (lane 3) and VLA-6 (lane 4) were immunoprecipitated from ^{125}I-labeled platelet lysates using mAbs A-1A5, 12F1, DIE5 and GoH3. Samples were analyzed on SDS-5% polyacrylamide gels, under nonreducing conditions and on a SDS-10% polyacrylamide gel under reducing conditions.

complex defined by mAb GoH3 (hereafter called VLA-6; Fig. 3), but not VLA-1, VLA-3 and VLA-4 (not shown). This is consistent with results of previous VLA phenotyping (6). The α subunit of VLA-2 is a single polypeptide that migrated at 160.000 Mr under nonreducing conditions and slightly increased in Mr value under reducing conditions. In contrast, the α subunits of VLA-5 and VLA-6 each consist of a heavy and a light chain linked together by disulfide bonding. The heavy chain of α^5 comigrated with the common β^1 subunit at the Mr 130.000 position and was somewhat larger than the α^6 heavy chain which migrated slightly in front of the common β^1 subunit. Although the β^1 subunits that are associated with α^2, α^5 and α^6 subunits are identical with respect to V-8 protease cleavage mapping and recognition by antibodies (6), a small difference in electrophoretic mobility between the β^1 subunit associated with α^2 on the one hand and the β^1 subunits associated with α^5 and α^6 on the other hand could be detected. It is possible that this difference is due to a different degree of glycosylation of the β subunits when they become associated with α subunits. Alternatively, the two light chain bands may be due to differential splicing of the β^1 mRNAs. If the latter is true, this finding would imply that there are β subunits specific for a particular α subunit. The fact that under reducing conditions the α^6 subunit is smaller than the α^5 subunit is due to the release of a larger light chain polypeptide from α^6 (Mr 31.000/30.000) than from α-5 (Mr 17.000). Notably, the light chain of α^6 migrates as a closely spaced doublet. This doublet is not due to differences in glycosylation (see below) but may reflect alternative proteolytic cleavage of the α^6 precursor during biosynthesis.

Carbohydrate analysis

VLA proteins are glycoproteins carrying large numbers of N-linked glycans. To determine the amount and types of glycans on the α^6 and β^1 subunits of the VLA-6 complex, digestions with neuraminidase (removes sialic acid residues from complex-type N-linked glycans and O-linked carbohydrates), endoglycosidase-H (removes high-mannose-type N-linked glycans) and endoglycosidase-F (removes both high mannose and complex-type N-linked glycans) were carried out on immunoprecipitates prepared with mAbs GoH3 and A-1A5. The native α^6 and β^1 polypeptides were separated in a 5% polyacrylamide gel under nonreducing conditions. As shown in Fig. 4, the α^6 subunit is susceptible to digestion with neuraminidase, endo-H and endo-F, indicating that it carries both high mannose and complex type-N-linked glycans. Since endo-F caused a much larger reduction in Mr value than endo-H, it is concluded that the majority of the N-linked glycans are of the complex-type. By analysis of the digestion products on 5% and 10% polyacrylamide gels under reducing conditions, it is possible to discriminate between glycans present on either the heavy or the light chain. The results show that most of the endo-F sensitive complex-type N-linked glycans reside on the heavy chain of the α^6 subunit. The α^6 light chain which migrates as a closely spaced doublet, consists of a population of heterogenously glycosylated molecules. A major part has one high mannose and one complex-type N-linked glycan, but a small part carries two high mannose N-linked glycans. No conversion of the slower migrating band into the faster

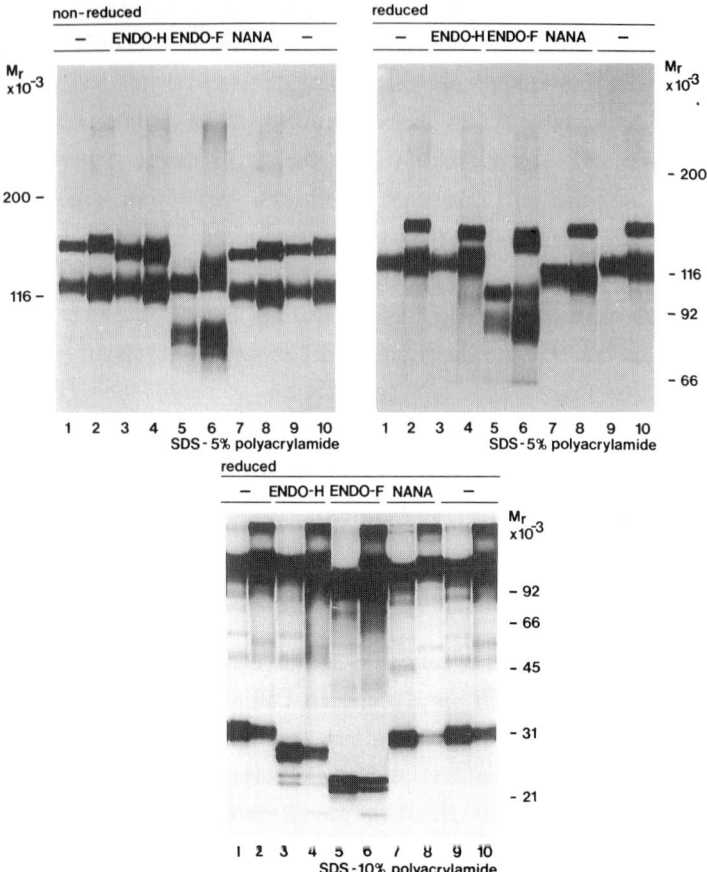

Fig. 4. Carbohydrate analysis of VLA-6 subunits. VLA-6 recognized by mAb GoH3 (lanes 1,3,5,7 and 9) and total VLA (lanes 2,4,6 and 8) recognized by mAb A-IA5 were immunoprecipitated from lysates of ^{125}I-labeled platelets. Immunoprecipitated proteins were subjected to digestion with 0.1 unit of endo-H/ml for 2 h at 37 °C, 20 units of endo-F/ml for 2 h at 37 °C and 5 units of neuraminidase/ml for 2 h at 37 °C. Control incubations were performed in the absence of enzymes. Samples were analyzed on SDS-5% polyacrylamide gels, under nonreducing and reducing conditions and on a SDS-10% polyacrylamide gel, under reducing conditions.

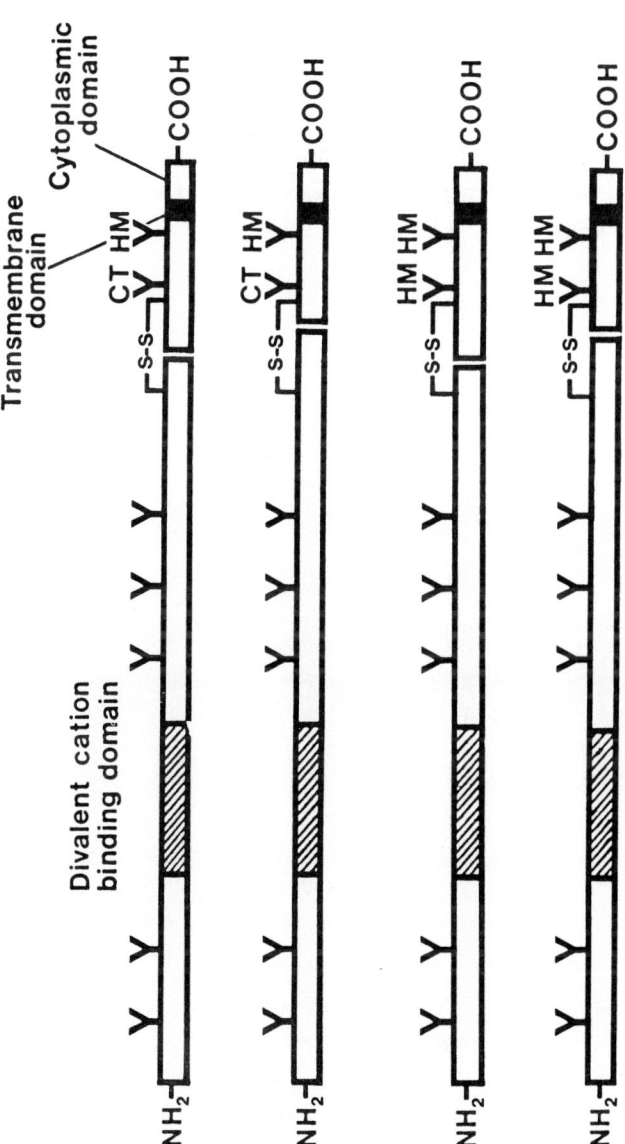

Fig. 5. Proposed structure of the α^6 subunits on platelets. The α^6 subunit is synthesized as a single polypeptide that is proteolytically cleaved into a heavy and a light chain. These two chains remain disulfide-linked to one another. It is suspected that cleavage of the α^6 precursor occurs at two sites, generating two distinct forms of the α^6 subunit. Both the heavy and light chain carry N-linked glycans (Y). The light chain consists of two differently glycosylated polypeptides. The major form has one high mannose (HM) and one complex-type (CT) N-linked glycan and a minor form has two high mannose N-linked glycans. The putative divalent cation binding domain is also given.

Fig. 6. Analysis of VLA proteins on platelets by preclearing. Lysate of ^{125}I-labeled platelets was precleared of VLA-5, VLA-6 and VLA-2 proteins by succesive incubations with mAbs BIE5 (three times), GoH3 (three times) and 12F1 (four times). Then, the mAb A-1A5 was used to immunoprecipitate any remaining VLA β-associated proteins from platelets. Samples were analyzed on SDS-5% polyacrylamide gels, under nonreducing and reducing conditions. Lanes 1 and 13, immunoprecipitations of total VLA from unprecleared platelet lysates with mAb A-1A5, lane 2-4, preclearing steps with mAb BIE5, lanes 4-7, preclearing steps with mAb GoH3, lanes 8-11, preclearing steps with mAb 12F1 and lane 12, immunoprecipitation of remaining VLA proteins from VLA-5, VLA-6, VLA-2 precleared lysate with mAb A-1A5.

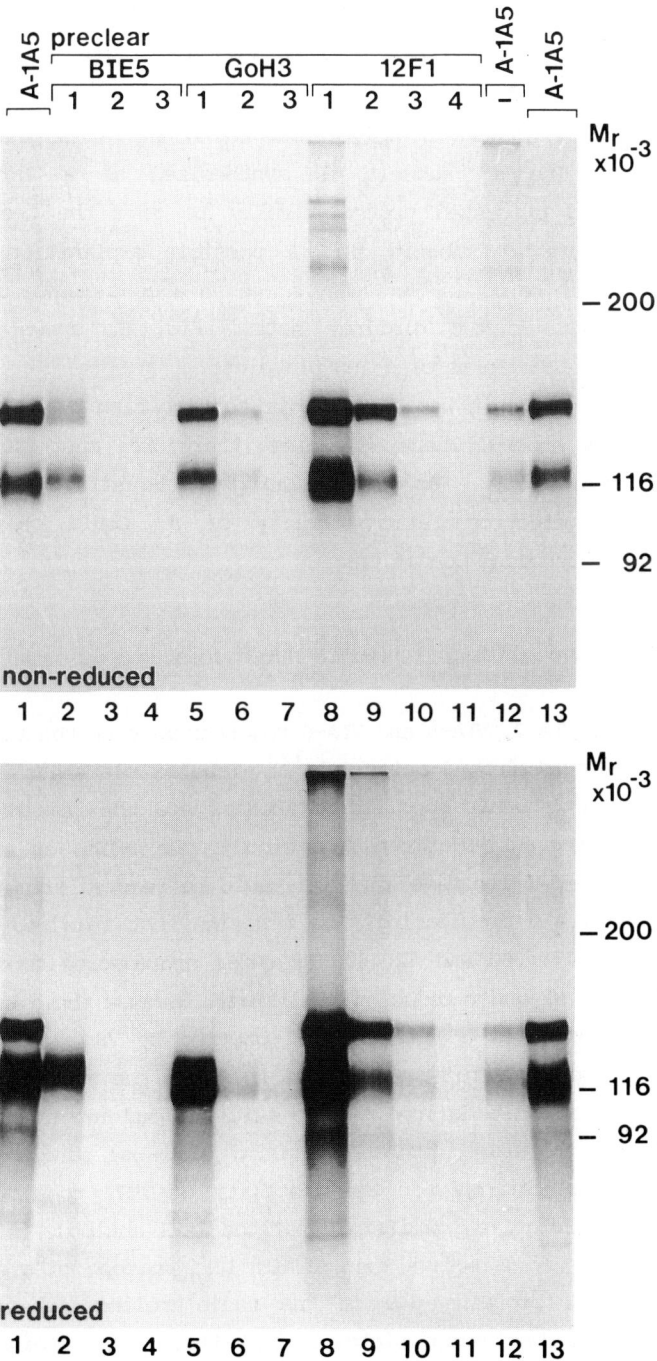

migrating band of the doublet was obtained by digestion with the various glycosidases. In addition, we could not demonstrate the presence of O-linked glycans on the α^6 light chains either by treatment with O-glycanase or by treatment with 0.1 M $NaBH_4$ in 0.1 M NaOH. Thus, the two bands comprising the doublet represent differences in polypeptide backbones rather than differences in glycosylation. The α^6 subunit is synthesized as a large precursor polypeptide that is processed proteolytically to give the heavy and light chains of the mature α^6 subunit (8). A possible explanation for the two different light chain bands is that they arise as a consequence of alternative proteolytic cleavage at two distinct sites. Fig. 5, shows the proposed structure of the various forms of α^6 on platelets.

The common VLA β^1 subunit was susceptible to digestion by neuraminidase and endo-F, but not by endo-H. These molecules, therefore, must contain complex-type N-linked glycans only. For reasons unknown, the effect of neuraminidase treatment on the electrophoretic mobility of β^1 could only be clearly demonstrated under reducing conditions.

Platelets do not have additional new VLA structures.

To examine whether VLA-2, VLA-5 and VLA-6 together make up the total VLA, these proteins were removed from lysates of ^{125}I-labeled platelets by preclearing with α^2, α^5 and α^6 subunit specific antibodies and the remaining lysate was precipitated with the anti-β^1 specific antibody, mAb A-1A5. As shown in Fig. 6 almost all of the A-1A5 reactive material could be removed from the lysates by VLA-2, VLA-5 and VLA-6 preclearing. The proteins that remained migrated as α and β subunits of 160.000 and 120.000 Mr under nonreducing conditions and of 165.000 and 130.000 Mr under reducing conditions. Because the α subunit of this protein complex resembled α^2, they were compared by V8 peptide mapping. As shown in Fig. 7 the α subunit seen by mAb A-1A5 in the precleared lysate and the classical α^2 subunit defined by mAb 12F1 yielded identical V8 digestion patterns. We are, therefore, probably dealing with one single protein: i.e. VLA-2. Possible explanations for the inability of 12F1 to remove all VLA-2 proteins are (1) a relative low affinity of the 12F1 antibody in comparison to that of A-1A5 and (2) selective loss of the 12F1 epitope on a small fraction of the total VLA-2 proteins due to the radiolabeling and preparation of platelet lysates. In conclusion, platelets have three VLA proteins, VLA-2, VLA-5 and VLA-6 and no additional VLA proteins.

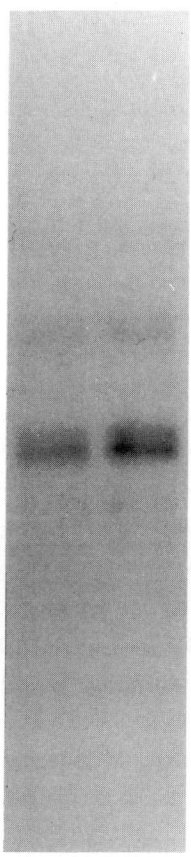

1   2

Fig. 7. Comparison of the α^2 subunit and the α subunit precipitated by mAb A-1A5 from precleared lysate by peptide mapping with V8 protease. Lysate of ^{125}I-labeled platelets was precleared using the mAbs 12F1 (for VLA-2), B1E5 (for VLA-5) and GoH3 (for VLA-6) and the remaining lysate was used for specific precipitations with A-1A5 (for the remaining VLA-β associated protein). The α^2 subunit precipitated by mAb 12F1 and the α subunit precipitated from the precleared lysate using the mAb A-1A5 were separated from β subunits by SDS-PAGE under nonreducing conditions (see Fig. 6), and then gel slices containing each α subunit was excised, placed on top of a second gel, and treated with 2 μg of V8 protease. The digested products were analyzed on a 15% polyacrylamide gel. Lane 1, peptide fragments of the α^2 subunit precipitated by mAb 12 F1 and lane 2, peptide fragments of the α subunit precipitated from the precleared lysate by mAb A-1A5.

Flow cytometric analysis of VIA proteins.

The expression of VIA proteins on platelets was quantitated using flow cytometry. As shown in Table 2, platelets express approximately equal amounts of the VIA-2 and VIA-6 proteins. VIA-5 expression on platelets was weak and not readily detectable by flow cytometry. The sum of the quantitated levels of the three VIA structures approximately equals that of total VIA.

VIA-6 functions as a specific receptor for laminin.

In adhesion assays, the mAb GoH3 has been shown to specifically block the binding of platelets to laminin, but not to fibronectin, collagen types I or III, or fibrinogen (27). As VIA-6 is the integrin recognized by the mAb GoH3 on platelets, it was concluded that this protein complex serves as a specific receptor for laminin. The binding of platelets to laminin is dependent on divalent cations. Specifically Mg^{2+}, but not Ca^{2+} supported platelet adhesion to laminin. A higher degree of adhesion to laminin could be obtained when, instead of Mg^{2+}, Mn^{2+} or Co^{2+} was included in the assay buffer. Whereas mAb GoH3 completely prevented the adhesion of platelets to laminin in the presence of Mg^{2+}, only partial inhibition by this antibody was seen in the presence of Mn^{2+} or Co^{2+}. The reason is for this incomplete blocking by GoH3 is not clear,

Table 2

Analysis of surface expression of VIA proteins on platelets by flow cytometry

Antibody	Receptor	MFI
A-1A5	VIA-β	74.2 ± 4.8
10G11	VIA-2	39.9 ± 0.5
B1E5	VIA-5	3.5 ± 3.2
GoH3	VIA-6	36.8 ± 7.7

Human blood platelets were fixed with paraformaldehyde, incubated with monoclonal antibodies, followed by FITC-conjugated goat-anti-mouse IgG, and fluorescence was analyzed by flow cytometry. Results are expressed as the mean ± SD of the mean fluorescence intensity (MFI) determined for platelets of 3 donors.

but it might be due to an increase in the affinity of VLA-6 for laminin. Alternatively, Mn^{2+} and Co^{2+} might expose laminin binding sites on other platelet proteins.

In contrast to adhesion to immobilized laminin, interaction of platelets with soluble laminin determined in a binding assay, only occurred when Mn^{2+} was present (Fig. 8). No binding could be demonstrated in the presence of Mg^{2+}, Ca^{2+} or EDTA. The Mn^{2+}-dependent binding appeared to be mediated by the VLA-6 protein as it can be blocked almost completely by the α^6-specific mAb GoH3. This finding supports the supposition that divalent cations indeed can affect the affinity of receptor-laminin interactions.

VLA-6 serves as a specific receptor for the elastase-derived fragment E8 of laminin.

Laminin has been cleaved into a number of distinct fragments using a variety of proteases. The localization of these fragments within the laminin molecule has been determined by electron microscopical and biochemical methods (for review see 28,29). Several of these proteolytic fragments have been shown to support cell adhesion. They include fragment E1-4, corresponding to the three short arms of laminin (30); fragment P1, which is identical to E1-4 except that it lacks a substantial portion at the ends of the short arms (31-33). The P1 cell-binding site is cryptic in intact laminin (34,35); fragment E8, which consists of the rod-like segment and of the proximal part of the globular domain on the long arm of laminin (30,33,36) and fragment E3, which represents the distal moiety of the globular domain on the long arm of laminin (37). Fragment E4 stems from the ends of the short arms of laminin and is inactive in promoting cell adhesion. Nidogen or entactin is a 150 kD dumbbell-shaped glycoprotein that strongly binds to laminin (38,39). When we tested the ability of platelets to bind to the various laminin fragments and to nidogen, specific binding (defined as binding that is significantly higher than that to fragment E4) was demonstrated to fragments P1 and E8 and to nidogen in the presence of Mn^{2+} (Fig. 9). In the presence Mg^{2+} binding was found with intact laminin, but with none of the fragments and nidogen. The mAb GoH3, in the presence of Mn^{2+} only blocked platelet adhesion to the fragment E8. Therefore, VLA-6 acts as a specific receptor for fragment E8.

In conclusion

In this report we have described the identification and characterization of a platelet membrane glycoprotein complex that is recognized by the rat mAb GoH3.

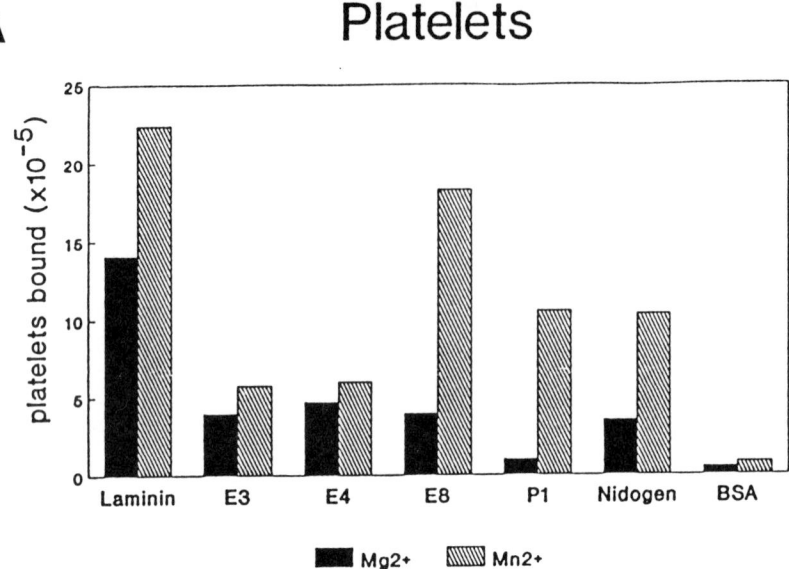

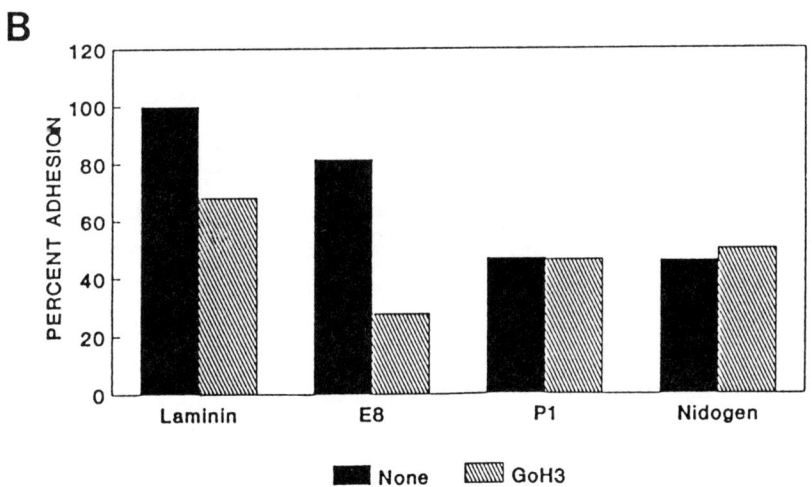

Fig. 8. Binding of ^{125}I-labeled laminin to platelets. Platelets at 1×10^8 per ml were incubated at room temperature with 8 µg/ml ^{125}I labeled laminin in the presence of 1 mM EDTA, MgCl$_2$, MnCl$_2$ or CaCl$_2$ and with or without monoclonal antibodies (1:100 dilution of ascitic fluid) as indicated. The antibodies were mAb GoH3, against the α^6 subunit of VLA-6 and mAb JsE3, a rat control antibody of the same IgG subclass as GoH3. The platelets were prepared by differential centrifugation and were suspended in Tyrode's buffer pH 7.2 containing 20 mg/ml albumin. Platelets and laminin were incubated for 1h at 37 °C. The platelet-

bound laminin was recovered by centrifugation of the platelet suspension through a cushion of 700 μl 20% sucrose. The pelleted material was dissolved in SDS sample buffer containg 10% mercaptoethanol, heated for 5 min at 95 °C and analyzed on a SDS-5% polyacrylamide gel.

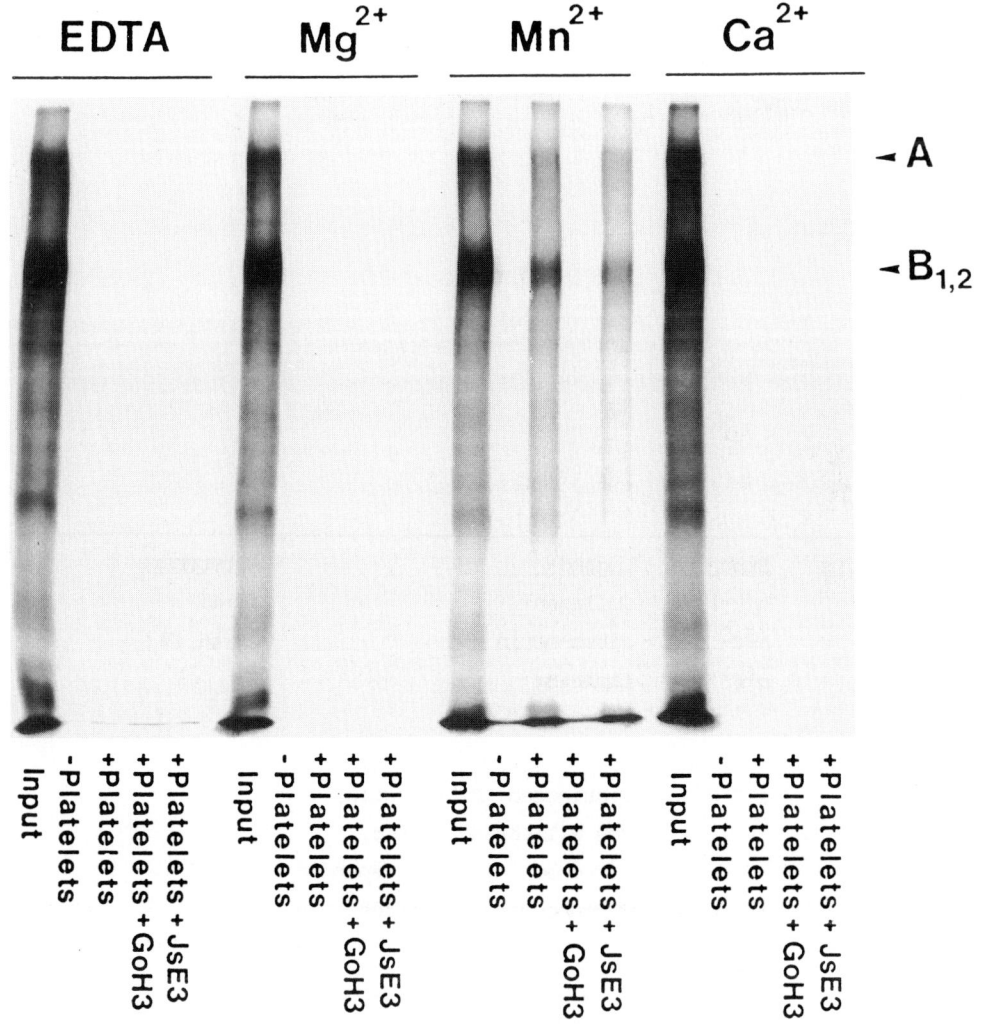

Fig. 9. Adhesion of platelets to laminin, fragments of laminin, nidogen or BSA in the presence of Mg^{2+} or Mn^{2+} and the effect of mAb GoH3. (A) Platelets were

labeled with ^{51}Cr, resuspended in Tyrode's buffer containing 2mM MgCl$_2$ (solid bars) or 2 mM MnCl$_2$ (shaded bars) and added to microtitre wells coated with 20 μg/ml laminin, fragments of laminin (E3, E4, E8 and P1), nidogen or BSA. Platelets were allowed to attach for 40 min at 37 °C. Then the microtitre wells were washed six times and the attached platelets were quantified by measuring the amount of radioactivity present in each well. (B) ^{51}Cr-labeled platelets were preincubated for 60 min at room temperature with a 100-fold dilution of ascitic fluid containing mAb GoH3 (shaded bar) or without antibody (solid bar) in the presence of 1 mM MnCl$_2$. Adhesion to wells coated with laminin, fragments of laminin (E8 and P1) or nidogen was determined in a 40 min adhesion assay. The number of platelets bound to laminin in the absence of antibody is indicated as 100%.

Table 3

Integrins			
VLA proteins	Subunits	Ligand	References
VLA-2	$\alpha^2\beta^1$	Collagen	40-45
VLA-5	$\alpha^5\beta^1$	Fibronectin	22,46,47
VLA-6	$\alpha^6\beta^1$	Laminin	27
Cytoadhesins			
GPIIbIIIa	$\alpha^{IIb}\beta^3$	Fibrinogen, Fibronectin, von Willebrand factor, Vitronectin, Thrombospondin	48-57
VNR	$\alpha^v\beta^3$	Thrombospondin, Vitronectin	23,57

Nonintegrins		
Receptor	Ligand	References
GPIb/IX	von Willebrand factor	17,48
GPIV	Thrombospondin Collagen?	58-61

We have presented evidence that this complex is in fact the platelet glycoprotein, Ic-IIa and that it is a member of the VLA subfamily of integrins (VLA-6). Furthermore, we showed that VLA-6 functions as a specific receptor for the E8 fragment of laminin. Various receptors have now been implicated in the initial adhesion of platelets to subendothelial matrix (see Table 3). Five of these receptors belong to the integrin family, whilst two do not. Obviously, there is a great diversity of receptors of different specificities to mediate this important adhesion process. This diversity of receptors ensures proper adhesion to subendothelial matrices, the composition of which may differ in various blood vessels.

Acknowledgements

We would like to thank Drs C. Damsky, V. Woods and M. Hemler for the antibodies to the integrin subunits, Mrs L. Admiraal for performing the FACS analysis, Drs. C.P. Engelfriet and A.E.G. Kr. von dem Borne for helpful comments on the manuscript and C. de Lint and W. Winkel for typing the manuscript.

References

1. Hynes, R.O. (1987) Cell 48, 549-554.
2. Ruoslahti, E., and Pierschbacher, M.D. (1987) Science 238, 491-497.
3. Hemler, M.E., Huang, C., and Schwartz, L. (1987) J. Biol. Chem. 262, 3300-3309.
4. Springer, T.A., Dustin, M.L., Kishimoto, T.K., and Martin, S.D. (1987) Ann. Rev. Immunol. 5, 223-252.
5. Ginsberg, M.H., Loftus, J.C., and Plow, E.F. (1988) Thromb. Hemost. 59,, 1-6.
6. Hemler, M.E., Crouse, C., Takada, Y. and Sonnenberg, A. (1988) J. Biol. Chem. 263, 7660-7665.
7. Vogel, B.E., Tarone, G., Giancotti, F.G., Gailit, J., and Ruoslahti, E. (1990) J. Biol. Chem., in press.
8. Sonnenberg, A., Hogervorst, F., Osterop, A., Veltman, F.E.M. (1988) J. Biol. Chem. 263, 14030-14038.
9. Hemler, M.E., Crouse, C. and Sonnenberg, A. (1989) J. Biol. Chem. 264, 6529-6535.
10. Kajiji, S., Tamura, R.N., and Quaranta, V. (1989) EMBO J. 8, 673-680.
11. Hogervorst, F., Kuikman, I., von dem Borne, A.E.G. Kr., and Sonnenberg, A. (1990) EMBO J., 9, 765-770.
12. Suzuki, S., and Naitoh, Y. (1990) EMBO J. 9, 757-763.
13. Horwitz, A.F., Duggan, K., Buck, C., Beckerle, M.C., and Burridge, K. (1986) Nature 320, 531-533.
14. Burridge, K., and Mangeat, P. (1984) Nature 308, 744-746.
15. Burridge, K., Fath, K., Kelly, T., Nuckolls, G., and Turner, C. (1988) Annul. Rev. Cell Biol. 4, 487-523.

16. Phillips, D.R., and Poh Agin, P. (1977) J. Biol. Chem. 252, 2121-2126.
17. Nurden, A.T., Dupuis, D., Kunicki, T.J., and Caen, J.P. (1981) J. Clin. Invest. 67, 1431-1440.
18. Clemetson, K.J, Capitanio, A., and Lüscher, E.F. (1979) Biochem. Biophys. Acta 553, 11-24.
19. McGregor, J.L., Clemetson, K.J., James, E., Capitanio, A., Greeland, T., Lüscher, E.F., and Dechavanne, M., (1981) Eur. J. Biochem. 116, 379-388.
20. Clemetson, K.J. (1985) in Platelet Membrane Glycoproteins (George, J.N., Nurden, A.T. and Phillips, D.R., eds.) pp 51-85, Plenum Press, New York.
21. Sonnenberg, A., Janssen, H., Hogervorst, F., Calafat, J., and Hilgers, J. (1987) J. Biol. Chem. 262, 10376-10383.
22. Piotrowicz, R.S., Orchekowski, R.P., Nugent, D.J., Yamada, K.Y., and Kunicki, T.J. (1988) J. Cell Biol. 106, 1359-1364.
23. Lam, S.C., Plow, E.F., D'Souza, S.E., Cheresh, D.A., Frelinger, A.L. III, Ginsberg, M.H. (1989) J. Biol. Chem. 264, 3742-3749.
24. Pischel, K.D., Bluestein, H.E., and Woods Jr., V.L. (1988) J. Clin. Invest. 81, 505-513.
25. Mourik, J.A. van, Leeksma, O.C., Reinders, J.H., Groot, P.G. de, and Zandbergen-Spaargaren, J. (1985) J. Biol. Chem. 260, 11300-11306.
26. McEver, R.P., and Martin, M.N. (1984) J. Biol. Chem. 259, 9799-9804.
27. Sonnenberg, A., Modderman, P.W., and Hogervorst, F. (1988) Nature 336, 487-489.
28. Timpl, R. (1989) Eur. J. Biochem. 180, 487-502.
29. Beck, K., Hunter, I., and Engel, J. (1990) FASEB J. 4, 148-160.
30. Goodman, S.L., Deutzmann, R., and Mark, K. von der (1987) J. Cell Biol. 105, 589-598.
31. Terranova, V.P., Rao, C.N., Kalebic, T., Margulies, I.M., and Liotta, L.A. (1983) Proc. Natl. Acad. Sci. USA 80, 444-448.
32. Barsky, S.H., Rao, C.N., Hyams, D., and Liotta, L.A. (1984) Breast Cancer Res. Treatm. 4, 181-188.
33. Aumailley, M., Nurcombe, V., Edgar, D., Paulsson, and Timpl, R. (1987) J. Biol. Chem. 262, 11532-11538.
34. Nurcombe, V., Aumailley, M., Timpl, R., and Edgar, D. (1989) Eur. J. Biochem. 180, 9-14.
35. Aumailley, M., Gerl, M., Sonnenberg, A., Deutzmann, R. and Timpl, R. (1990) FEBS Lett., in press.
36. Edgar, D., Timpl, R., and Thoenen, H. (1984) EMBO J. 3, 1463-1468.
37. Sonnenberg, A., Linders, C.J.T., Modderman, P.W., Damsky, C.H., Aumailley, M., and Timpl, R. (1988) J. Cell Biol., in press.
38. Carlin, B.E., Durkin, M.E., Bender, B., Jaffer, R., and Chung, A.E. (1983) J. Biol. Chem. 258, 7729-7737.
39. Paulsson, M., Deutzmann, R., Dziadek, M., Nowack, H., Timpl, R., Weber, S., and Engel, J. (1986) Eur. J. Biochem. 156, 467-478.
40. Santoro, S.A. (1986) Cell 46, 913-920.
41. Santoro, S.A., Rajpara, S.M., Staatz, W.D., and Woods Jr., V.L. (1988) Biochem. Biophys. Res. Commun. 153, 217-223.
42. Staatz, W.D., Rajpara, S.M., Wayner, E.A., Carter, W.G, and Santoro, S.A. (1989) J. Cell Biol. 108, 1917-1924.
43. Kunicki, T.J., Nugent, D.J., Staats, S.J., Orchekowski, R.P., Wayner, E.A., and Carter, W.G. (1988) J. Biol. Chem. 263, 4516-4519.
44. Coller, B.S., Beer, J.H., Scudder, L.E., and Steinberg, M.H. (1989) Blood 74, 182-192.
45. Kirchhofer, D., Languino, L.R., Ruoslahti, E., and Pierschbacher, M.D. (1990) J. Biol. Chem. 265, 615-618.
46. Wayner, E.A., Carter, W.G., Piotrowicz, R.S., and Kunicki, T.J. (1989) J. Cell Biol. 109, 877-889.
47. Giancotti, F.G., Languino, L.R., Zanetti, A., Peri, G., Tarone, G., and Dejana, E. (1987) Blood 69, 1535-1538.

48. Ruggeri, Z.M., De Marco, L., Gatti, L., Bader, R., and Montgomery, R.R. (1983) J. Clin. Invest. 72, 1-12.
49. Nachman, R.L., and Leung, L.L.K. (1982) J. Clin. Invest. 69, 263-269.
50. Bennet, J.S., Vilaire, G., and Cines, D.B. (1982) J. Biol. Chem. 257, 8049-8064.
51. Plow, E.F, McEver, R.P., Coller, B.S., Woods Jr., V.L., Marguerie, G.A., and Ginsberg, M.H. (1985) Blood 66, 724-727.
52. Thiagarajan, P. and Kelly, K.L. (1988) J. Biol. Chem. 263, 3035-3038.
53. Gardner, J.M., and Hynes, R.O. (1985) Cell 42, 439-448.
54. Pytela, R., Pierschbacher, M.D., Ginsberg, M.H., Plow, E.F., and Ruoslahti, E. (1986) Science 231, 1559-1562.
55. Parise, L.V., and Phillips, D.R. (1985) J. Biol. Chem. 260, 10698-10707.
56. Ginsberg, M., Pierschbacher, M.D., Ruoslahti, E., Marguerie, G., and Plow, E. (1985) J. Biol. Chem. 260, 3931-3936.
57. Lawler, J. and Hynes, R.O. (1989) Blood 74, 2022-2027.
58. Asch, A.S., Barnwell, J., Silverstein, R.L., Nachman, R.L. (1987) J. Clin. Invest. 79, 1054-1061.
59. McGregor, J.L., Catimel, B., Parmentier, S., Clezardin, P., Dechavanne, M., and Leung, L.L.K. (1989) J. Biol. Chem. 264, 501-506.
60. Barnwell, J.W., Ockhenhouse, C.F., and Knowles, D.M., (1985) J. Immunol. 135, 3494-3497.
61. Tandon, N.N., Kralisz, U., Jamieson, G.A. (1989) J. Biol. Chem. 264, 7576-7583.

Résumé

Le complexe glycoprotéique (GP) plaquettaire humain GPIc-IIa est reconnu par l'anticorps monoclonal (MAb) de rat GoH3 qui est spécifiquement dirigé vis-à-vis de la GPIc. Ce complexe est identifié comme étant le VLA-6, de la famille protéique des Very Late Activation antigens (VLA), car il est détecté par un Mab (A-1A5) dirigé contre la sous-unité beta-1. Ce complexe (VLA-6) n'est pas reconnu par des Mab dirigés contre la sous-unité alpha-5. Les plaquettes expriment 4 formes de VLA-6 qui se distinguent par des différences structurales au niveau des sous-unités alpha 6. Le VLA-6 fonctionne comme un récepteur spécifique de la laminine alors que le VLA-2 et le VLA-5 fonctionnent respectivement comme des récepteurs du collagène et de la laminine. Ces trois récepteurs (VLA-2, VLA-5 et VLA-6) permettent l'adhésion des plaquettes au sous-endothélium vasculaire.

Effects of monoclonal antibodies on the platelet receptors – Regulation of platelet-vessel wall interactions

Effets des anticorps monoclonaux sur les récepteurs plaquettaires. Régulation des interactions plaquette-paroi capillaire

A monoclonal antibody against platelet GPIIb/IIIa interacts with a calcium binding site and induces fibrinogen binding and platelet aggregation

M.J. Rabiet, C. Boudignon, D. Gulino, J.J. Ryckewaert, A. Andrieux and G. Marguerie

INSERM U 217, DRF/Laboratoire d'Hématologie, Centre d'Etudes Nucléaires, Avenue des Martyrs, BP 85X, F38041 Grenoble Cedex, France

SUMMARY

Among the various members of the integrin family, platelet GPIIbIIIa is unique since the expression of its adhesive properties depends upon an induction reaction. The monoclonal antibody D33C, specific for platelet GPIIb, behaves as a GPIIbIIIa activator, inducing fibrinogen binding and platelet aggregation. This activity is similar to that observed when ADP is used as platelet agonist. However, activation of platelet by D33C is independant of the secretion reaction and is not inhibited by PGE1. Several peptides, corresponding to potential antigenic sequences, have been synthesized. Only one of them was found to inhibit D33C activity. Its sequence corresponds to a putative calcium binding site on GPIIb. This antibody may prove to be a valuable tool to study the mechanisms involved in the induction of a functional adhesive GPIIbIIIa.

INTRODUCTION

A number of critical vascular functions such as permeability, cell migration in wound healing and developpement, thrombosis and angiogenesis are influenced by the ability of vascular cells to attach to each other as well as to the underlying extracellular matrix in cell-cell or cell-substratum adhesion.

A group of cell adhesion receptors important for platelet and endothelial cell interactions are the integrins which constitute a family of heterodimeric proteins composed of non covalently linked α and β subunits. Each subfamily is defined by a common β subunit while substrate specificity is determined by the particular combination of α and β subunits (Hynes, 1987).

Among the various members of the integrin family, platelet GPIIbIIIa and the leucocyte adhesion molecule LFA1 have a unique feature since their adhesive properties depend upon an activation reaction. GPIIbIIIa functions as a receptor for fibrinogen, fibronectin and von Willebrand factor and is involved in platelet spreading and aggregation (Marguerie et al., 1987, Plow et al., 1987). In blood vessels, platelets must circulate freely and ligand binding must be controlled to prevent massive thrombosis. GPIIbIIIa is exposed at the surface of platelet but in an inactive state and does not interact with its adhesive ligands. Stimulation by a variety of physiological agonists transforms platelet into an aggregative cell. While numerous informations have recently been accumulated on the structure and the function of GPIIbIIIa, little is known about the molecular bases that control receptor induction. Both modification of the microenvironment (Coller et al., 1986) and conformational changes have been postulated (Parise et al., 1987, and Frelinger et al., 1988) but the precise structural basis for the induction reaction has not yet been identified.

We have produced and characterized several monoclonal antibodies which have the interesting properties to induce or inhibit fibrinogen binding and platelet aggregation and could represent valuable reagents to investigate the nature of the molecular events leading to an adhesive GPIIbIIIa. This paper describes the characterization of a monoclonal antibody, D33C, inducing fibrinogen binding and platelet aggregation, and the localization of its epitope on GPIIb.

PRODUCTION AND CARACTERISATION OF MONOCLONAL ANTIBODY D33C

A series of monoclonal antibodies specific for GPIIbIIIa were produced by fusing the murine myeloma cell line SPO2 AG14 with splenic lymphocytes from mice immunized with purified human GPIIb or GPIIIa. Hybridoma culture supernatants were screened for antiplatelet reactivity in a solid phase immunoassay. One of the positive clones, designated D33C, produced an IgG1 type antibody. In ELISA, D33C reacted only with platelet membranes or purified GPIIbIIIa. Immunofluorescence studies and alkaline phosphatase labelling indicated that D33C was reactive with platelets but did not label endothelial cells or monocytic cell lines. This antibody immunoprecipitated two proteins from surface labeled platelets, with electrophoretic mobilities compatible with the molecular weights of GPIIb and GPIIIa. Finally, after platelet lysate separation by SDS-PAGE, D33C antibody immunoblotted only the heavy chain of purified GPIIb (Fig. 1).

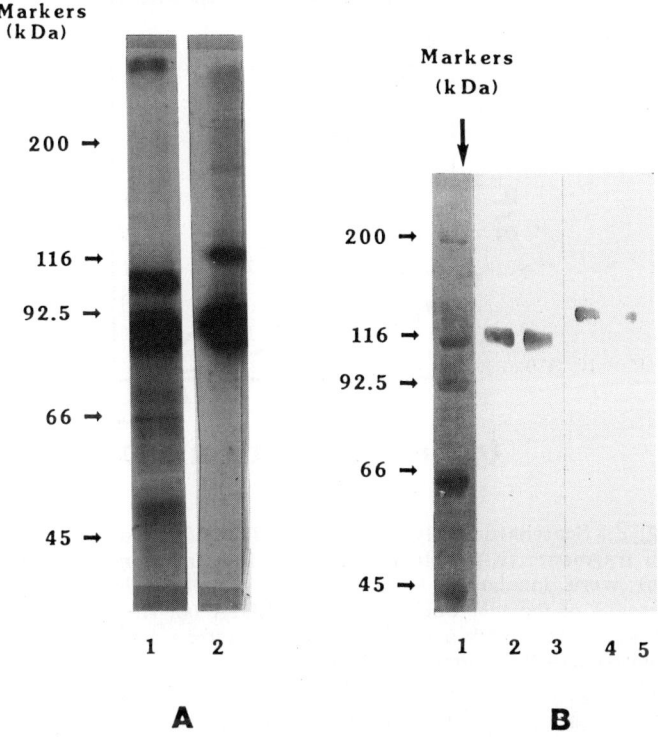

Fig. 1 : Monoclonal antibody D33C specificity for GPIIb. A. Autoradiography of radiolabeled reduced (lane 1) and non reduced (lane 2) GPIIbIIIa complex immunoprecipitated by monoclonal antibody D33C. B. Immunoblots of platelet lysates and purified GPIIb in their reduced (lane 2 and 3) or non reduced forms (lane 4 and 5).

DIRECT BINDING OF D33C TO PLATELETS

The direct binding of D33C antibody was examined using radioiodinated Fab fragments prepared from purified D33C IgGs. In the presence of 1mM $CaCl_2$, their interaction with non stimulated platelets was a slow reaction but was saturable with time. Statchard analysis of the binding isotherms (Fig 2) was compatible with only one class of binding sites. Saturation was reached at a 1mM concentration of ^{125}I D33C. Fab fragments and intact IGgs bound to 44 000 ± 20 000 sites on platelet. Binding was inhibited by an excess of non labelled IgGs. The presence of 1 mM EDTA did not affect the number of Fab fragments bound per cell but decreased the dissociation constant (Kd) from 0.8 µM to 0.17 µM.

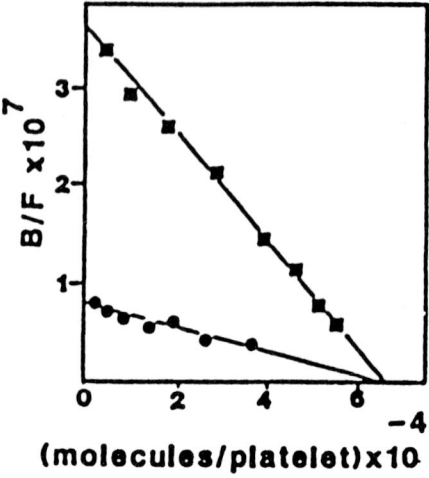

Fig. 2 : Scatchard analysis of the binding of radiolabeled D33C Fab fragments to platelets. 125I D33C Fab fragments (1.2 x 10^{-7} Mm) were incubated with platelets (2 x 10^8 cells/ml) in the presence of 0.5 mM $CaCl_2$ (●) or 1 M EDTA (■). At selected time points samples were centrifuged over a sucrose dense solution to separate free from bound ^{125}I Fabs.

IDENTIFICATION OF D33C EPITOPE

Purified GPIIb was digested by lysine endopeptidase with a 1/50 enzyme to substrate ratio and the derived fragments were separated by SDS-PAGE and immunoblotted on PVDF membrane with D33C monoclonal antibody. The major and smaller fragment recognized by the antibody was a 15 000 molecular weight peptide. Its N-terminal amino acid sequence, determined by automatic Edman degradation directly on the PVDF membrane blotted fragment (Matsudaira, 1987) begins with the sequence KLAEVGRVYLFLQPR corresponding to residue 321 to 335 in GPIIb. GPIIb contains multiple potentiel cleavage sites for lysine endopeptidase. cleavage at lysine 321 and lysine 455 (or lysine 471) would generate such a 15 000 molecular weight fragment. In addition, potent antigenic sites were predicted from the amino acid sequence of GPIIb using the algorithm method of Parker et al. (1986). Several sequences were selected, synthesized, and their capacity to inhibit the binding of D33C IgGs to platelets was examined. The different peptides are listed in Table 1.

	Numbers	Amino acid sequences	Residues	IC_{50}
GPIIb	IIb$_1$	DIDDNGYPDLIV	426-437	350 μM
	IIb$_{1-9}$	DNGYPDLIV	429-437	500 μM
	IIb$_{1-8}$	NGYPDLIV	430-437	> 5mM
	IIb$_{1-7}$	GYPDLIV	431-437	> 5mM
	IIb$_{1-6}$	YPDLIV	432-437	> 5mM
	IIb$_{1-5}$	PDLIV	433-437	> 5mM
	IIb$_2$	EGLRSRPSQVLD	397-408	> 5mM
	IIb$_3$	SKNSQNPNS	725-733	> 5mM
	IIb$_4$	DVNGDGRHDLLV	297-308	> 5mM
	IIb$_5$	DLDRGYNDIAN	365-376	> 5mM
	IIb$_6$	EFDGDLNTTEYV	243-254	> 5mM

Table I : Various peptides used as competitors in ELISA and preincubated with D33C IgGs prior to the antibody binding to platelet membrane lysates. Ic50 values correspond to half of the maximal inhibition concentration.

IIb1, IIb4, IIb5 and IIb6 correspond to the four putative calcium binding sites whereas IIb2 and IIb3 correspond to non calcium related potential antigenic sites. IIb1 was the only peptide which was found to produce a complete inhibition of the binding of D33C IGgs to platelets with an IC50 of 350 μM. IIb10 which contains half of the IIb1 amino acid sequence and has an extension towards the N-terminus, was not active. A detailed analysis indicated that the minimum sequence for which a relevant dose dependant inhibition was measurable correspond to the peptide IIb 1-9 with the sequence DNGYPDLIV. Peptides corresponding to adjacent sequences had no effect. Peptides corresponding to other putative calcium binding site were also inactive.

INDUCTION OF THE GPIIbIIIa RECEPTOR FUNCTIONS

This monoclonal antibody has the interesting property of inducing fibrinogen binding and platelet aggregation. Addition of D33C IgGs or Fab fragments of D33C antibody (2 μM) to stirring platelets in the presence of fibrinogen induced an aggregation response comparable to that obtained with 10 μM ADP (Fig. 3). D33C induced aggregation was not inhibited by 1 µM PGE1, a concentration that produced a complete inhibition of ADP induced aggregation, suggesting that activation of adenylate cyclase is not involved in the stimulation of platelets by the antibody. Activation of platelets by 2 µM D33C did not induce a significant secretion of ^{14}C serotonin.

Binding of fibrinogen to platelets was analyzed as a function of fibrinogen concentration using different concentrations of D33C IgGs or Fabs (Fig 4). Binding with respect to both antibody and fibrinogen concentrations was saturable with a maximum of 30 000 ± 10 000 fibrinogen molecules bound per platelet and a Kd value of 0.8 µM. These numbers are consistent with the values obtained in the presence of ADP and with a one to one stoechiometry for the activation of GPIIbIIIa by monovalent Fab fragments. In addition, D33C induced aggregation did not occur in the absence of fibrinogen, providing an additional correlation between stimulation of the receptor, binding of fibrinogen and platelet aggregation.

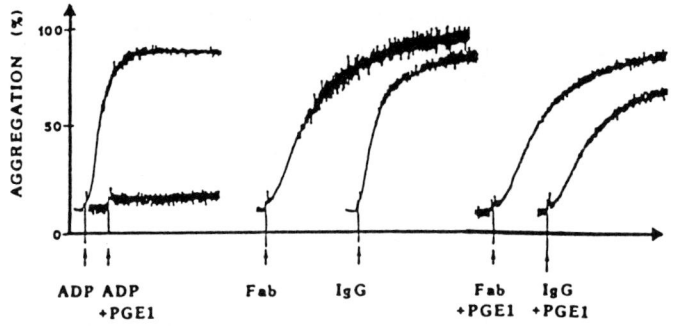

Fig. 3 : Platelet aggregation induced by D33C IgG and Fab fragments. Washed platelets (2 10^8 cells/ml) were stimulated with 2 µM D33C IgGs, 2 µM D33C Fabs, or with 10 µM ADP in the presence of 1 µM fibrinogen and 0.5 mM $CaCl_2$. PGE1 was used at a concentration of 1 µM and was added to the platelet suspension with fibrinogen prior to the agonist addition.

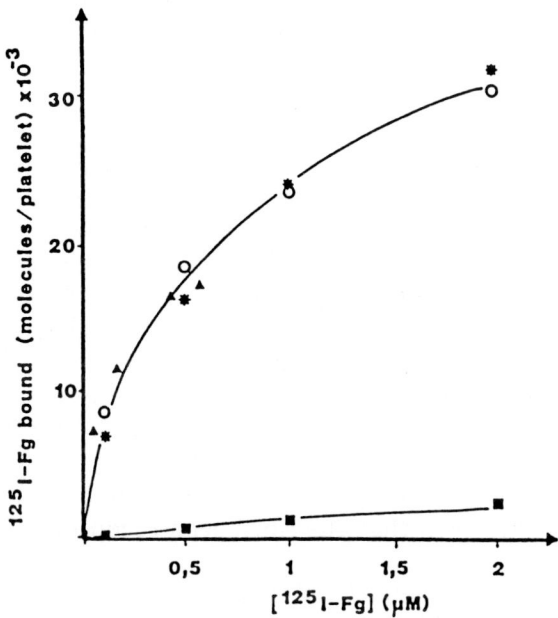

Fig. 4 : Fibrinogen binding to D33C stimulated platelets. Washed platelets (2 x 10^8 cells/ml), in the presence of various concentrations of radiolabeled fibrinogen, were stimulated with D33C IgGs (0 = , 0.50 µM =) or with D33C Fabs (0.5 µM =) or with 10 µM ADP ( ). The bound radiolabeled fibrinogen was separated from the free ligand by centribugation through a 20 % sucrose solution.

SPECIFICITY OF D33C ANTIBODY FOR PLATELETS

The sequence of the dodecapeptide IIb1 is highly conserved among the α subunits of various integrins. However, in immunofluorescence experiments, this antibody interacted only with platelets and failed to label endothelial cells which exhibit vitronectin (VnR) and fibronectin (FnR) receptors at their surface. This suggest that an homologous sequence that may function as a calcium binding site within the three different integrins is differently exposed at the surface of the two cells. Thus cellular-specific signals may influence the exposure of similar structure and modulate the specificity of the different integrins.

DISCUSSION

Recently, a number of anti-GPIIbIIIa monoclonal antibodies have been described which, upon binding, stimulate platelet activation and aggregation (Bachelot et al., Kouns et al., Morel et al., Yu et al., 1989). For most of them, only intact monoclonal antibodies or F(ab')2 binding can induce the fibrinogen receptor GPIIbIIIa, suggesting a possible role for Fc mediated or surface crosslinking mediated activation.

However, D33C antibody, specific for GPIIb, and a monoclonal antibody, specific for GPIIIa, described by Kouns et al. (1989), can expose the GPIIbIIIa fibrinogen receptor when their Fab fragments are used. The activity of D33C resemble ADP induced platelet aggregation but did not stimulate the secretion reaction, as evaluated by the measurement of serotonin release and was not inhibited by PGE1. This suggests that the mechanism involved in platelet activation by ADP and D33C are somewhat different. Binding of D33C may induce a conformational change in the GPIIb such that the fibrinogen receptor is exposed.

In that respect, D33C monoclonal antibody could potentially be used as a tool to stimulate GPIIbIIIa into a fibrinogen receptor in a non platelet environment. The availability of full length cDNA encoding for GPIIb and GPIIIa allows the expression of recombinant proteins. The lack of platelet agonists specific transduction signals may be critical in using transfected cells to study the molecular events controlling the receptor function. This problem could be avoided using D33C antibody to stimulate the receptor.

REFERENCES

Bachelot, C., Rendu, F. and Levy-Toledano, S. (1989) : Activation of platelets induced by mAb P256 specific for glycoprotein IIbIIIa : evidence for a role for IIbIIIa in membrane signal transduction. Thromb. Haemost. 62, abstract 820.

Coller, B.S. (1989) : Activation affects access to the platelet receptor for adhesive glycoproteins. J. Cell. Biol. 103, 451-456.

Frelinger, A.L., Lam, C.T., Plow, E.F., Smith, M.A., Loftus, J.C. and Ginsberg, M.H. (1988) : Occupancy of an adhesive glycoprotein receptor modulates expression of an antigenic site involved in cell adhesion. J. Biol. Chem. 263, 12397-12402.

Hynes, R.O. (1987) : Integrins : a family of cell surface receptors. Cell 48, 459-554.

Kouns, W.C., Fox, C.F., Lamoreaux, W.J., Coons, L.R. and Jennings, L.K. (1989) : Activation-independant exposure of the GPIIbIIIa fibrinogen receptor. Blood 74, abstract 336.

Marguerie, G., Ginsberg M.H.,and PLOW, E.F. (1987) : The platelet fibrinogen receptor. In "Platelets biology and pathology" J.Gordon Ed, Elsevier Science Publishers, pp.95-121.

Morel, M.C., Lecompte, J., Champeix, P., Favier, R., Potevin, F., Samama, M., Salmon, C. and Kaplan, C. (1989) : PL2-49, a monoclonal antibody against glycoprotein IIb which is a platelet activator. Brit. J. Haematol 71, 57-63.

Matsudaira, P. (1987) : Sequence from picomole quantities of proteins electroblotted onto polyvinylidene difluoride membranes. J. Biol. Chem. 21, 10035-10038.

Parise, L.V., Helgerson, S.L.; Steiner, B., Nannizzi, L. and PHILLIPS D.R. (1987) : Synthetic peptides derived from fibrinogen and fibronectin change the conformation of purified platelet glycoprotein IIbIIIa. J. Biol. Chem. 262, 12597-12602.

Parker, J.M., Guo, D. and Hodges, R.S. (1986) : New hydrophilicity scale derived from high performance liquid chromatography peptide retention data : correlation of predicted surface residus with antigenicity and X-ray derivided accessible sites. Biochem. 25, 5425-5432.

Plow, E.F., Marguerie, G. and Ginsberg, M.H. (1987) : Interaction of adhesive proteins with platelets : common features with distinct differences. In perspertives in inflammation, Heoplasia and vascular Cell Biology, New York, D.R. Liss Inc., pp. 267-275.

Yu, A.X., Li, J.Z. and Liam, E.C.Y. (1986) : A murine monoclonal antibody which binds platelet membrane glycoprotein IIbIIIa complex induces aggregation. Thromb. Haemostas. 62, abstract 339.

Résumé

Parmi les differents membres de la famille des intégrines, la GPIIbIIIa plaquettaire possède l'unique propriété de n'être fonctionnelle qu'après une réaction d'induction. L'anticorps monoclonal D33C, spécifique de la GPIIb, induit la fixation du fibrinogène sur son récepteur et l'agrégation plaquettaire. Cette activité est similaire à celle observée lorsque l'ADP est utilisé comme agent inducteur. Cependant, l'activation des plaquettes par le D33C est indépendante de toute sécrétion et n'est pas inhibée par la PGE1. Plusieurs peptides correspondant à des sites antigéniques potentiels sur la GPIIb, ont été synthétisés. Un seul inhibe l'activité du D33C. Sa séquence correspond à l'un des sites potentiels de fixation du calcium sur la GPIIb. Cet anticorps pourrait se révéler être un outil appréciable pour l'étude de la réaction d'induction des fonctions adhésives de la GPIIbIIIa.

Anti-platelet monoclonal activating or inhibitory antibodies to probe the functions and regulations of the glycoprotein IIb-IIIa complex

T. Lecompte*, R. Favier*, F. Potevin*, M.-C. Morel**, S.-K. Luo*, C. Kaplan** and M.M. Samama*

*Laboratoire central d'hématologie, Hôtel-Dieu, 1, place du Parvis-Notre-Dame, 75004 Paris, France
** INTS, 6 rue Alexandre Cabanel, 75015 Paris, France

ABSTRACT

Monoclonal antibodies directed at the glycoprotein IIb-IIIa complex of the platelet membrane (the inducible receptor for fibrinogen required for aggregation) inhibit aggregation with or without inhibition of fibrinogen binding, or induce aggregation, or have no detectable functional effect. The variety of the effects suggests the presence of different functional domains in the complex. We found the anti- GP IIIa antibodies to be the most potent inhibitors of aggregation. Platelet-activating antibodies are truly complex specific (6C9), or directed at an epitope located on GP IIb, the appropriate conformation for the binding depending on the presence of calcium and/or on the association of GP IIb to GP IIIa (PL2-49). The mechanisms of platelet activation induced with such antibodies are not fully understood, but might differ, at least in part, from those corresponding to CD9 antibodies. In both cases however, the binding of the Fc domain to the Fc gamma receptor type II, which follows the binding of the Fab domain to its specific epitope, is required. Although there are still uncertainties about the membrane molecule that carries the transduction of the activating signal brought by the antibodies, GP IIb-IIIa probably plays a role in physiological platelet activation.

The first monoclonal antibodies (MoAbs) against human platelets were reported in the early eighties (see Coller, 1984). They brought additional clues to elucidate the roles of the two main glycoprotein (GP) heterodimers of the platelet membrane, and their molecular mechanism: GPIb-IX binds von Willebrand factor and is involved in platelet adhesion onto the sub-endothelium; GPIIb-IIIa binds fibrinogen and is involved in platelet-platelet adhesion, namely aggregation. Several MoAbs with unequivocal epitope location on either complex were demonstrated to inhibit both the ligand binding and the respective function. Since then however many more MoAbs have been obtained with various functional effects, and with different epitopes belonging to the two above-mentioned complexes, or to other proteins of the platelet membrane. It took less than 10 years to realize that the functional changes brought by the incubation of platelets with a MoAb could result from more sophisticated mechanisms than the antagonism with ligand binding by binding site occupancy.

The aim of this paper is not to provide an exhaustive review on the functional effects of the large number of reported anti-platelet MoAbs. Starting from our own data and critically analyzing some works carried out by other groups, we rather would like to discuss some controversial issues and to outline the subjects of ongoing and future research. The effects of MoAbs directed at the glycoproteins Ib, IX, and IV (or IIIb), or at proteins expressed on the platelet surface only after activation, are beyond the scope of this review.

HISTORICAL BACKGROUND

Our interest in this field stemmed from the results of a functional screening of murine hybridoma-derived antibodies generated after immunization with human whole platelets. One MoAb, called PL2-49, was unique since it could trigger platelet aggregation. Much to our surprise PL2-49 was directed against an epitope in the GP IIb-IIIa complex (Morel et al., 1988).

At that time all the well described platelet-activating MoAbs were directed at the CD9 (ninth cluster of leucocytes differentiation antigens) molecule. The pioneering work of Boucheix and coworkers (1983) indicated that a MoAb such as ALB6 could bind to the platelet surface and induce platelet aggregation. The epitope was unrelated to GP IIb-IIIa, and was clearly localized on a distinct low molecular weight protein, the CD9 molecule. The role of the CD9 molecule was unknown at that time (and remains so in 1990), and since most of the MoAbs to CD9 shared the same property it was speculated that the CD9 molecule could be involved in platelet activation. Shortly thereafter (Jennings et al., 1985) a set of platelet-activating MoAb was claimed to bind to the light chain (previously known as ß-chain) of GP IIb.

The immunogen was supposed to be purified GP IIb, but now there are some lines of evidence that at least one of these MoAbs belongs to CD9 (Jennings et al., 1990). However it has not been submitted to any workshop on hematopoietic cell differentiation antigens (see below). Such a mistake emphasizes the advantage of the unambiguous assignment of any MoAb to a cluster by means of a workshop.

As reviewed for instance by Plow and Ginsberg (1989), several MoAbs generated against GP IIb-IIIa were reported in 1983 to inhibit platelet aggregation and fibrinogen binding, in keeping with the hypothesis that GP IIb-IIIa was the receptor for fibrinogen (Bennett, 1985). It was much more surprising that a MoAb could bind to the same GP complex and trigger the opposite response, that is aggregation. Such a finding had been briefly mentioned before (Bai et al., 1984; Boucheix et al., 1987). When our paper

describing the MoAb PL2-49 was in press (and it was eventually published in early 1989 - Morel et al , 1989), we became aware in mid 1988 of a similar, but probably not identical (see below for the detailed comparison), MoAb called 6C9 and later also CLB-thromb/7 (Modderman et al. , 1988).
All the known responses to platelet stimuli we have looked for with PL2-49 were found to exist (Table 1). The still missing pieces of the picture are: the

TABLE 1
The responses to the MoAb PL2-49

Response	Evidenced by means of ...
shape change	changes in light transmission (LT) (decrease in LT with dampening of the high frequency oscillations) observation with phase microscope occurs after a lag phase
aggregation	same tools and inspection with the naked eye inhibition of the increase in LT with the RGDS peptide *
release from dense granules	ATP-dependent luminescence with the luciferin-luciferase mixture platelets loaded with labeled serotonin *
release from alpha granules	indirect evidence for the release of fibrinogen (inhibitory effect of RGDS on aggregation) *
thromboxane synthesis	inhibitory effect of the cyclo-oxygenase inhibitors aspirin and diclofenac (partial) radioimmunoassay for TXB2 *
raise in cytoplasmic Ca^{++}	aequorin probe fluorescent dye (fura-2) *
protein phosphorylation	whole platelets loaded with ^{32}P, and stimulated; protein lysate run on SDS-PAGE followed by autoradiography *

The results summarized in this table are taken from Morel et al. (1989) and Favier et al. (1989a); those published only as an abstracted form (Favier et al., 1990) are indicated by (*). Calcium changes were also evidenced by means of the luminescent probe aequorin with the following MoAbs: VI-Pl3 (Favier et al. , 1989a), and 6C9 and P256 (Favier et al. , unpublished data).

release of the content of the lysosomes, which is documented for CD9 MoAbs; the exposure of procoagulant activities; the breakdown of phosphatidyl-inositides; the alcalinization of the cytoplasm through the sodium-proton exchange.
We have been carrying out our research along the following lines:
(i) the comparison of different MoAbs directed at the GP IIb-IIIa complex with various, and even opposite, functional effects;
(ii) the comparison of different MoAbs directed at different molecules but with the same functional effect, namely platelet activation.

DIVERSITY OF THE MoAbs AGAINST THE GP IIb-IIIa COMPLEX

Inhibition of aggregation and of fibrinogen binding.

As pointed above, inhibition of platelet aggregation was the expected result of the incubation of platelets with MoAbs directed at GP IIb-IIIa, and was easy to understand. This effect was called the induction *in vitro* of a thrombasthenic-like state of incubated normal platelets, since it mimicks the behaviour of the platelets prepared from patients with type I Glanzmann's thrombesthenia: these platelets profoundly deficient in GP IIb-IIIa exert upon activation all their functions but aggregation. With the MoAb called A2A9 for instance, a competitive antagonism of fibrinogen binding was also evidenced, and thus it was concluded that the MoAb prevented the access of fibrinogen to its binding site on GP IIb-IIIa, and thereby was able to inhibit platelet aggregation (Bennett *et al.*, 1983). Recently the same MoAb was shown to inhibit the binding of a synthetic hexapeptide containing the RGDS sequence to purified GP IIb-IIIa (Steiner *et al.*, 1989). Plow and Ginsberg (1989) stressed that many of the inhibitory MoAbs were demonstrated to be of the "calcium / complex-dependent" variety; the binding of these MoAbs and that of fibrinogen have the same dependence upon the maintenance of the calcium-dependent heterodimeric structure of GP IIb-IIIa, but the latter, and not the former, requires platelet activation and a change in the state of GP IIb-IIIa or in its micro-environment.

Other effects and their significance.

More complex effects of MoAbs directed at GP IIb-IIIa on platelet functions were reported however. Thus Di Minno *et al.* (1983) found that normal platelets incubated with their MoAb (B59.2) had a defect in the release reaction upon stimulation with arachidonic acid (thromboxane synthesis being preserved). Arguing that their results were at variance with the reported behaviour of thrombasthenic platelets, they concluded that the GP IIb-IIIa complex could be involved both in aggregation and secretion. Yamaguchi *et al.* (1987) also reported that a MoAb against GP IIb-IIIa (TM83) could modify the aequorin-detected calcium changes in platelets stimulated with thrombin.
However it should be recalled that platelets with a deficient ability to bind fibrinogen, and to aggregate, whether they are obtained from a trombasthenic patient, or from a normal subject but are incubated with a MoAb impairing the

binding of fibrinogen, or are prevented to aggregate by omitting the stirring, may also have deficient release from storage granules, deficient thromboxane synthesis ..., merely as the result of the sole, above-mentioned, basic defect in platelet aggregation. This is ascribed to the amplifying effect of close platelet-platelet contacts on platelet activation (Holmsen, 1977), which is required to obtain complete activation when intrinsically weak agonists, or low concentrations of strong agonists, are used. As discussed below, this secondary activation signal could be transduced by the GP IIb-IIIa complex, both sub-units being integral components of the plasma membrane. We have also recently demonstrated (Lecompte et al. , 1990) by means of the aequorin probe for calcium that platelets prepared from patients with type I thrombasthenia could normally change their intracellular calcium concentration in response to a high concentration of thrombin, but the second, delayed change in response to ADP was absent. To conclude this part it should be kept in mind that an inhibitory effect of MoAbs to GP IIb-IIIa on another platelet function than aggregation does not imply that GP IIb-IIIa is directly involved in that particular function; on the contrary a more likely explanation is that defective aggregation in the presence of the MoAb under study can slow down activation; in turn this leads to a very indirect impairment of that platelet function.

There is another way to misinterpret the inhibitory effect of some MoAbs to GP IIb-IIIa: they may inhibit by steric hindrance the functioning of a membrane component which is spatially related to, but distinct from, GP IIb-IIIa. Powling & Hardisty (1985) for instance demonstrated that the incubation of normal platelets with a MoAb to GP IIb-IIIa (M148) led to the impairment of intracytoplasmic calcium changes upon stimulation. But since thrombasthenic platelets profoundly deficient in GP IIb-IIIa had a similar pattern of calcium changes as compared to control, non-incubated platelets, they hypothesized that the putative calcium channel of the platelet plasma membrane was not the GP IIb-IIIa complex, but could be closely adjacent to it. As discussed also by Phillips et al. (1988), MoAbs to GP IIb-IIIa were reported to inhibited thrombospondin binding to platelets, but again it was also shown that thrombospondin binds normally to thrombasthenic platelets, and even does not bind to purified GP IIb-IIIa, suggesting that the thrombospondin receptor could be ajacent to GP IIb-IIIa.

Murine IgG have a high molecular mass, which is comparable to that of each sub-unit of the GP IIb-IIIa complex, but it should not be inferred that any inhibitory effect of MoAbs to GP IIb-IIIa is due to non specific steric hindrance, rather than to a specific effect due to the binding to a discrete epitope (a few amino-acids). First, some MoAbs were shown to bind to GP IIb-IIIa but to have no inhibitory effect, such as the Tab antibody (McEver et al. , 1980), and also 3B2 (Varon & Karpatkin, 1983). Thus, if the binding of these MoAbs is not down regulated after platelet activation, one GP IIb-IIIa complex can simultaneously bind one 160 kDa molecule of murine IgG and one 320 kDa molecule of fibrinogen. Second the binding of the same amount of MoAbs with

distinct epitopes on GP IIb-IIIa, as discussed here, may have various functional consequences.
Finally to further add to the complexity, C 15, a MoAb directed at GP IIb-IIIa, was reported to inhibit platelet aggregation, but not fibrinogen binding (Tetteroo et al., 1983). In another work (Newman et al., 1987), two MoAbs which individually did not inhibit ADP-induced fibrinogen binding or aggregation were used: the above-mentioned Tab, and AP3, specific for GP IIb and GP IIIa, respectively. The combination of both MoAbs completely abolished aggregation and release in response to ADP, whereas fibrinogen binding remained apparently unaffected.

The fourth workshop on hematopoietic cell differentiation antigens.
We thought that the fourth workshop on "leucocyte" differentiation antigens provided a good opportunity to see whether the effect on platelet aggregation could be related to the location of the epitopes of the MoAbs of the platelet panel. The effects of these antibodies were blindly investigated after a selection on the basis of their binding to GP IIb-IIIa, by incubating them with human normal platelets washed according to a slightly modified procedure from Mustard et al. (1972). These platelets do not undergo the release reaction when stimulated with ADP: ADP-induced aggregation requires the addition of exogenous fibrinogen. By contrast a strong agonist such as thrombin triggers the release reaction and aggregation is supported by fibrinogen released from the alpha-granules and is inhibitable by the tetrapeptide RGDS, the common recognition site of many of the so-called adhesive proteins (Ruoslahti & Pierschbacher, 1987; Harfenist et al., 1988). In parallel different biochemical tests were performed to localize the epitopes: among them western blotting, and immuno-precipitation of ^{125}I surface labeled platelet lysates as described by Morel et al. (1989).
We identified (Favier et al., 1989) three submitted MoAbs, studied under the respective code numbers, as able to trigger aggregation on their own, including the MoAb PL2-49 we had previously characterized (Morel et al., 1989), and the MoAb (6C9) published by Modderman et al. (1988); there was also in this group an as yet unpublished one, called TP80. In agreement with our results, these three MoAbs were classified among the "aggregators" by Powling et al. during the same workshop (1989). At variance with various claims, we found that platelet aggregation induced with these MoAbs started after a lag phase and a clearly noticeable shape change, as ALB6-induced aggregation does. In other experiments we found that both the release of ATP from the dense granules, and intra-platelet calcium changes detected with the aequorin probe, occured after a similar lag phase.
The inhibitory effect of the other MoAbs of the platelet panel of the workshop were assessed as follows (Favier et al., 1989). Washed platelets were incubated with the MoAb (1:100 dilution) during 3 minutes at 37°C under constant stirring in the cuvette of the aggregometer, and then stimulated with thrombin (0.1 U/mL). The inhibitory effect (Fig. 1) was said to be slight when the maximal increase in light transmission was unaffected, but the slope was

less steep and/or the high frequency oscillations at completion of aggregation had a smaller amplitude: curve B in Fig. 1; maximal when no platelet clumps could be seen at inspection with the naked eye although usually a slight increase in light transmission persisted: curve D (the same holds true when the peptide RGDS or a calcium chelator such as EDTA is added); and finally partial when intermediate results were obtained: curve C.
As shown in Fig. 1,

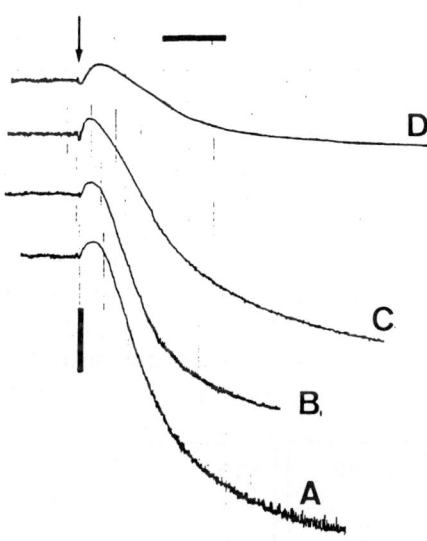

Fig. 1: Typical tracings showing the effects of different MoAbs of the platelet panel of the 4th workshop on leucocyte differentiation antigens against thrombin (0.1 U/mL)-induced aggregation of washed human platelets.
The MoAbs were blindly studied under their code numbers as follows: thrombin was added at the time indicated with the arrow. The horizontal bar indicates 1 minute on the time scale, the vertical one a 10 per cent change in light transmission. The release of ATP was continuously monitored by adding a mixture of luciferin and luciferase (luminescent tracings not shown), and the results mentioned here refer to the maximal release calculated as the concentration of ATP reached in the surrounding milieu (platelet count = 300,000/µL).
A: after a 3-minute incubation with 4 µL of the buffer or the MoAb 5.6E (P 090, anti-GPIIa'); maximal release = 7.2 µM.
B: after incubation with the MoAb MB9 (P 063, anti-GP IIb); maximal release (expressed as the percentage of the value in A - control experiment) = 70 %.
C: with the MoAb PBM 6.4 (P 007, anti-complex); ATP release = 71 %.
D: with the MoAb Y2/51 (P 036, anti-GP IIIa); ATP release = 68 %.

the most potent inhibitors of aggregation are directed against GP IIIa (Favier et al. , 1989b). This is in agreement with the literature, since for instance the C17 MoAb was reported to strongly inhibit aggregation (Tetteroo et al. , 1983). The MoAbs the epitopes of which could be localized to the GP IIb sub-unit had the least effect, and this is again in agreement with the literature, since for instance the Tab antibody, directed at GP IIb as proved by means of crossed immunoelectrophoresis, was shown to have no effect against ADP-induced platelet aggregation and fibrinogen binding (McEver et al. , 1980 & 1983).

Such a work has surely several weaknesses, despite the worldwide collection of several MoAbs from different laboratories. As a matter of fact we were surprised that the complex-specific antibodies were poor inhibitors of aggregation, in disagreement with the literature we have reviewed. There might be a selection bias. The precise concentrations of the MoAbs were not known, neither were their affinities, so that some of them could have been studied under unfavourable conditions. With these limits kept in mind, one can conclude that a fairly coherent pattern emerged from our study (Fig. 2) and (i) the GP IIIa moiety seems to play a crucial role in the binding of fibrinogen; (ii) the epitopes of the platelet-activating MoAbs are not evenly distributed within the GP IIb-IIIa complex, but are rather probably closely related. The MoAb 6C9 seemed to be truly calcium / complex-specific, whereas our MoAb PL2-49, and TP80 as well, were demonstrated to have their

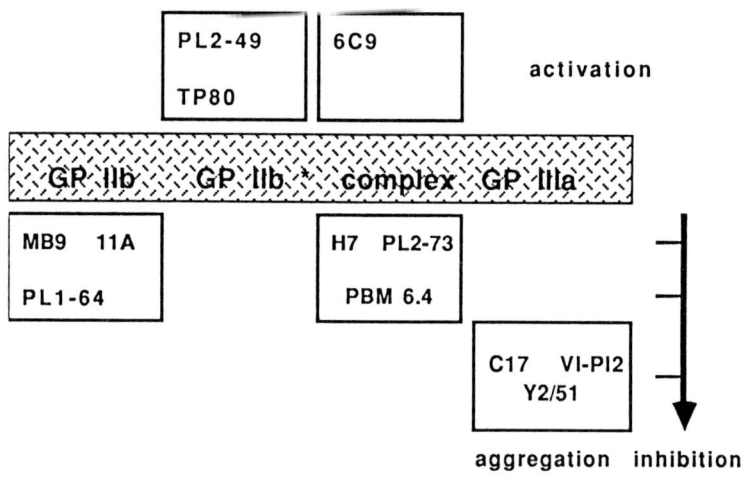

Fig. 2: Classification of the MoAbs of the 4th workshop that we have studied, according to the location of their epitopes, and their functional effect. As described in the text and examplified in Fig. 1, the inhibitory effect (downwards) defined three subgroups of MoAbs with increasing potencies. The horizontal scale defines the whole spectrum of epitopes, and GP IIb* refers to an epitope entirely located on GP IIb, the conformation of which is calcium / complex dependent.

epitopes on GP IIb, but to bind it only when GP IIb is associated to GP IIIa, in the presence of calcium (Favier et al. , 1989b). The same experiment has to be done with the MoAbs P256 and VI-P13. Although this remains a controversial issue, our data are compatible with a model of this integrin where the ß sub-unit, shared with the vitronectin receptor, bears the RGD recognition site, and the alpha sub-unit, which has calcium-binding sites, would control the exposure of the binding sites for the adhesive proteins (Ruoslahti & Pierschbacher, 1987; Plow & Ginsberg, 1989). This model recieved further support from results obtained with one peculiar MoAb called PMI-1. Its epitope was shown to be regulated by divalent cations, in that at millimolar concentrations of calcium or magnesium it was unavailable (Ginsberg et al. , 1986), and was elegantly localized in the heavy chain of GP IIb, near its carboxy terminus, as a continuous stretch of 17 amino-acids (Loftus et al. , 1987).

The era of the clinical use of the MoAbs is now nearly opened. If the greater potency of MoAbs against GP IIIa than that of the other MoAbs against GP IIb or the complex is confirmed, this could have therapeutic implications. However the broader distribution of the vitronectin receptor (comprising the ß3 sub-unit) would also imply broader and perhaps unwarranted clinical effects. On the other hand since the vitronectin receptor is present on the platelet membrane, and since there is an endogenous pool of vitronectin (Asch & Podack, 1990), the potent effects of anti-GP IIIa MoAbs may be explained by the inhibition of both the binding of fibrinogen to GP IIb-IIIa and that of vitronectin to its specific receptor.

PLATELET-ACTIVATING MoAbs

The platelet-activating MoAbs that are directed at low molecular weight proteins (not all of them were proved to belong to CD9), and for which detailed functional studies are available, are listed in the Table 2.

The activation induced with three MoAbs against GP IIb-IIIa has been the subject of detailed reports (Modderman et al. , 1988; Morel et al. , 1989; Favier et al. , 1989a; Bachelot et al. , 1990).

Finally a unique platelet-activating MoAb, called LeoA1 (an IgG1), was recently characterized as binding to a platelet membrane glycoprotein of about 67 kDa, and expressed as 1,200 copies per platelet (Scott et al. , 1989). The antigen, termed PTA1, belongs to a protein which was not identified before, and which is also found on T lymphocytes.

What does an increase in light transmission mean: agglutination, aggregation with or without platelet activation, lysis ?

All the MoAbs so far described trigger both platelet aggregation and activation. When aggregation can be suppressed by metabolic inhibitors (aggregation requires ATP production), and by agents that elevates cytoplasmic cAMP, such iloprost, a chemically stable analogue of prostacyclin,

TABLE 2
Platelet-activating MoAbs directed at low molecular weight proteins.

Name	Isotype	Assigned to CD9 *	First publication
ALB6	G1	yes (3rd)	Boucheix et al., 1983
TP82	G1	yes (4th)	Higashihara et al., 1985
FMC 56	G1	yes (3rd and 4th)	Gorman et al., 1985
AG-1	G1	no	Miller et al., 1986
50H.19	G2	no, but very likely	Seehafer et al., 1988
PMA2	G1	no, but very likely	Hato et al., 1988
SYB-1	G1	CD9 panel (3rd)	Caroll et al., 1990a

(*) Assignment during the 3rd or the 4th workshop on leucocyte differentiation antigens.

aggregation is probably one of the consequences of activation. Whether or not some MoAbs directed at GP IIb-IIIa can induce the exposure of fibrinogen binding sites without activation, by a purely intramolecular change in the complex, will be discussed below. Iloprost blocks all the responses to the MoAb PL2-49 we have studied, suggesting that cAMP acts at an early, common step of activation of these responses. In most instances agglutination and cell lysis were ruled out with the appropiate tools. Agglutination is a passive phenomenon which does not require ATP production, which is not inhibitable by prostaglandins, and which also occurs with fixed platelets (as agglutination induced with von Willebrand factor in the presence of ristocetin). A small agglutination, barely detectable with the aggregometers, can trigger activation and aggregation, but we did not detect such small agglutinates before or during the shape change in response to PL2-49 (Morel et al., 1989). Platelet lysis usually corresponds to typical curves of changes in light transmission and is easily recognized by inspection of the cuvette with the naked eye (Caroll et al., 1990b). It is worth however to check that point also by measuring the LDH release into the supernatant after the incubation with the MoAb, as compared to maximal lysis in the presence of Triton X-100. A recent thorough investigation (Caroll et al., 1990b) regarding this topic was carried out with several CD9 MoAbs using the release of ^{51}Cr from labeled platelets as a sensitive index of lysis.

CD9 MoAbs-induced activation: established facts.

The threshold concentrations of MoAbs able to elicit a platelet response are around 1 µg/mL. There is a general agreement on the following points: (i) dose-dependent lag phase, whereas aggregation is always maximal; (ii) simultaneous release of the content of the different platelet granules (Higashihara *et al.*, 1985b; Rendu *et al.*, 1987); (iii) no requirement of exogenous fibrinogen for aggregation; (iv) partial inhibitory effect only of aspirin or ADP scavengers, at least when high concentrations of MoAbs are used; (v) induction of a calcium mobilization from the internal storage sites. Although Higashihara *et al.* (1985b), using the fluorescent dye quin 2, failed to evidence intracellular calcium changes with the MoAb TP-82, we demonstrated for the first time that ALB6 was able to induce a calcium rise, using aequorin-loaded platelets (Favier *et al.*, 1989). This result was confirmed by our further studies with the fluorescent dye fura 2 (Favier *et al.*, 1990), and by other groups with ALB6 (Caroll *et al.*, 1990) or with PMA2 (Hato *et al.*, 1990). The calcium rise was shown to occur even in the virtual absence of external calcium (Favier *et al.*, 1989; Hato *et al.*, 1990), in keeping with the remaining shape change and release reaction (at the begining not clearly evidenced - for instance see Higashihara *et al.*, 1985a), and the reportedly unaffected phosphorylation of the P20, namely myosin light chain kinase (Rendu *et al.*, 1987).

CD9 MoAbs can be classified among the strong platelet activating molecules such as thrombin, since (i) the blockade of thromboxane synthesis has only a slight effect on the other responses; (ii) the MoAbs induce the release of the content of the lysosomes and an almost complete release from the dense granules; (iii) and thromboxane synthesis and serotonin release still occur under non-stirring conditions (Hato *et al.*, 1988).

There are several indirect lines of evidence collected with various MoAbs indicating that they trigger the phospholipase C- controlled PIP_2 breakdown (Haslam, 1987): calcium mobilization from the internal stores, presumably mediated by inositol-trisphosphate; phosphorylation of P40-47 proteins, substrates for protein kinase C (Higashihara *et al.*, 1985b; Rendu *et al.*, 1987; Favier *et al.*, 1990). Phosphoinositide turnover was directly evidenced by Rendu *et al.* (1987) with ALB6.

All these data make CD9 MoAbs very similar to the prototype strong agonist thrombin, except fot the lag phase. However Rendu *et al.* (1987) had noticed slight differences in the kinetics of the release of the 3 platelet granules, in the presence or in the absence of EDTA, between ALB6 and thrombin.

CD9 MoAbs-induced activation: controversies.

There are also several highly disputed issues that preclude any firm conclusion regarding the mechanisms of platelet activation induced by CD9 MoAbs. First aggregation was claimed by several investigators to be "almost" completely suppressed with the combination of an inhibitor of thromboxane synthesis and a scavenger of ADP, and the same would hold true for calcium changes (Hato *et al.*, 1990). We do not agree with these findings (Favier *et al.*,

1989), and we have recently confirmed our data with another calcium probe (Favier et al., 1990). Aspirin in combination with apyrase was also recently shown by Carroll et al. (1990) to only partially inhibit aggregation and release reaction in response to ALB6. Furthermore a residual activation and even a slight aggregation are shown in the paper of Slupsky et al. (1989), although these authors stated they observed a total inhibition with the combination of aspirin with CP/CPK. The latter ADP scavenger might have non specific effects, as compared to the one that we used, namely apyrase, and further experiments should be carried out with ADP antagonists such as ATP and non hydrolyzable analogues. The GP IIb-IIIa was said to play a role in transduction of the activating signal (Slupsky et al., 1989), since some MoAbs against GP IIb-IIIa were found to actually block any response to CD9 MoAbs (Hato et al., 1988; Favier et al., 1989b). Hato et al. (1988) had also demonstrated that a blocking anti-GP IIb-IIIa MoAb did not inhibit the binding of the MoAb PMA2, which is presumably directed at the CD9 molecule. The MoAb 50H.19 was shown, by a combination of a homobifunctional cross-linking reagent and immunoprecipitation of surface labeled proteins, to induce the association of the CD9 molecule with the GP IIb-IIIa complex (Slupsky et al., 1989). We have also reached a similar conclusion by means of the MAIPA-test (Favier et al., 1989b). Since the association could not be prevented with the combination of aspirin and CP/CPK, Slupsky et al. (1989) concluded that an antibody-imposed conformational change in the CD9 molecule exposed a binding site for GP IIb-IIIa, resulting in intra-platelet signalling. Unfortunately no experiments were carried out with strong platelet inhibiting molecules such as prostacyclin. Moreover it should be pointed out that thrombasthenic platelets profoundly deficient in GP IIb-IIIa were repeatedly found to be activated with CD9 MoAbs (Boucheix et al., 1983; Higashihara et al., 1985a; Hato et al., 1988; our unpublished data). Therefore the association of the CD9 molecule with GP IIb-IIIa is not a prerequisite for CD9 MoAbs-induced platelet activation, but of course the GP IIb-IIIa complex is required for aggregation. Thus the inhibitory effect of anti-GP IIb-IIIa MoAbs might be related to the alteration of the interaction of the CD9 MoAbs with a third partner of the platelet membrane still to be identified.

Intracellular calcium changes monitored with the fluorescent dye fura-2 was claimed to be "amost completely" mediated by the aspirin-sensitive thromboxane pathway (Caroll et al., 1990), but our data are in total disagreement with those results (Favier et al., 1989a and 1990). The discrepancies between the findings of the different groups may be related to the different concentrations of MoAbs which are used; thrombin-induced platelet activation is also well-known to be much more dependent on thromboxane and ADP at low than at high concentration. There may be also due to differences between the MoAbs, to the experimental conditions used to obtain platelets separated from the plasma, and finally to the kind of probe for intracellular calcium.

The functional effects of fragments lacking the Fc domain of CD9 MoAbs are far from clear. Fab fragments of ALB6 were reported to be unable to trigger activation but to inhibit aggregation induced by non immune agonists (Boucheix et al., 1983). Fab fragments prepared from the AG-1 antibody also failed to induce aggregation, and inhibited the response to the intact antibody but not those to non immune agonists (Miller et al., 1986). On the other hand F(ab')2 fragments of TP82 were claimed to induce aggregation (Higashihara et al., 1985a). Platelet activation in response to the CD9 MoAbs ALB6 and SYB-1 was however recently demonstrated (Worthington et al., 1990) to be totally blocked by another MoAb (IV-3) directed at the Fc gamma receptor type II present in the platelet membrane (Rosenfeld et al., 1985), and we have obtained identical results with ALB6 and PL2-49 as well (Favier et al., 1990; Luo et al., manuscript in preparation).

Platelet activation induced with MoAbs directed at GP IIb-IIIa.
Three platelet-activating MoAbs directed at GP IIb-IIIa have been the subject of detailed studies: 6C9 (Modderman et al., 1988); PL2-49 (Morel et al., 1989; Favier et al., 1989a & 1990); P256 (Bachelot C. et al., 1990).
They have common features (see also the Table 1). The number of binding sites for 6C9 and PL2-49 and for fibrinogen are roughly similar, around 40,000 per platelet. Aggregation with intact MoAbs of platelets separated from plasma does not require the addition of fibrinogen. The exposure of fibrinogen binding sites was documented for 6C9 and P256, and aggregation is inhibited by the addition of the RGDS peptide. Thus aggregation in response to these MoAbs appears to depend on the release of endogenous fibrinogen from the alpha granules, as aggregation in response to CD9 MoAbs and to thrombin does. It was indeed also demonstrated that these anti-GP IIb-IIIa MoAbs, when intact, are able to trigger the release reaction, even under non stirring, non aggregating conditions, whereas proteolytic fragments lacking the Fc domain do not. The responses are partially inhibited, and not blocked, by incubating the platelets with aspirin or a scavenger of ADP. We demonstrated that even the combination of both agents cannot abolish the activation to PL2-49. Thus again thromboxane synthesis and ADP release seem to play the role of amplifying feed back loops, but not of the initial signalling.
There are also discrepant results. We showed (Morel et al., 1989) that F(ab')2 fragments bind to the platelets, do not induce any response even in the presence of exogenous fibrinogen, but block the responses to the intact immunoglobulin. Furthermore, the MoAb IV-3 also blocks the responses to PL2-49 (Favier et al., 1990). Thus we concluded (Fig. 3) that the exposure of fibrinogen binding sites is the result of platelet activation (PL2-49 acting as indicated for "MoAb 2" in the Fig. 3), and not of a change directly induced by the MoAb in the state of the GP IIb-IIIa complex. We postulate that PL2-49 has the same activating effects as those of fibrinogen binding, perhaps by inducing the interaction of GP IIb-IIIa with the cytoskeleton (see Ruoslahti & Pierschbacher, 1987; Phillips et al., 1988). As we mentioned above, platelets deficient in GP IIb-IIIa, or normal platelets prevented to aggregate, have an altered pattern of intracellular calcium changes in response to ADP (Lecompte et al., 1990). Thus GP IIb-IIIa may have a role in physiological activation. On

the other hand, F(ab')2 fragments of 6C9 and P256 were reported to induce aggregation, although slow and slight as compared to the responses of the corresponding intact immunoglobulins (Modderman *et al.*, 1988; Bachelot *et al.*, 1990). Thus these MoAbs could behave, at least in part, as indicated for "MoAb 1" in Fig. 3, but it should be recalled that the Fc domain is required for the release reaction to occur. Moreover it is difficult to understand how RGDS-sensitive aggregation can occur in the absence of exogenous fibrinogen and release reaction (which would have provided endogenous fibrinogen), as reported by Bachelot *et al.* (1990).

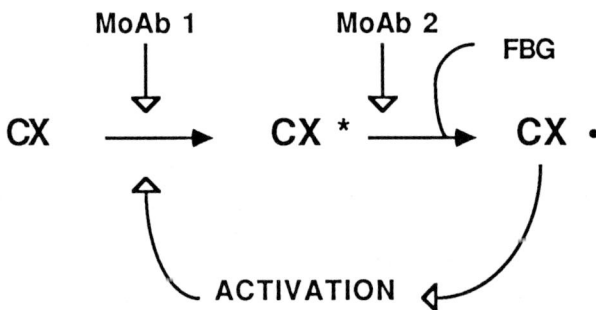

Fig. 3: Mechanisms of the exposure of fibrinogen binding sites in the presence of anti-GP IIb-IIIa MoAbs. The MoAb 1 would induce this exposure by a purely intra-molecular mechanism, mimicking the <u>result</u> of platelet activation induced with physiological agents; activation would be prevented by prostacyclin but aggregation still would occur if fibrinogen were present in the external milieu. The MoAb 2 (such as PL2-49), by contrast, induces the exposure of fibrinogen binding sites by triggering the process of activation, perhaps mimicking one of the effects of fibrinogen binding under physiological circumstances; fibrinogen comes from the alpha granules through the release reaction. In contrast to fibrinogen however, the MoAb PL2-49 binds to the "unactivated" complex.

We have for the first time compared in the same sets of experiments activation in response to a CD9 MoAb (ALB6) and to an anti-GP IIb MoAb (PL2-49). Although in both cases the blocking effect of MoAb IV-3 suggests that the interaction of the Fc domain with the Fc gamma type II receptor is required for activation, we have found differences between the responses to these 2 MoAbs, and this suggest that the Fc receptor might not always, or solely, transduce the activating signal, as suggested by Worthington *et al.* (1990). The main difference between ALB6 and PL2-49, in our hands, is the occurence of a calcium mobilization from the internal strorage sites in response to the former, but not to the latter, as evidenced with aequorin-loaded platelets (Favier et al. , 1989a). Further studies (Favier et al. , 1990) confirmed that there is still an activation in the absence of external calcium, but under these experimental conditions, intracellular calcium changes monitored by means of the fluorescent probe fura-2 are very low, and it remains doubtful that they might account for platelet activation. This is partly in agreement with the recent report of Bachelot et al. (1990), since these authors failed to evidence the breakdown of PIP_2 and the generation of inositol-trisphosphate, the likely second messenger for calcium mobilization. It is difficult however to explain why they observed such a low difference in P256-induced calcium changes, monitored with the indo-1 probe, in the presence or in the absence of EGTA.

In conclusion the mechanisms of platelet activation in response to MoAbs directed at the CD9 molecule and at GP IIb-IIIa remains to be elucidated. Experiments with the different available MoAbs should be repeated under the same, carefully defined, experimental conditions, in order to see whether the differences lie in the experimental conditions or in the epitopes.

The very first steps of the reaction can be depicted as follows: specific binding to the epitope, which allows the binding of the Fc domain with the Fc gamma receptor type II. This receptor has a very low affinity for monomeric immunoglobulins in solution. We think that both bindings at the surface of the same platelet, as also reported for the B lymphocyte (Sinclair & Panoskaltis, 1987), play a role in signal transduction through the membrane. Whether the CD9 molecule has indeed a physiological role in platelet activation is not yet proven, whereas several lines of evidence favour such a role for the GP IIb-IIIa complex. MoAb-induced platelet activation may also be relevant to some clinical settings where immunoglobulins, whether auto-antibodies (Sugiyama et al. , 1987; Pfueller et al. , 1990) or drug-dependent anti-platelet antibodies (Chong et al. , 1989), could trigger activation *in vitro* as well as *in vivo*.

REFERENCES

Asch, E. & Podack, E. (1990): Vitronectin binds to activated human platelets and plays a role in platelet aggregation. *J. Clin. Invest.* 85, 1372-1378

Bachelot, C., Rendu, F., Boucheix, C., Hogg, N. & Levy-Toledano, S. (1990): Activation of platelets induced by mAb P256 specific for glycoprotein IIb-IIIa. Possible evidence for a role for IIb-IIIa in membrane signal transduction. *Eur. J. Biochem.* 190, 177-183

Bai, Y., Durbin, H. & Hogg, N. (1984): Monoclonal antibodies specific for platelet glycoprotein react with human monocytes. *Blood* 64, 139-146

Bennett, J.S., Hoxie, J.A., Leitman, S.F., Vilaire, G. & Cines, D.B. (1983): Inhibition of fibrinogen binding to stimulated platelets by a monoclonal antibody. *Proc. Natl. Acad. Sci. USA.* 80, 2417-2421

Bennett, J.S. (1985): The platelet-fibrinogen interaction. In *Platelet membrane glycoproteins*, ed. J.N. George, A.T. Nurden & D.R. Phillips, pp. 193-214. Plenum New-York.

Boucheix, C., Soria, C., Mirshahi, M., Soria, J., Perrot, J.-Y., Fournier, N., Billard, M. & Rosenfeld, C. (1983): Characteristics of platelet aggregation induced by the monoclonal antibody ALB6 (acute lymphoblastic leukemia antigen p 24). *FEBS Lett.* 161, 289-295

Boucheix, C., Benoit, P., Billard, M., Mishal, Z., Azzarone, B., Rendu, F., Esnouf, J., Hermant, L., Bredoux, R., Levy-Toledano, S., Soria, C., Perrot, J.-Y., Mirshahi, M., Giannoni, F., Bernadou, A. & Soria, J. (1987): Platelet aggregation induced by CD9 mAbs. Mechanisms and comparison with platelet aggregating properties of mAbs directed against other membrane antigens. In *Leucocyte typing III*, ed. A.J. McMichael, pp.780-782. Oxford University Press.

Caroll, R.C., Worthington, R.E. & Boucheix, C. (1990) Stimulus-response coupling in human platelets activated by monoclonal antibodies to the CD9 antigen, a 24 kDa surface-membrane glycoprotein. *Biochem. J.* 266, 527-535

Caroll, R.C., Rubinstein, E., Worthington, R.E. & Boucheix, C. (1990): Extensive C1q-complement initiated lysis of human platelets by IgG subclass murine monoclonal antibodies to the CD9 antigen. *Thromb. Res.* in press

Chong, B.H., Fawaz, I., Chesterman, C.N. & Berndt, M.C. (1989): Heparin-induced trhombocytopenia: mechanism of interaction of the heparin-dependent antibody with platelets. *Br. J. Haematol.* 73, 235-240

Coller, B.S., Peerschke, E.I., Scudder, L.E. & Sullivan, C.A. (1983): A murine monoclonal antibody that completely blocks the binding of fibrinogen to platelets produces a thrombasthenic-like state in normal platelets and binds to glycoproteins IIb and/or IIIa. *J. Clin. Invest.* 72, 325-338

Coller, B.S. (1984): Report of the working party on hybridoma-derived monoclonal antibodies to platelets. *Thromb. Haemostas.* 51, 169-173

Di Minno, G., Thiagarajan, P., Perussia, B., Martinez, J., Shapiro, S., Trinchieri, G. & Murphy, S. (1983): Exposure of platelet fibrinogen binding sites by collagen, arachidonic acid and ADP: inhibition by a monoclonal antibody to the glycoprotein IIb-IIIa complex. *Blood* 61, 140-148

Favier, R., Lecompte, T., Morel, M.-C., Potevin, F., Benoit, P., Boucheix, C., Kaplan, C. & Samama, M. (1989): Calcium rise in human platelets elicited by anti-CD9 and -CD41 murine monoclonal antibodies. *Thromb. Res.* 55, 591-599

Favier, R., Morel, M.-C., Potevin, F., Kaplan, C. & Lecompte, T. (1989): The glycoprotein IIb/IIIa complex contains very distinct epitopes and may be associated with the CD9 molecule within the platelet plasma membrane. In *Leucocyte typing IV* , ed. W. Knapp, pp. 1006-1008. Oxford University Press.

Favier, R., Renesto, P., Baudet, V., Morel, M.-C., Kaplan, C., Toulec, D., Chignard, M. & Lecompte, T. (1990): Mechanisms of platelet activation induced by a CD41 monoclonal antibody (PL2-49): comparison with ALB6 (CD9). *Fibrinolysis* 4 (suppl. 1), 14

Ginsberg, M.H., Lightsey, A.L., Kunicki, T.J., Kaufman, A., Marguerie, G.A. & Plow, E.F. (1986): Divalent cations regulation of the surface orientation of platelet membrane glycoprotein IIb: correlation with fibrinogen binding function and definition of a novel variant of Glanzmann's thrombasthenia. *J. Clin. Invest.* 78, 1103-1111

Gorman, D.J., Castaldi, P.A., Zola, H. & Berndt, M.C. (1985): Preliminary functional characterization of a 24,000 dalton platelet surface protein involved in platelet activation. *Nouv. Rev. Fr. Hématol.* 27, 255-259

Harfenist, E.J., Packham, M.A. & Mustard, J.F. (1988): Effects of the cell adhesion peptide, Arg-Gly-Asp-Ser, on responses of washed platelets from humans, rabbits, and rats. *Blood* 71, 132-136

Haslam, R.J. (1987): Signal transduction in platelet activation. In *Thrombosis and Haemostasis* , ed. M. Verstraete, J. Vermylen, R. Lijnen, J. Arnout, pp. 147-174, Leuven University Press Publishers

Hato, T., Ikeda, K., Yasukawa, M., Watanabe, A. & Kobayashi, Y. (1988): Exposure of platelet fibrinogen receptors by a monoclonal antibody to CD9 antigen. *Blood* 72, 224-229

Hato, T., Sumida, M., Yasukawa, M., Watanabe, A., Okuda, H. & Kobayashi, Y. (1990): Induction of platelet calcium influx and mobilization by a monoclonal antibody to CD9 antigen. *Blood* 75, 1087-1091

Higashihara, M., Maeda, H., Shibata, Y., Kume, S. & Ohashi, T. (1985): A monoclonal anti-human platelet antibody: a new platelet aggregating substance. *Blood* 65, 382-391

Higashihara, M., Maeda, H., Yatomi, Y., Takahata, K., Oka, H. & Kume, S. (1985): The platelet protein phosphorylation induced by a monoclonal antibody against human platelets (TP82). *Biochem. Biophys. Res. Comm.* 133, 306-313

Holmsen, H. (1977): Prostaglandin endoperoxide thromboxane synthesis and dense granule secretion as positive feed back loops in the propagation of platelet responses during the basic platelet reaction. *Thromb. Haemostas.* 38, 1030-1040

Jennings, L.K., Phillips, D.R. & Walker, W.S. (1985): Monoclonal antibodies to human platelet glycoprotein IIbß that initiate distinct platelet responses. *Blood* 65, 1112-1119

Jennings, L.K., Fox, C.F., Kouns, W.C., McKay, C.P., Ballou, L.R. & Schultz, H.E. (1990): The activation of human platelets mediated by anti-human platelet p24/CD9 monoclonal antibodies. *J. Biol. Chem.* 265, 3815-3822

Lecompte, T., Potevin, F., Champeix, P., Morel, M.-C., Favier, R., Hurtaud, M.-F., Schlegel, N., Samama, M.M. & Kaplan, C. (1990): Aequorin-detected calcium changes in stimulated thrombasthenic platelets. Aggregation-dependent calcium movement in response to ADP. *Thromb. Res.* 58, 561-570

Loftus, J.C., Plow, E.F., Frelinger, A.L.III, D'Souza, S.E., Dixon, D., Lacy, J., Sorge, J. & Ginsberg, M.H. (1987): Molecular cloning and chemical synthesis of a region of platelet GP IIb involved in adhesive function. *Proc. Natl. Acad. Sci. USA* 84, 7114-7118

McEver, R.P., Baenziger, N.L. & Majerus, P.W. (1980): Isolation and quantitation of the platelet membrane glycoprotein deficient in thrombasthenia using a monoclonal hybridoma antibody. *J. Clin. Invest.* 66, 1311-1318

McEver, R.P., Bennett, E.M. & Martin, M.N. (1983): Identification of two structurally and functionally distinct sites on human platelet membrane glycoprotein IIb-IIIa using monoclonal antibodies. *J. Biol. Chem.* 258, 5269-5275

Miller, J.L., Kupinski, J.M. & Hustad, K.O. (1986): Characterization of a platelet membrane protein of low molecular weight associated with platelet activation following binding by monoclonal antibody AG-1. *Blood* 68, 743-751

Modderman, P.W., Huisman, H.G., van Mourik, J.A., & van dem Borne, A.E.G.Kr. (1988): A monoclonal antibody to the human platelet glycoprotein IIb/IIIa complex induces platelet activation. *Thromb. Haemostas.* 60, 68-74

Morel, M.-C., Favier, R., Champeix, P., Lecompte, T., Potevin, F., Samama, M. & Kaplan, C. (1988): Characterization of an anti-IIb/IIIa monoclonal antibody which is a platelet activator. In *Current Studies in Hematology and Blood Transfusion*, ed C. Kaplan-Gouet & C. Salmon, vol. 55, pp 53-63. Basel: Karger.

Morel, M.-C., Lecompte, T., Champeix, P., Favier, R., Potevin, F., Salmon, C., Samama, M. & Kaplan, C. (1989): PL2-49, a monoclonal antibody against glycoprotein IIb which is a platelet activator. *Br. J. Haematol.* 71, 57-63

Mustard, J.F., Perry, D.W., Ardlie, N.G. & Packham, M.A. (1972): Preparations of suspensions of washed platelets from humans. *Br. J. Haematol.* 22, 193-204

Newman, P.W., McEver, R.P., Doers, M.P. & Kunicki, T.J. (1987): Synergistic action of two murine monoclonal antibodies that inhibit ADP-induced platelet aggregation without blocking fibrinogen binding. *Blood* 69, 668-676

Pfueller, S.L., David, R., Firkin, B.G., Bilston, R.A., Cortizo, W.F. & Raines, G. (1990): Platelet aggregating IgG antibody to platelet surface glycoproteins associated with thrombosis and thrombocytopenia. *Br. J. Haematol.* 74, 336-341

Phillips, D.R., Charo, I.F., Parise, L.V. & Fitzgerald, L.A. (1988): The platelet membrane glycoprotein IIb-IIIa complex. *Blood* 71, 831-843

Plow, E.F. & Ginsberg M.H. (1989): Cellular adhesion: GPIIb-IIIa as a prototypic adhesion receptor. In *Progress in Hemostasis and Thrombosis*, ed. B.C. Coller, vol. 9, pp 117-156. W.B. Saunders Company.

Powling, M.J. & Hardisty, R.M. (1985): Glycoprotein IIb-IIIa complex and calcium influx into stimulated platelets. *Blood* 66, 731-734

Powling, M.J., Cox, A.D., Goodall, A.H. & Hardisty, R.M. (1989): The functional and phenotypic heterogeneity of CD41, CD61 and CD42 antibodies. In *Leucocyte typing IV*, ed. W. Knapp, pp. 1003-1004. Oxford University Press

Rosenfeld, S.I., Looney, R.J., Leddy, J.P., Phipps, D.C., Abraham, G.N. & Anderson, C.L. (1985): Human platelet Fc receptor for immunoglobulin G. Identification as a 40,000-molecular-weight membrane protein shared by monocytes. *J. Clin. Invest.* 76, 2317-2322

Ruoslahti, E. & Pierschbacher, M.D. (1987): New perspectives in cell adhesion: RGD and integrins. *Science* 238, 491-497

Rendu, F., Boucheix, C., Lebret, M., Bourdeau, N., Benoit, P., Maclouf, J., Soria, C. & Levy-Toledano, S. (1987): Mechanisms of the mAb ALB6 (CD9) induced human platelet aggregation: comparison with thrombin. *Biochem. Biophys. Res. Comm.* 146, 1397-1404

Scott, J.L., Dunn, S.M., Jin, B., Hillam, A.J., Walton, S., Berndt, M.C., Murray, A.W., Krissansen, G.W. & Burns, G.F. (1989): Characterization of a novel membrane glycoprotein involved in platelet activation. *J. Biol. Chem.* 264, 13475-13482

Seehafer, J.G., Slupsky, J.R., Tang, S.-C. & Shaw, A.R.E. (1988): The functional cell surface glycoprotein CD9 is distinguished by being the major fatty acid acylated and a major iodinated cell-surface component of the human platelet. *Biochim. Biophys. Acta* 952, 92-100

Sinclair, N.R.StC. & Panoskaltsis, A. (1987): Immunoregulation by Fc signals. A mechanism for self-non self discrimination. *Immunology Today* 8, 76-79

Slupsky, J.R., Seehafer, J.G., Tang, S.-C., Masellis-Smith, A. & Shaw, A.R.E. (1989): Evidence that monoclonal antibodies against CD9 antigen induce specific association between CD9 and the platelet glycoprotein IIb-IIIa complex. *J. Biol. Chem.* 264, 12289-12293

Steiner, B., Cousot, D., Trzeciak, A., Gillessen, D. & Hadvary, P. (1989): Calcium-dependent binding of a synthetic Arg-Gly-Asp (RGD) peptide to a single site on the purified platelet glycoprotein IIb-IIIa complex. *J. Biol. Chem.* 264, 13102-13108

Sugiyama, T., Okuma, M., Ushikubi, F., Sensaki, S., Kanaji, K. & Uchino, H. (1987): A novel platelet aggregating factor found in a patient with defective collagen-induced platelet aggregation and autoimmune thrombocytopenia. *Blood* 69, 1712-1720

Tetteroo, P.A.T., Lansdorp, P.M., Leeksma, O.C. & von dem Borne, A.E.G.Kr. (1983): Monoclonal antibodies against human glycoprotein IIIa. *Br. J. Haematol.* 55, 509-522

Varon, D. & Karpatkin, S. (1983): A monoclonal anti-platelet antibody with decreased reactivity for autoimmune thrombocytopenic platelets. *Proc. Natl. Acad. Sci. USA* 80, 6992-6995

Worthington, R.E., Carrol, R.C. & Boucheix, C. (1990): Platelet activation by CD9 monoclonal antibodies is mediated by the Fc gamma II receptor. *Br. J. Haematol.* 74, 216-222

Yamaguchi, A., Yamamoto, N., Kitagawa, H., Tanoue, K. & Yamazaki, H. (1987): Calcium influx mediated through the GPIIb/IIIa complex during platelet activation. *FEBS Lett.* 225, 228-232

Résumé

La fixation d'anticorps monoclonaux sur le complexe glycoprotéique IIb-IIIa de la membrane plaquettaire (qui est le récepteur inductible pour le fibrinogène, impliqué dans l'agrégation), a des conséquences fonctionnelles variables, incluant même l'induction de l'agrégation. Dans une certaine mesure elles peuvent être corrélées avec la localisation des épitopes, et suggèrent l'existence de différents domaines fonctionnels. Les mécanismes de l'activation induite par certains anticorps (anti-GP IIb-IIIa ou dirigés contre la molécule CD9) ne sont pas encore bien compris. Cependant il est établi que l'interaction du domaine Fc avec le récepteur Fc gamma de type II, qui succède à la liaison spécifique de l'anticorps avec son épitope, joue un rôle important. Le vecteur de la transduction du message n'est pas déterminé, mais dans le cas des anticorps anti-GP IIb-IIIa, il pourrait s'agir de ce complexe. Il existe d'autres faits expérimentaux qui indiquent que l'intervention du complexe GP IIb-IIIa dans les processus physiologiques de l'activation est vraisemblable.

Regulation of platelet-vessel wall interactions by the fibrinolytic system

A.I. Schafer

Baylor College of Medicine, Medical Service, Veterans Affairs Medical Center, 2002 Holcombe Blvd, Houston, TX 77030 USA

The fibrinolytic protease plasmin has been considered to exert its antithrombotic actions on the digestion of fibrin. Several lines of investigation in recent years have demonstrated that plasmin also has important effects on platelet function and platelet-vessel wall interactions. We and others have shown that plasmin directly activates platelets as an agonist to stimulate phospholipase C-specific hydrolysis of inositol phospholipids, calcium mobilization and protein kinase C activation, leading to platelet secretion and aggregation. Plasmin also inhibits PGI_2 (prostacyclin) synthesis by cultured vascular endothelial cells. The net effect of these activities is to promote platelet thrombus formation. However, at lower concentrations, plasmin is also a potent inhibitor of platelet activation and thromboxane A_2 production, and acts synergistically with PGI_2 to block platelet function. In vivo studies have demonstrated that thrombolytic agents (which generate plasmin in the circulation) can either promote or inhibit platelet-dependent thrombosis, depending on experimental conditions. Further elucidation of the important effects of the fibrinolytic system on platelet-vessel wall interactions will permit more rational and safer application of thrombolytic therapy in patients with vascular occlusive disease.

The formation of a hemostatic plug at a site of vascular injury is now known to occur by reciprocal interactions between platelets and thrombin. Platelets activated by thrombin expose surface receptors that support the rapid conversion of prothrombin to thrombin; thrombin thus generated on platelet surfaces then activates additional platelets, resulting in the rapid formation of a thrombus composed of platelets and fibrin. The fibrinolytic protease plasmin has been generally considered to be targeted simply at the digestion of fibrin, and little was known until recently about its possible interactions with platelets. We have considered that, in a manner analogous to the reciprocal activation of thrombin and platelets to promote clot formation, plasmin and platelets may interact to regulate clot dissolution.

Platelets can support and localize fibrinolysis by facilitating clot retraction (Carroll et al, 1982), binding plasminogen, and potentiating plasminogen activation (Miles & Plow, 1985). Our laboratory has been interested in the actions of plasmin on platelets. Niewiarowski et al (1973) originally showed that streptokinase injection into rabbits causes thrombocytopenia, associated with prolongation of the bleeding time, in vivo platelet degranulation, and inhibition of ex vivo platelet responsiveness to collagen. Greenberg et al (1979) subsequently reported that platelets exposed to plasmin ex vivo have shortened survival when infused into rabbits, and hypothesized that this was due to plasmin-induced changes in platelet membrane glycoproteins.

In vitro studies of plasmin effects on platelet function in our laboratory demonstrated that the protease can directly activate washed human platelets, causing aggregation and release at plasmin concentrations $\geq$ 1.0 caseinolytic units (CU)/ml (Schafer et al, 1986). The biochemical mechanism of plasmin-induced platelet activation was further investigated. We found that plasmin stimulates a dose- and time-dependent phosphorylation of the platelet 47,000-kD protein that has been identified as the substrate for protein kinase C (PKC). In addition, plasmin also induces phosphorylation of the platelet 20,000-kD protein, suggesting calmodulin-dependent activation of myosin light chain kinase. PKC activation in platelets generally indicates that diacylglycerol has been formed by phospholipase C (PLC)-dependent breakdown of inositol phospholipids. We confirmed this by demonstrating that plasmin stimulates diacylglycerol (and phosphatidic acid) production in platelets in a dose- and time-dependent manner that parallels PKC activation. Myosin light chain kinase is activated by an increase in cytosolic calcium concentration, and we confirmed that plasmin raises cytosolic calcium in either quin2 or aequorin-loaded platelets. Despite this evidence of plasmin stimulation of platelet PLC-specific inositol phospholipid turnover, we were unable to show significant plasmin-induced synthesis of thromboxane A_2 (TXA_2). Only small amounts of this eicosanoid were detected late in the time course after plasmin stimulation. The conclusion of this series of studies was that plasmin causes platelet aggregation and secretion associated with calcium mobilization, PLC and PKC activation, but these events are dissociated from TXA_2 formation for unclear reasons.

It has been recently shown that platelets isolated from the blood of experimental animals (Ohlstein et al, 1987) or human subjects (Fitzgerald et al, 1988) receiving thrombolytic agents may be hyperreactive to certain stimuli. Furthermore, Fitzgerald et al (1988) have reported that the administration of intravenous streptokinase to patients with acute myocardial infarction is associated with a marked increase in the urinary excretion of 2,3-dinor-thromboxane B_2 and plasma levels of 11-dehydro-thromboxane B_2, the major in vivo enzymatic metabolites of TXA_2. Similar findings were subsequently reported in patients receiving tissue plasminogen activator (tPA) (Kerins et al, 1989). Since platelets are the major source of TXA_2, these findings were considered to reflect in vivo platelet activation after coronary thrombolysis with streptokinase or tPA. It was suggested that possible mechanisms might include the release of active thrombin from the lysed clot (Francis et al, 1983; Fitzgerald & Fitzgerald, 1989) or, as we had previously found, the activation of platelets by the local formation of high concentrations of plasmin during thrombolytic therapy.

We considered that another possible explanation for the finding of apparent in vivo platelet hyperreactivity associated with the administration of thrombolytic agents may be plasmin-mediated impairment of the thromboresistant properties of vascular endothelium. As is the case with platelet, endothelial cells have specific binding sites for plasminogen (Hajjar et al, 1986) and tPA (Hajjar et al, 1987), thus providing a surface for the assembly of proteins of the fibrinolytic system on which enhanced plasmin generation can proceed. We have therefore examined the effects of plasmin on PGI_2 (prostacyclin) synthesis by cultured endothelial cells (Schafer et al, 1989).

Plasmin was found to cause little or no direct stimulation of PGI_2 formation by cultured human umbilical vein (HUVEC) or bovine aortic (BAEC) endothelial cells. However, preincubation of endothelial cells with plasmin produces time- and concentration-dependent inhibition of ionophore A23187-, thrombin-, and histamine-induced PGI_2 synthesis. A smaller inhibitory effect of plasmin is found on arachidonate- and endoperoxide (PGH2)-induced PGI_2 synthesis, suggesting that the major inhibitory action of plasmin on PGI_2 production is directed at the phospholipase-mediated release of endogenous arachidonic acid. Incubation of HUVEC or BAEC with tPA and a physiologic concentration of plasminogen generates tPA dose-dependent plasmin activity that exceeds that generated in the absence of endothelial cells, confirming the original observations of Hajjar et al (1986, 1987). In the presence of a constant physiologic concentration of plasminogen, tPA also causes a tPA dose-dependent inhibition of thrombin- and ionophore A23187-stimulated PGI_2 production. The PGI_2 inhibitory plasmin activity is generated within the concentration range of tPA achieved in plasma during pharmacologic therapy with tPA. These findings suggested that vascular endothelial cells not only regulate activation of the fibrinolytic system but may also be targets of plasmin action. Inhibition of PGI_2 production by plasmin may cause loss of the thromboresistant properties of endothelium, thereby potentially contributing to the previously observed in vivo activation of platelets under certain conditions of thrombolytic therapy.

While all of the lines of evidence described above suggested that plasmin (and thrombolytic agents that generate plasmin) interacts with platelets as an activating stimulus, we and others have also observed an inhibitory effect of plasmin on platelet function under certain conditions. Adelman et al (1984) reported that plasmin treatment of platelets in vitro leads to a loss of platelet membrane glycoprotein Ib, a surface receptor for von Willebrand factor, with an associated inhibition of ristocetin-induced platelet agglutination. This would be theoretically expected to cause a platelet adhesion defect in vivo, although such an abnormality has yet to be demonstrated experimentally. Subsequently it was found that plasmin may also hydrolyze the platelet membrane glycoprotein IIb/IIIa complex (Stricker et al, 1986).

We have reported (Schafer & Adelman, 1985) that preincubation of washed human platelets with low concentrations of plasmin (<1 CU/ml) that are insufficient to directly activate the cells, causes a dose- and time-dependent inhibition of platelet aggregation in response to thrombin, ionophore A23187, and collagen. Complete loss of aggregation is found with 0.1 to 0.5 CU/ml of plasmin. In a parallel dose-dependent manner, plasmin likewise blocks platelet TXA_2 synthesis in response to the same stimuli. In contrast, neither aggregation nor TXA_2 formation induced by exogenous arachidonate is inhibited by plasmin pretreatment of the platelets. In the same series of studies, we found that plasmin blocks thrombin-induced release of endogenous arachidonic acid from platelet membrane phospholipids. Simultaneous measurements of intracellular cyclic AMP demonstrated that the inhibition of arachidonic acid release by plasmin is not mediated by an increase in platelet cyclic AMP. These results suggested that plasmin inhibits platelet function, at least in part, by blocking the phospholipase-mediated mobilization of arachidonic acid from membrane phospholipid pools. Loscalzo & Vaughan (1987) subsequently reported that tPA can actually promote the disaggregation of platelets in plasma. They postulated that this is due to kinetically selective proteolysis of platelet-cohesive fibrinogen by plasmin.

Since the inhibitory effects of plasmin on platelet function are not mediated by cyclic AMP, we next investigated possible interactions between plasmin and cyclic AMP on platelet activation (Schafer et al, 1987). We found that PGI_2, the potent endothelium-derived activator of platelet adenyl cyclase, and plasmin cause synergistic inhibition of thrombin- and ADP-induced aggregation of washed platelets. Inhibition by PGI2 is similarly potentiated by tPA added to platelets in plasma (to generate plasmin). Thrombin-stimulated increases in platelet cytosolic calcium (measured in these studies by fura2 fluorescence) and TXA_2 formation are likewise synergistically blocked by PGI2 and plasmin. Under the same conditions, plasmin neither increases nor potentiates PGI2-stimulated increases in platelet cyclic AMP. Thus, PGI2 and plasmin cause synergistic inhibition of platelet activation by both cyclic AMP-depended and independent mechanisms. We have proposed that this synergistic interaction between two different endothelium-derived products may play an important role in localizing the hemostatic plug to a site of vascular injury by preventing further thrombin-mediated accrual of platelets.

To test this synergistic interaction in thrombolysis in vivo, we measured rates of thrombolysis induced by tPA in the presence and absence of coinfusion with PGE_1, in a rabbit jugular vein model of thrombosis (Vaughan et al, 1989). PGE_1 acts like PGI2 as a potent inhibitor of platelet aggregation by stimulating platelet adenyl cyclase following occupancy of the same platelet receptors (Schafer et al, 1979). Rates of lysis were quantified by measuring the half-time for lysis of the thrombus. At all concentrations of tPA used, we found that PGE_1 markedly reduces the half-time for clot lysis and enhances the overall extent of thrombolysis, without significantly affecting either the degree of fibrinogen depletion or the animals' mean arterial pressures. Platelet function studies performed ex vivo demonstrated that treatment with the combination of tPA and PGE_1 attenuates the maximal platelet aggregation rate when compared with that seen in animals receiving tPA alone.

It can be concluded from the several lines of investigation summarized above that plasmin exerts significant effects on platelet function, in addition to its previously known action in lysing fibrin. However, both platelet activation and platelet inhibition have been observed when plasmin-platelet interactions are examined in vitro under various conditions. Furthermore, the effects of plasmin (or thrombolytic agents that generate plasmin) in vivo have not been clearly demonstrated. Rudd et al (1988) have begun to address these issues by studying the temporal effects of tPA infusion on platelet aggregation ex vivo. They infused tPA intravenously in rabbits for 3 hours and concomitantly measured both net plasmin activity generated in the plasma of animals treated with tPA and ex vivo aggregability of platelets induced by ADP. They found that within the first 30 minutes following initiation of tPA infusion, plasmin activity in plasma reached 1.6 CU/ml, a concentration we had previously shown to stimulate platelet activation in vitro. Consistent with our in vitro studies (Schafer et al, 1986), they noted hyperreactivity of platelets in response to ADP at this point. However, 3 hours after initiation of tPA infusion, plasmin activity in plasma had declined to 0.5 CU/ml. Again, consistent with our previous in vitro observations that preincubation of platelets with <1 CU/ml plasmin causes inhibition of platelet activation (Schafer et al, 1985), they observed that concomitant ex vivo platelet responsiveness to ADP was significantly diminished. These data suggest that the effects of tPA on platelet function in vivo are complex and depend on the time and concentration of exposure to plasmin generated.

To further investigate the actions of plasmin formed in vivo on platelet function, we have tested the effects of the thrombolytic agent streptokinase on platelet dependent vasocclusion in a well established canine model of experimental coronary artery stenosis (Folts et al, submitted for publication). This animal model involves the placement of an external plastic cylinder around the outside of an exposed coronary artery, which produces subtotal occlusion of the vessel and intimal damage at the site of occlusion (Folts et al, 1976). Occlusive thrombi consisting purely of platelets develop in the stenosed lumen periodically and then embolize distally. The periodic development of these platelet thrombi causes cyclic reductions in the blood flow within the vessel being studied. These cyclical flow reductions (CFR's) in coronary arterial blood flow are therefore indications of an in vivo platelet-dependent vascular occlusive process. To test the hypothesis that plasmin effects in vivo platelet thrombus formation, we studied the effects of intravenous infusion of streptokinase on the formation of acute platelet thrombi in dogs with stenosed coronary arteries.

Infusion of the thrombolytic agent into 22 dogs at doses sufficient to cause a systemic lytic state leads to complete abolition of CFR's at sites of coronary artery injury in all cases. This inhibition of coronary platelet occlusion is associated with marked prolongations of the bleeding time (from 3.2 ± 0.6 min before to 14 ± 5 min after streptokinase infusion, mean $\pm$ SD, n = 22). Despite the striking effects of streptokinase on in vivo platelet-vessel wall interactions, only platelet aggregation is response to collagen was diminished among the ex vivo parameters of platelet function that were studied simultaneously. TXA_2 production, monoclonal antibody binding to platelet membrane glycoprotein IIb/IIIa, glycoprotein Ib-dependent botrocetin-induced platelet aggregation, and platelet levels of cyclic AMP are not significantly altered. We have concluded that thrombolysis appears to cause important inhibitory effects on in vivo platelet reactivity with injured vascular intimal surfaces, possibly due to localized changes in platelet aggregate formation in the microenvironment of exposed sub-endothelium. These findings have suggested that plasmin generated by thrombolytic agents exhibits platelet inhibitory activity, and that this effect may be important in re-establishing blood flow in certain forms of platelet-mediated arterial thromboses. Studies are underway to attempt to reproduce these findings with thrombolytic agents other than streptokinase.

The various lines of investigation described in this report have shed new light on the role of the fibrinolytic system in hemostasis and thrombosis. Whereas the fibrinolytic protease plasmin was previously considered to exert its antithrombotic actions entirely on the digestion of fibrin, we now recognize that is also has important effects on platelet activation and platelet-vessel wall interactions. The clinical implications of these findings are that alterations in platelet function may play a critical role in the beneficial effects of thrombolytic agents on coronary artery thrombosis, a predominantly platelet-mediated occlusive event. At the same time, however, the effects of plasmin and thrombolytic agents on platelet function are also likely to be involved in the bleeding complications and reocclusive problems that may accompany this form of treatment. Elucidation of the precise mechanisms of this "double-edged sword" involved in the actions of the fibrinolytic system on platelet-vessel wall interactions will permit the application of more rational and safer uses of antithrombotic therapy.

REFERENCES

Adelman, B., et al (1984): Plasmin effect on platelet glycoprotein Ib-von Willebrand's factor interaction. Blood 65, 32-40.

Carroll, R.C., et al (1982): Plasminogen, plasminogen activator, and platelets in the regulation of clot lysis. J. Lab. Clin. Invest. 100, 986-996.

Fitzgerald, D.J., et al (1988): Marked platelet activation in vivo after intravenous streptokinase in patients with acute myocardial infarction. Circulation 77, 142-150.

Fitzgerald, D.J. & Fitzgerald, G.A. (1989): Role of thrombin and thromboxane A_2 in reocclusion following coronary thrombolysis with tissue-type plasminogen activator. Proc. Natl. Acad. Sci. USA. 86, 7585-7589.

Folts, J.D., et al (1976): Platelet aggregation in partially obstructed vessels and their elimination with aspirin. Circulation. 54, 365-370.

Folts, J.D., et al (submitted for publication): Strepto-kinase inhibits acute platelet thrombus formation in stenosed dog coronary arteries.

Francis, C.W., et al (1983): Thrombin activity of fibrin thrombi and soluble plasmic derivatives. J. Lab. Clin. Med. 1102,220-230.

Greenberg, J.P., et al (1979): Survival of rabbit platelets treated in vitro with chymotrypsin, plasmin, trypsin, or neuraminidase. Blood 53, 916-927.

Hajjar, K.A., et al (1986): Binding of plasminogen to cultured human endothelial cells. J. Biol. Chem. 261, 11656-11662.

Hajjar, K.A., et al (1987): Binding of tissue plasminogen activator to cultured human endothelial cells. J. Clin. Invest. 80, 1712-1719.

Kerins, D.M., et al (1989): Platelet and vascular function during coronary thrombolysis with tissue-type plasminogen activator. Circulation. 80, 1718-1725.

Loscalzo, J. & Vaughan, D.E. (1987): Tissue plasminogen activator promotes platelet disaggregation in plasma. J. Clin. Invest. 79, 1749-1755.

Miles, L.A. & Plow, E.F. (1985): Binding and activation of plasminogen on the platelet surface. J. Biol. Chem. 260, 4303-4311.

Niewiarowski, S.A., et al (1973): Plasmin-induced platelet aggregation and platelet release reaction. J.Clin. Invest. 52, 1647-1659.

Ohlstein, E.H., et al (1987): Tissue-type plasminogen activator and streptokinase induce platelet hyperaggregability in the rabbit. Thromb. Res. 46, 575-585.

Rudd, M.A., et al (1988): Temporal effects of tissue plasminogen activator infusion on platelet aggregation ex vivo. Blood. 72(suppl), 374a.

Schafer, A.I., et al (1979): Identificaiton of platelet receptors for prostaglandin I_2 and D_2. J. Biol. Chem. 254, 2914-2917.

Schafer, A.I. & Adelman, B. (1985): Plasmin inhibition of platelet function and of arachidonic acid metabolism. J. Clin. Invest. 75, 456-461.

Schafer, A.I., et al (1986): Platelet protein phosphorylation, elevation of cytosolic calcium, and inositol phospholipid breakdown in platelet activation induced by plasmin. J. Clin. Invest. 78, 73-79.

Schafer, A.I., et al (1987): Synergistic inhibition of platelet activation by plasmin and prostaglandin I$_2$. Blood. 69, 1504-1507.
Schafer, A.I., et al (1989): Inhibition of vascular endothelial cell prostacyclin synthesis by plasmin. Blood. 74, 1015-1020.
Stricker, R.B., et al (1986): Activation of plasminogen by tissue plasminogen activator on normal and thrombasthenic platelets: Effects on surface proteins and platelet aggregation. Blood. 68, 275-280.
Vaughan, D.E., et al (1989): PGE$_1$ accelerates thrombolysis by tissue plasminogen activator. Blood. 73, 1213-1217.

Résumé

L'action antithrombotique de la plasmine est liée à son action fibrinolytique. Des investigations menées sur plusieurs années ont démontré que la plasmine a un effet majeur sur les fonctions plaquettaires ainsi que sur l'interaction plaquette-paroi des vaisseaux. Ainsi que d'autres équipes, nous avons montré que la plasmine agissait directement comme un agoniste pour stimuler l'hydrolyse spécifique des phosphatidyl inositol par la phospholipase C, la mobilisation du calcium et l'activation de la protéine kinase C qui mène à la sécrétion et l'agregation des plaquettes. La plasmine inhibe aussi la synthèse de la prostacycline (PGI$_2$) par les cellules endothéliales en culture. La finalité de l'activité de la plasmine est de promouvoir la formation des thrombus plaquettaires. Cependant, à de faible concentration, la plasmine est aussi un puissant inhibiteur de l'activation plaquettaire et de la production du thromboxane A$_2$ et agit en synergie avec la PGI-2 pour bloquer les fonctions plaquettaires. Des études in vivo ont montré que des agents thrombolytiques (qui génèrent de la plasmine en circulation) peuvent promouvoir ou inhiber des thromboses plaquette-dépendantes, selon les conditions expérimentales utilisées. Des études plus poussées de l'effet du système fibrinolytique sur l'interaction-plaquettes-parois vasculaires devront permettre une application plus rationnelle et plus sûre des thérapeutiques thrombolytiques chez des malades souffrant de maladies occlusives des vaisseaux.

Inherited thrombopathies

Thrombopathies héréditaires

Glanzmann's thrombasthenia : a general introduction with comments on specific cases

A.T. Nurden, M. Pico*, D. Fournier**, V. Jallu, D. Lacaze and P. Hourdillé

Section pathologie cellulaire de l'hémostase, Hôpital Cardiologique, Avenue Magellan, 33604 Pessac, France
*Hospial Vall d'Hebron, Barcelona, Spain
**INSERM U 150, Hôpital Lariboisière, 6, rue Guy Patin, 75475 Paris cedex 10, France

ABSTRACT

Glanzmann's thrombasthenia (GT) is an inherited bleeding disorder resulting from an absent platelet aggregation induced by physiologic agonists. In most cases, clot retraction is also defective. The molecular lesion is an absence or severe to moderate deficiency of GP IIb-IIIa complexes, the platelet receptor for fibrinogen and the other adhesive proteins which mediate platelet aggregation. Recently, patients with qualitative defects of GP IIb-IIIa have also been described. In this chapter, we will detail the functional and molecular defects which characterize this disorder. Our text will be illustrated by reference to individual patients who have been personally studied by us. In particular, we will review the studies on patients who have formed isoantibodies in response to the transfusion of blood or platelet concentrates from normal donors. We will also describe some preliminary experiments on megakaryocytes isolated from GT patients.

BACKGROUND INFORMATION

Glanzmann's thrombasthenia (GT) was first described in 1918 by Glanzmann who noted the failure of platelets to clump on a blood smear or retract a clot. The platelet function defect is now well characterized. GT patients have a long bleeding time arising from an inability of their platelets to aggregate in response to ADP and all physiologic agonists. Clot retraction is also nearly always defective but the extent of this particular lesion varies between patients. GT is an autosomal recessive inherited disease. Bleeding occurs because in the absence of thrombus formation the haemostatic plug cannot form. It is a rare disorder and its occurrence is most common within ethnic groups where consanguinity is a feature. Bleeding is usually noted from birth and is often most severe during childhood. It primarily occurs from small blood vessels in mucocutaneous tissues. Purpura, epistaxis, gingival bleeding, and menorrhagia are the most prominent symptoms. The clinical aspects of GT were reviewed in detail by Bellucci et al (1983) and more recently by George et al (1990).

It is now well established that the primary molecular lesion in GT is an absence, severe deficiency, or qualitative defect of GP IIb-IIIa complexes (see Nurden, 1990). Much is now known about the structure of this complex. GP IIb is composed of two subunits: GP IIbα (Mr=132,000) and IIbβ (Mr=23,000) while GP IIIa is a single chain polypeptide (Mr=99,000) characterized by the presence of many intramolecular disulphides (see Phillips et al., 1988). GP IIb and GP IIIa are coded for by different genes and, interestingly, both localize to the 17q21-23 region of chromosome 17 (Sosnoski et al., 1988). GP IIb-IIIa complexes are an inducible receptor and on <u>activated</u> platelets bind the adhesive protein cofactors which mediate the platelet aggregation response. Normal circulating platelets express about 50,000 copies of this complex and an internal pool of about the same size is externalized after platelet activation by agonists which induce secretion (Woods et al., 1986). Structural studies have shown that GP IIb-IIIa complexes belong to the integrin family of cell surface receptors where, with the vitronectin receptor (VnR), they constitute the subclass termed "cytoadhesins". Each integrin is composed of two subunits coded for by different genes. These are termed the α- and β-subunits and for each subclass the β-subunit is constant while the α-subunit varies in structure and gives the functional specificity of the complex in question. In the cytoadhesins, GP IIIa is the β-subunit. GP IIb-IIIa complexes are exclusive to cells of the megakaryocytic lineage. In contrast, VnR has been located in many tissues including endothelial cells, chondrocytes, smooth muscle cells and fibroblasts. Platelets also express the VnR but in small amounts as compared to GP IIb-IIIa complexes (estimated as ~1,500 complexes by Lawler and Hynes, 1989). Further information on the structure and function of GP IIb-IIIa complexes and of their relationship to other integrins is to be found in the reviews of Phillips et al. (1988) and Newman (1989).

Early studies on Glanzmann's thrombasthenia including those which led to the discovery and characterization of the GP IIb-IIIa lesion have been reviewed in detail elsewhere (see Nurden, 1990). The object of this manuscript is to discuss the clinical implications of a deficiency of GP IIb-IIIa complexes in the light of our present knowledge. The personal experience of one of us (ATN) relates back to 1973, when the initial discovery of the glycoprotein lesion in GT platelets was made (Nurden and Caen, 1974). In the period up to 1988, platelets of a large number of GT patients were examined at the Unité 150 INSERM, Hôpital Lariboisière, Paris (Dir: Prof. JP Caen) and glycoprotein analyses performed. Recently, George et al (1990) have reviewed data on 113 published GT cases and supplemented this with details of 64 patients studied at the hôpital Lariboisière. Table I summarizes some of the molecular and platelet function data presented on these 64 patients.

Table I. Glanzmann's thrombasthenia: Review of 64 patients

Sub-group	GP IIb-IIIa content	Platelet fibrinogen	Platelet aggregation	Clot retraction
Type I (75 % of patients)	< 5 % (GP IIIa < 10 %)	strongly reduced	absent	minimal
Type II (16 % of patients)	5 - 25 %	variable (30 - 70 %)	absent	normal or moderately reduced
Variants				
C.M. M.S.	100 %, 60 % (unstable to EDTA)	absent	absent	minimal
R.P.	40 %	normal	absent	normal
C.G.	60 %	strongly reduced	absent	minimal
A.P.	40% / 18 % total / surface	50 %	variable	normal

PLATELET FUNCTION DEFECTS

As stated above, a common characteristic of GT is a defective platelet aggregation in response to ADP and other physiologic agonists. This is sometimes stated as being a defective "macroscopic" platelet aggregation for the aggregation response may not always be nil. The formation by some (but not all) patients of small clusters of platelets in response to collagen or thrombin was first noted by Caen et al (1966) and recently detailed for a single patient by McGregor et al (1989). One possibility is that such interactions are mediated by residual GP IIb-IIIa complexes for a total absence of GP IIb and GP IIIa in thrombasthenic platelets is rare (see below). Surface-bound thrombospondin, adhesive proteins bound to other membrane receptors, or the newly described PECAM-1 glycoprotein (see Newman et al., 1989), are possible alternative mediators of such interactions. Nonetheless, the physiologic relevance of the GP IIb-IIIa deficiency is shown by the fact that thrombus formation on subendothelium is greatly reduced (see Weiss et al., 1986). Other receptor-mediated interactions such as platelet shape change and secretion occur normally, although a decreased thromboxane synthesis has been reported. Platelet attachment to subendothelium occurs readily, and this is in line with the normal expression by GT platelets of GP Ib, GP Ia-IIa and GP Ic-IIa, adhesion receptors for von Willebrand factor, collagen and fibronectin respectively. However, although the attached GT platelets become activated, and secrete their granule contents, there is a reduced spreading of the platelets on the subendothelium (Weiss et al., 1986), an abnormality that is accentuated at high shear rates (Sakariassen et al. 1986). This suggests an additional role for GP IIb-IIIa complexes in the platelet-vessel wall interaction. A more complete review of the platelet function defects in GT is given by Nurden (1987, 1989).

HETEROGENEITY IN GLANZMANN'S THROMBASTHENIA

Caen (1972) was the first to highlight heterogeneity in GT when he defined two subgroups of patients. The type I subgroup represents those patients with absent platelet aggregation and minimal clot retraction, while in the type II subgroup a reduced to normal clot retraction was observed despite the continued defective platelet aggregation. Another difference was that platelet fibrinogen was found to be severely decreased or lacking from the platelets of the type I patients whereas it was present in the platelets of the type II patients. Evaluation of the 64 patients described above was first made in terms of the the type I and type II nomenclature.

Type I subgroup: Table I shows that the majority of patients fitted into the type I category and substantiates previous claims that type I patients are those with minimal amounts of residual GP IIb-IIIa complexes (see Nurden, 1987). Western blot analysis showed that residual GP IIIa could be detected in the platelets of most type I patients, and amounts of up to 10 % of normal platelet levels were occasionally revealed (illustrated by Nurden et al., 1985; and in Figs. 2 and 3). GP IIb was sometimes also present, but at levels which were lower than would be expected if the normal 1:1 ratio of GP IIb to GP IIIa was maintained. One explanation for the presence of residual GP IIIa is that it is complexed to the VnR α-subunit. The amounts of VnR in platelets or other cells of our patients have yet to be determined. Previous reports have signalled an altered fibroblast (Donati et al., 1977) or monocyte function in GT (Altieri et al., 1986) suggesting that the VnR can be modified in some patients. That this is not a general phenomenon was shown by Giltay et al (1987, 1989), who detected the normal presence of GP IIIa in endothelial cells, smooth muscle cells and fibroblasts cultured from the umbilical cord of a child belonging to the type I subgroup. The normal presence of LFA-1, Mac-1 and p150/95 in leukocytes from two type I patients has also been described (see Nurden, 1989).

Type II subgroup: Table II confirms that the rarer type II patients possessed platelets with readily detectable amounts of GP IIb-IIIa complexes which, in our experience, reached a maximum of 25 % of normal platelet levels. It should be emphasized that the dividing line between the two subgroups, the possession of more or less than 5 % of the normal platelet content of GP IIb-IIIa, has been arbitrarily chosen. The GT phenotype is given by a spectrum of genetic defects that range from a complete lack of GP IIb-IIIa to the presence of a reduced content of these complexes. The term "type II subgroup" is simply a way of describing a group of the latter patients. All of the type II patients possessed at least a limited α-granule pool of fibrinogen. Flow cytometry has established that the residual complexes of such patients are evenly distributed throughout the total platelet population and this is illustrated for patient (A.D.) in Fig. 1. Similar findings have been reported for other type II patients by Johnston et al. (1984) and by Jennings et al. (1986). Recent evidence points to the fact that fibrinogen is taken up from their environment by megakaryocytes and platelets and translocated to the α-granules (see Harrison et al., 1989). The results from the survey shown in Table I suggest that there is a correlation between the presence of residual GP IIb-IIIa in the platelet membrane and the presence of fibrinogen in the α-granules of the type II patients. This might be taken as evidence that GP IIb-IIIa complexes mediate the uptake. However, some caution has to be taken in this interpretation, for the amount of fibrinogen present in the granules (30 % - 70 % of normal) exceeds the amount of residual GP IIb-IIIa that is present (5 % - 25 % of normal).

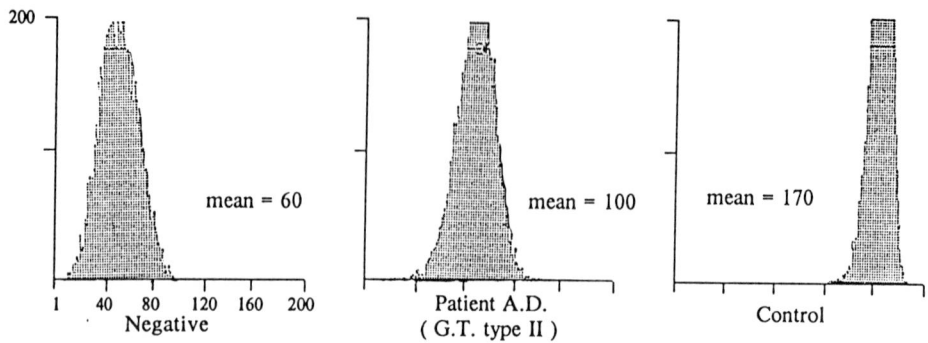

Fig. 1. Analysis of monoclonal antibody binding to normal platelets and those isolated from a patient with type II thrombasthenia using flow cytometry. Washed, formaldehyde-fixed, normal human platelets (control) and those isolated from the patient (A.D.) were incubated with AP-2, a monoclonal antibody to GP IIb-IIIa complexes (see Nurden et al., 1987), followed by fluorescein (FITC)-labelled goat antibody to mouse IgG. A maximum of 10,000 cells were analyzed using a Spectrum III flow cytometer (Ortho, USA). The negative represents control platelets analyzed in the absence of primary antibody. Fluorescence was expressed using a logarithmic scale. Note the decreased binding of AP-2 to (A.D.) platelets and the symmetrical nature of the histogram showing that the total population of platelets was affected. The mean channel fluorescence is given. x axis = FITC fluorescence, y axis = number of cells.

ISOANTIBODY FORMATION

One consequence of a GP IIb-IIIa deficiency is the risk of antibody formation following transfusion, when the patient is exposed to platelets carrying a normal complement of GP IIb-IIIa complexes.

Patient (L.) is a 62 year old man who belongs to the type I subgroup. Western blotting showed that his platelets contain readily detectable amounts of GP IIIa but no GP IIb (Fig.2). Diagnosis of GT occurred relatively late in life, when he was 27 years old, and this is a rare occurrence for bleeding is most often first observed early in life. Patient (L.) received transfusions of whole blood in 1966 and 1973 for bleeding episodes connected with the presence of a duodenal ulcer. The second transfusion was followed by the formation of an isoantibody that has been much studied, and which was termed the IgG L (see Nurden, 1987). In brief, the antibody binds to the surface of normal platelets and, in so doing, blocks platelet aggregation. Figure 2 shows that in Western blotting the antibody recognizes GP IIb, the glycoprotein lacking from the patient's own platelets. Previous studies performed using crossed immunoelectrophoresis (CIE) had shown that the antibody binds to GP IIb-IIIa complexes (see Rosa et al., 1984). The results shown here suggest that this is due to the presence of anti-GP IIb specificity, although the additional presence of antibodies to complex-dependent determinants cannot be ruled out.

Patient (A.F.) also belongs to the type I subgroup. Western blotting showed that her platelets contained but trace amounts of GP IIb and GP IIIa. She is a 27 year old Spanish woman whose first child was born with a severe thrombocytopenia. Figure 2 shows that her serum contains a strong anti-GP IIIa antibody. The antibody somewhat surprisingly reacted with trace amounts of residual GP IIIa in her own platelets. This result suggests that the antibody is not directed against an alloantigen absent from the mother's own platelets, as is the case in neonatal alloimmune thrombocytopenia. Further testing confirmed that the antibody reacted independently of the PlA or

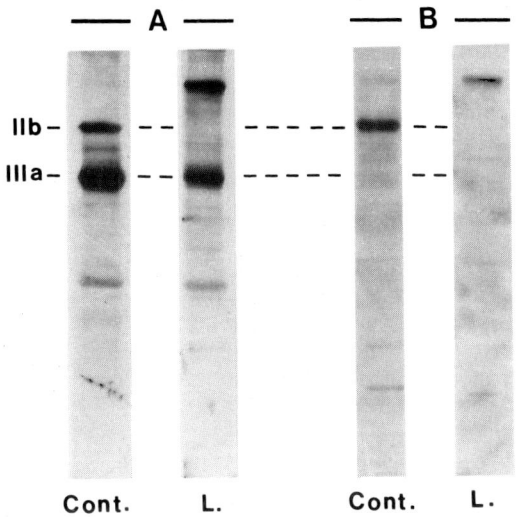

Fig. 2. Western blot analysis showing the reactivity of (L.) serum with GP IIb and GP IIIa of autologous and control platelets. In A, control and (L.) platelet proteins were incubated with a mixture of 1:20 dilutions of rabbit antisera to GP IIb and GP IIIa. Note the presence of residual GP IIIa (but not GP IIb) in (L.) platelets. In B, control and (L.) platelet proteins were incubated with a 1:5 dilution of (L.) serum. Note the reactivity of this serum with GP IIb of normal platelets and the absence of reactivity with his own platelets. SDS-polyacrylamide gel electrophoresis of platelet proteins, transfer to nitrocellulose membrane, incubation with antibody, and detection of bound IgG using ^{125}I-labelled Protein A were all performed as described by Nurden et al. (1985). The upper band located on the patients's pattern in A is platelet IgG, unusually absent from that of the control.

Pen specificities (Nurden et al., 1989). The origin of the antibody rests obscure. The patient had received multiple transfusions during early life when sensitization could have occurred. Alternatively, the antibody could have been formed during the gestation period as a result of a direct immunization by the neonatal platelets. Two years after the birth of the child the antibody remains in the mother's circulation. These two patients illustrate one of the risks of GT. Yet, although nearly all patients have received several transfusions, the formation of isoantibodies is a relatively rare event. This may be due to the presence of residual amounts of the defective glycoproteins in their platelets, although this did not prevent the formation of an anti-GP IIIa antibody by (A.F). To the best of our knowledge, there are two other reports where antibodies reactive with GP IIIa in immunoblotting have been detected in GT patients (Kunicki et al., 1987; Bierling et al., 1988). The production of antibodies to GP IIIa is curious, in view of the presence of GP IIIa as the β-subunit of VnR in endothelial and several other cell types (see above). Perhaps the conformation(s) recognized by the antibodies in in vitro test systems are only expressed by platelets in vivo, or, that they are simply not accessible to circulating antibodies in tissue cells.

NEWLY DESCRIBED VARIANTS

These represent a newly defined category of patient with thrombasthenia-like functional defects, but where platelet GP IIb-IIIa levels are those normally expected to support platelet aggregation. Historically, the first such report was by Lightsey et al. (1981) who studied three members of a family from Guam. Both GP IIb and GP IIIa were normally radiolabelled with ^{125}I during lactoperoxidase-catalyzed iodination and exhibited a normal pI during isoelectric focusing. However, a thrombasthenia-like trait was present and the platelets failed to bind fibrinogen or fibronectin when

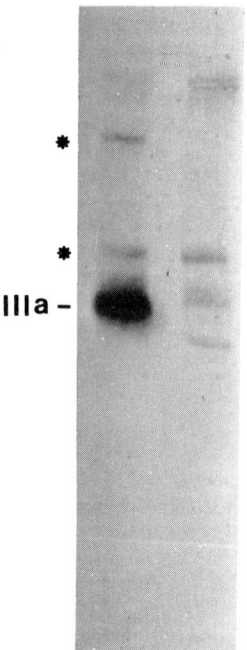

Fig. 3. Western blot analysis showing the reactivity of (A.F.) serum with control and her own platelets. Note the reactivity of this serum with GP IIIa of normal platelets (Cont.) and the presence of abnormally migrating residual antigen in her own platelets. Experimental details were as given in the legend to Fig. 2 except that bound IgG was detected using an anti-mouse IgG antibody adsorbed to gold particles (Janssen Pharmaceutica, Beerse, Belgium) followed by silver enhancement performed according to the manufacturers instructions.

stimulated. Interestingly, both platelet aggregation and clot retraction were modified. Subsequent studies confirmed the presence of a near-normal platelet content of GP IIb-IIIa complexes but revealed a virtual absence of platelet fibrinogen (Ginsberg et al., 1986). An altered reactivity of the patients platelets with the monoclonal antibody PMI-1, which binds to GP IIbα, suggested a structural or organizational defect of GP IIb-IIIa complexes. Recently, the defective platelet function in this family has been shown to involve a loss of Arg-Gly-Asp (RGD) binding function of GP IIb-IIIa which in turn was related to a single base substitution (aspartic acid/tyrosine) in GP IIIa (Loftus et al., 1989).

We have described in detail another variant (C.M.) who also associates an absent platelet aggregation, minimal clot retraction, and a severely decreased level of platelet fibrinogen, with a normal platelet content of GP IIb-IIIa complexes (Nurden et al., 1987; and Table I). The key findings for this patient were (i) an increased facility for the complexes to be dissociated with EDTA and (ii) an inability of the complexes to bind fibrinogen in an in vitro test system in which Triton X-100 soluble platelet extracts were electrophoresed through an agarose gel containing ^{125}I-labelled ligand. These findings point to the presence of a structural or organizational defect in GP IIb-IIIa. Patient (M.S.) featured in Table I presents a similar type of abnormality, but with an apparent decrease in the total level of GP IIb-IIIa complexes in her platelets. A third patient with GP IIb-IIIa complexes unstable to EDTA was recently reported by Fournier et al. (1989). The location of several patients with unstable GP IIb-IIIa complexes suggests a special category of thrombasthenic variant with related genetic defects. As this affects the stability of GP IIb-IIIa to chelating agents, abnormalities in the Ca^{2+}-binding region of the complex might be suggested. It should be noted that GP IIbα contains four repeating units responsible for binding Ca^{2+} to the complex (see Fitzgerald and Phillips, 1989).

It should be noted that of the variants cited in Table I, four (M.S., R.P., C.G., and A.P.) possess intermediate levels of GP IIb-IIIa complexes. The presence of additional defects affecting the function or repartition of the complexes suggests that these variants may, in fact, be double heterozygotes. Patient (R.P.) is particularly interesting for, while failing to bind fibrinogen when stimulated with

ADP, his platelets contain normal amounts of the α-granule pool of fibrinogen and support a normal clot retraction. Furthermore, part of this intracellular pool of fibrinogen is expressed on the platelet surface following platelet stimulation with α-thrombin (Legrand et al., 1989). This suggests that at least some of the residual GP IIb-IIIa complexes in his platelets are capable of functioning normally. One possibility is that the basic defect may lie in the transmission of the message (G proteins ?) which results in conformational changes in GP IIb-IIIa complexes in the plasma membrane during platelet activation. In contrast, in (C.G.) platelets a functional defect in GP IIb-IIIa can be hypothesized for here α-granule fibrinogen is greatly reduced and clot retraction severely diminished.

The monoclonal antibody PAC1 binds to an epitope close to the RGD-binding site on GP IIb-IIIa (Taub et al. 1989). Figure 4 shows that PAC1 (kindly provided by Dr. S. Shattil) binds to GP IIb-IIIa in crossed immunoelectrophoresis, although with intact platelets it's binding is activation-dependent (Shattil et al., 1987). The binding of ^{125}I-PAC1 to the GP IIb-IIIa complexes of platelets of variants (C.M.),(R.P.) and (C.G.) was assessed using the crossed immunoelectrophoresis system illustrated in Fig. 4 and detailed by Nurden et al. (1987). PAC1 failed to bind to the GP IIb-IIIa complexes of patient (C.M.), but bound to the residual complexes of (R.P.) and (C.G). This result confirms the probable heterogeneity in the genetic defects of the variants and provides additional evidence for a structural defect in (C.M.) platelets.

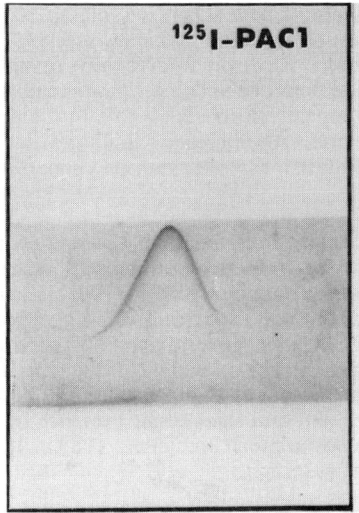 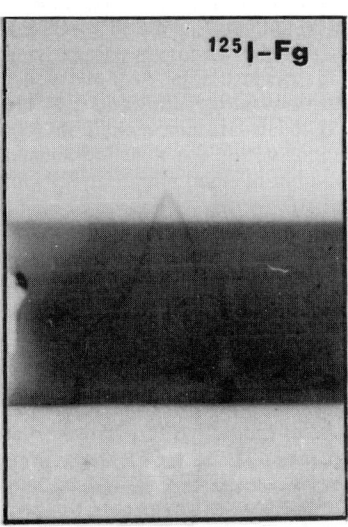

Fig. 4. Analysis of the binding of PAC1 and fibrinogen to GP IIb-IIIa complexes of normal platelets in vitro. The IgM monoclonal antibody PAC1 and purified fibrinogen were radiolabelled with ^{125}I by the chloramine T method and incorporated into the intermediate gel of the crossed immunoelectrophoresis system described by Nurden et al. (1987). Purified GP IIb-IIIa complexes (2 ug) were applied to the sample well and precipitated by the immunoglobulin fraction of a rabbit antiserum raised to whole platelets and incorporated into the upper gel of the second dimension. Bound antibody was detected by autoradiography.

The final variant included in Table I, patient (A.P.), represents a particularly unusual case. Crossed immunoelectrophoresis revealed that his platelets contained of the order of 50 % of the normal platelet content of GP IIb-IIIa complexes. Yet, surface-labelling procedures and monoclonal antibody-binding studies showed that the surface pool of GP IIb-IIIa was reduced to ≈18 % of normal (Hardisty et al., 1987). When (A.P.) platelets were stimulated with thrombin, the internal pool of complexes was normally expressed on the platelet surface. It appears that there is an abnormal organization of GP IIb-IIIa within the platelet with a disproportionate deficiency of the surface pool. Interestingly, ADP-induced aggregation of (A.P.) platelets in citrated platelet-rich plasma is severely diminished whereas that induced by collagen or thrombin is less affected. It will be most interesting to identify the genetic defect responsible for the lesion in the platelets of this patient. Meanwhile, he raises some interesting questions concerning the definition of the GT phenotype. Does this cover partial deficiencies of GP IIb-IIIa ? Does it include aggregation defects restricted to one or more agonists ?

MEGAKARYOCYTES

Relatively few studies have been performed on megakaryocytes of GT patients owing to the difficulty of performing bone marrow punctures on patients with a hereditary bleeding syndrome. In 1986, we reported immunofluorescence studies on marrow cells isolated from (A.M.), a type I patient who had been hospitalized for surgery (Hourdillé et al., 1986). Western blotting revealed the presence of trace amounts of GP IIb and GP IIIa in her platelets, with the latter having an abnormal migration (Nurden et al., 1990). Acetone-permeabilized marrow cells were incubated in double-staining experiments with a rabbit antibody to von Willebrand factor (vWF) and with AP-2, a murine monoclonal antibody to GP IIb-IIIa complexes. Cells from the megakaryocyte lineage, identified by their positive immunofluorescence with the anti-vWF, were mostly negative with AP-2. The presence of an occasional cell positive with AP-2 was an unexpected finding and showed that, for this patient, there was heterogeneity amongst the megakaryocytes concerning their ability to synthetize GP IIb-IIIa. It is not known whether this finding is unique to this particular patient, who has received multiple blood transfusions in the past (see also Nurden, 1989). Electron microscopy revealed a normal megakaryocyte morphology, and confirmed the usual presence of demarcation membranes within the mature cells. GP IIb-IIIa complexes, therefore, appear not to play a role in the development of membrane systems within the maturing megakaryocyte. An interesting finding with this patient was an increased number of small immature cells in the marrow aspirate, perhaps a sign of recent bleeding by the patient.

A marrow aspirate was also obtained by sternal puncture from the type II patient (A.D.) (described above). Cells were again examined by electron microscopy or by immunofluorescence following fixation and permeabilization with acetone. A decreased staining with anti-GP IIb-IIIa antibodies was apparent with residual immunofluorescence detected throughout the megakaryocyte population. This finding is illustrated in Fig. 5. Such a result is in good agreement with the flow cytometry experiments illustrated in Fig. 1 and suggests that the chief characteristic of the type II subgroup is a decreased biosynthesis of GP IIb-IIIa complexes. Standard electron microscopy confirmed the normal structure of the bulk of the megakaryocytes, but also showed the presence of an occasional cell full of vacuoles and showing signs of immune destruction (Pico et al., 1989). This was despite the fact that her last transfusion was approximately 3 years ago.

CONCLUSIONS

As stated above, George et al. (1990) have recently examined the case histories of 64 GT patients and found no correlation between the extent of the GP IIb-IIIa deletion and the frequency of the bleeding episodes. Patients with nearly undetectable GP IIb-IIIa can have mild disease while patients with platelet GP IIb-IIIa that is 10-15 % of normal can have recurrent severe haemorrhagic disease. This conclusion can be illustrated using the patients individually described in the present manuscript. For example, patient (G.L.) (see Fig. 2) has received but two transfusions and these to prevent bleeding from an intestinal complaint. He lives a relatively normal life. Yet, Western blot analysis shows a total absence of GP IIb. In contrast, patient (A.D.) (see Figs. 1 and 5) possesses platelets with ≈12 % residual complexes which are functional in that they bind fibrinogen after platelet stimulation (Pico et al., 1989). This patient experienced frequent epistaxes in early childhood. She was hospitalized at menarche and suffered from serious haemorrhage and bleeding during and after the birth of her first child. She has received multiple transfusions. Although two well-characterized examples have been illustrated in this text, the development of isoantibodies following transfusion is a relatively rare event. However, when it does occur, antibodies can be formed to GP IIb or GP IIIa despite the presence of the latter as part of the VnR in different cell types.

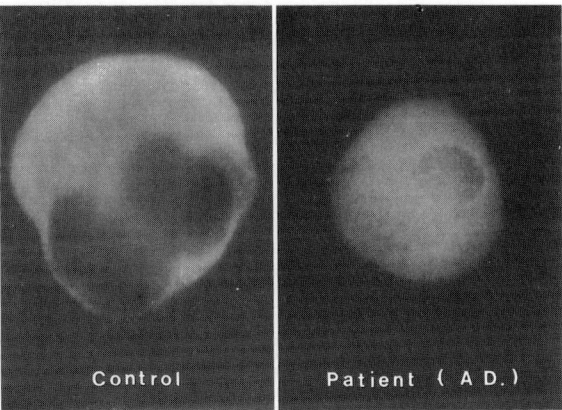

Fig. 5. Immunofluorescence labelling of acetone-permeabilized megakaryocytes from patient (A.D.) with type II thrombasthenia. Megakaryocytes were identified on glass smears by their positive labelling with tetramethylrhodamine-conjugated IgG of a goat anti-vWF antibody (not shown). GP IIb-IIIa complexes were located with AP-2, which was detected with FITC-conjugated F(ab')$_2$ fragments of a rabbit antibody to mouse IgG. The patient's megakaryocytes clearly showed detectable fluorescence with AP-2.

Amongst the 64 patients, significant clot retraction was only detected when residual GP IIb-IIIa complexes were present in the platelets. There was also a close correlation between the ability of platelets to retract a clot and the presence of fibrinogen in the α-granules. This could indicate either a role for secreted fibrinogen in clot retraction, or that the residual GP IIb-IIIa complexes mediate this process. It is tempting to speculate that the low density distribution of GP IIb-IIIa on the surface of type II platelets is sufficient to bind enough fibrin molecules to permit a modified clot retraction to occur. It should be recalled that in this process, GP IIb-IIIa complexes serve to link surface-bound fibrin with the platelet cytoskeleton (see Cohen, 1985). Platelet aggregation is a somewhat different process. Fibrinogen binding to stimulated platelets is followed by the clustering of occupied GP IIb-IIIa receptors and this process appears to be a prerequisite for aggregation (Isenberg et al.,1989). One possibility is that cluster formation increases the affinity of the bound fibrinogen for unoccupied GP IIb-IIIa complexes on adjacent platelets a process that permits platelet aggregation in plasma where the fibrinogen concentration is in the region of 3 mg/ml (see George et al., 1984). The low density of GP IIb-IIIa complexes on type II platelets may not allow cluster formation and, as a consequence, no significant platelet aggregation occurs.

It is well documented that obligate heterozygotes for type I GT contain intermediate amounts of GP IIb-IIIa complexes and that these levels are sufficient to support a normal platelet aggregation and clot retraction. The data accumulated by George et al. (1990) and summarized in Table I suggest that the threshold level of GP IIb-IIIa complexes required for normal platelet aggregation lies between 18 % (patient A.P.) and the 50 % levels of the heterozygotes.

FINAL COMMENTS

The observations made on GT have important implications for our understanding of haemostasis. Firstly, although GT is a haemorrhagic disorder, the fact that normal haemostasis can be preserved for long periods in some type I patients in spite of a virtual total deficiency of GP IIb-IIIa complexes and, therefore, in the absence of fibrinogen binding to activated platelets, means that either (i) other platelet-dependent mechanisms can compensate for this deficiency or (ii) that platelet aggregation, as it is studied in vitro, only becomes an essential process under special circumstances. Important questions which remain include an explanation as to why bleeding occurs more in certain GT patients than others, and as to what factors determine the onset of haemorrhage. In this regard, it will be interesting to evaluate whether genetic defects of GP IIIa result in deficiencies of the VnR, and, therefore, of functional defects in other cells (see above). Furthermore, in the absence of normal GP IIb-IIIa complex formation is there, in some patients, a compensatory increase in the platelet content of VnR.

As detailed in the chapter of Seligsson et al. (this volume), the detailed mapping of the genetic defects responsible for the GT phenotype has started. The fact that Western blot experiments frequently reveal the presence of traces of GP IIb and/or GP IIIa in platelets of type I patients suggest that large gene mutations will be rare. Presumably, for the GT phenotype to be expressed the mutation must affect either (i) GP IIb-IIIa complex formation or (ii) an active site on one or other of the two glycoproteins. This raises the possibility that many structural abnormalities or polymorphisms of GP IIb or GP IIIa may go undetected in the absence of modified platelet function.

The clinical experience in GT also has implications in other domains. For, if an absence of GP IIb-IIIa complexes does not always give rise to regular bleeding episodes, then the presence of drug- or immune-induced defects of platelet function may also escape detection unless there is a specific haemostatic requirement for GP IIb-IIIa-mediated thrombus formation, or another manifestation of the condition such as the onset of thrombocytopenia. Furthermore, thrombasthenia tells us that children may be an exception to this rule. In contrast, the use of anti-thrombotic therapy based on the inhibition of GP IIb-IIIa receptor function may be an important development, for bleeding complications may be predicted to be infrequent in most who receive it.

ACKNOWLEDGEMENTS

ATN acknowledges the members of his previous research group at the Unité 150 INSERM (Dir. Professor JP Caen): Dominique Didry, Dominique Pidard, Jean-Philippe Rosa, Maria del Cunto, Chantal Legrand, Véronique Dubernard, Magali Houssaye and Colette Bouillot, who played a key role in the studies on GT patients performed in his group in Paris during the period 1976-1988. ATN also acknowledges the roles played by Professor JN George (University of Oklahoma Medical School) and Dr. S. Bellucci who documented the medical histories of many of the patients who formed the basis of Table I. Finally, ATN would like to thank all of the MDs who kindly referred their patients for study over the years and without whose help none of the above data would have been accumulated.

REFERENCES

Altieri, D.C., Mannuccio, P.M. and Capitanio, A.M. (1986): Binding of fibrinogen to human monocytes. J. Clin. Invest. 78, 968-976.
Bellucci, S., Tobelem, G. and Caen, J.P. (1983): Inherited platelet disorders. Prog. Hematol. 131, 223-263.
Bierling, P., Fromont, P., Elbez, A., Duedari, N. and Kieffer, N. (1988): Early immunisation against platelet glycoprotein IIIa in a newborn Glanzmann type I patient. Vox Sang. 55, 109-113.
Caen, J.P., Castaldi, P.A., Leclerc, J.C., Inceman, S., Larrieu, M.J., Probst, M. and Bernard, J. (1966): Congenital bleeding disorders with long bleeding time and normal platelet count. I. Glanzmann's thrombasthenia. Amer. J. Med. 41, 4-26.
Caen, J.P. (1972): Glanzmann's thrombasthenia. Clin. Haematol. 1, 383-392.
Cohen, I. (1985): The mechanism of clot retraction. In Platelet Membrane Glycoproteins, ed J.N. George, A.T. Nurden, D.R. Phillips, pp 299-326, New York, Plenum Press.
Donati, M.B., Balconi, G., Remuzzi, G., Borgia, R., Morasco, L. and de Gaetano, G. (1977): Skin fibroblasts from a patient with Glanzmann's thrombasthenia do not induce fibrin clot retraction. Thromb. Res. 10, 173-174.
Fitzgerald, L.A. and Phillips, D.R. (1989): Structure and Function of Platelet Membrane Glycoproteins. In Platelet Immunobiology. Molecular and Clinical Aspects, ed. T.J. Kunicki, J.N. George, pp 9-30, Philadelphia, J.B. Lippincott.

Fournier, D., Kabral, A., Castaldi, P.A. and Berndt, M.C. (1989): A variant of Glanzmann's thrombasthenia characterized by abnormal glycoprotein IIb/IIIa complex formation. Thromb. Haemostas. 62, 977-983.
Giltay, J.C., Leeksma, O.C., Breederveld, C. and van Mourik, J.A. (1987): Normal synthesis and expression of endothelial IIb/IIIa in Glanzmann's thrombasthenia. Blood 69, 809-812.
Giltay, J.C., Brinkman, H.-J.M., von dem Borne, A.E.G.Kr. and van Mourik, J.A. (1989): Expression of the alloantigen Zwa (or PlA1) on human vascular smooth muscle cells and foreskin fibroblasts: A study on normal individuals and a patient with Glanzmann's thrombasthenia. Blood 74, 965-970.
George, J.N., Caen, J.P. and Nurden A.T. (1990): Glanzmann's thrombasthenia: The spectrum of clinical disease. Blood 75, 1383-1395.
George, J.N., Nurden, A.T. and Phillips, D.R. (1984): Molecular Defects of the vessel-wall interaction causing hemorragic disease. New Engl. J. Med. 311, 1089-1098.
Ginsberg, M.H., Lightsey, A., Kunicki, T.J., Kaufmann, A., Marguerie, G. and Plow, E.F. (1986): Divalent cation regulation of the surface orientation of platelet membrane glycoprotein IIb. Correlation with fibrinogen binding function and definition of a novel variant of Glanzmann's thrombasthenia. J. Clin. Invest. 78, 1103-1111.
Glanzmann, E. (1918): Hereditäre hämorrhagische thrombasthenie. Ein beitrag zür pathologie der blütplättchen. Jahr. Kinderheilkd. 88, 113-141.
Hardisty, R.M., Panocchia, A., Mahmood, N., Noakes, T.J.C., Pidard, D., Bouillot, C., Legrand, C. and Nurden, A.T. (1987): Partial platelet function defect in a variant of Glanzmann's thrombasthenia with intermediate levels of GP IIb-IIIa. Thrombos. Haemostas. 58, 526 (abstr.).
Harrison, P., Wilbourn, B., Debeli, N., Vainchenker, W., Breton-Gorius, J., Lawrie, A.S., Masse, J-M., Savidge, G.F. and Cramer, E.M. (1989): Uptake of plasma fibrinogen into the alpha granules of human megakaryocytes and platelets. J. Clin. Invest. 84, 1320-1324.
Hourdillé, P.H., Fialon, P., Belloc, F., Namur, M., Boisseau, M.R. and Nurden, A.T. (1986): Megakaryocytes from the marrow of a patient with Glanzmann's thrombasthenia lacked GP IIb-IIIa complexes. Thromb. Haemostas. 56, 66-70.
Isenberg, W.M., McEver, R.P., Phillips, D.R., Shuman, M.A. and Bainton, D.F. (1989): Immunogold-surface replica study of ADP-induced ligand binding and fibrinogen receptor clustering in human platelets. Am. J. Anat. 185, 142-148.
Jennings, L.K., Ashman, R.A., Wang, W.C. and Dockter, M.E. (1986): Analysis of human blood platelet glycoproteins IIb-IIIa and Glanzmann's thrombasthenia in whole blood by flow cytometry. Blood 68, 173-179.
Johnston, G.I., Heptinstall, S., Robins, R.A. and Price, M.R. (1984): The expression of glycoproteins on single blood platelets from healthy individuals and from patients with congenital bleeding disorders. Biochim. Biophys. Res. Commun. 123, 1091-1098.
Kunicki, T.J., Furihata, K., Bull, B. and Nugent, D.J. (1987): The immunogenicity of platelet membrane glycoproteins. Trans. Med. Rev. 1: 21-33.
Lawler, J. and Hynes, R.O. (1989): An integrin receptor on normal and thrombasthenic platelets that binds thrombospondin. Blood 74, 2022-2027.
Legrand, C., Dubernard, V. and Nurden, A.T. (1989): Studies on the mechanism of expression of secreted fibrinogen on the surface of activated human platelets. Blood 73, 1226-1234.
Lightsey, A.L., Plow, E.F., McMillan, R. and Ginsberg, M.H. (1981): Glanzmann's thrombasthenia in the absence of GP IIb and IIIa deficiency. Blood 58, 199 (abstr.).
Loftus, J.C., O'Toole, T.E., Plow, E.P. and Ginsberg, M.H. (1989): Identification of a GP IIb-IIIa mutation in a Glanzmann's variant associated with loss of RGD binding function. Blood 74, Suppl 1, 58 (abstr.).
McGregor, L., Sayegh, A., Calvette, J.J., Trzeciak, M.C., Ville, D., Catimel, B., Viala, J.J., Dechavanne, M. and McGregor, J.L. (1989): Aggregation to thrombin and collagen of platelets from a Glanzmann thrombasthenia patient lacking glycoproteins IIb and IIIa. Thromb. Haemostas. 62, 962-967.
Newman, P.J. (1989): Phylogeny and tissue distribution of platelet antigens. In Platelet Immunobiology. Molecular and Clinical Aspects, ed. T.J. Kunicki, J.N. George, pp 148-165, Philadelphia: J.B. Lippincott.
Newman, P.J., Gorski, J., White II, G.C. and Lyman S. (1989): PECAM-1: A new member of the immunoglobulin gene superfamily found on platelets and endothelial cells that shares structural motifs with neuronal cell adhesion molecules. Thrombos. Haemostas. 62, 360 (abstr.).

Nurden, A.T. and Caen, J.P. (1974): An abnormal glycoprotein pattern in three cases of Glanzmann's thrombasthenia. Br. J. Haematol. 28, 253-260.

Nurden, A.T., Didry, D., Kieffer, N. and McEver, R.P. (1985): Residual amounts of glycoproteins IIb and IIIa may be present in the platelets of most patients with Glanzmann's thrombasthenia. Blood 65, 1021-1024.

Nurden, A.T. (1987): Abnormalities of platelet glycoproteins in inherited disorders of platelet function. In Platelets in Biology and Pathology III, ed E. MacIntyre and J.L. Gordon, pp 37-94, Amsterdam, Elsevier.

Nurden, A.T. (1989): Congenital abnormalities of platelet membrane glycoproteins. In Platelet Immunobiology. Molecular and Clinical Aspects, ed. T.J. Kunicki, J.N. George, pp 63-96, Philadelphia: J.B.Lippincott.

Nurden, A.T., Jallu, V., Pico, M., Kaplan, C., Christie, D. and Kunicki, T.J. (1989): Evidence for multiple antibodies in the sera of two patients with immune thrombocytopenia of different origins. Thrombos. Haemostas. 62, 565 (abstr.).

Nurden, A.T., Pico, M., Heilmann, E., Jallu, V.and Hourdillé, P. H.(1990): Inherited disorders of platelets and megakaryocytes. In Molecular Biology and Differentiation of Megakaryocytes eds J. Breton-Gorius, J. Levin, A.T. Nurden and N. Williams, pp 333-346, New York, Wiley-Liss.

Phillips, D.R., Charo, I.F., Parise, L.V. and Fitzgerald, L.A. (1988): The platelet membrane glycoprotein IIb-IIIa complex. Blood 71, 831-843.

Pico, M., Hourdillé, P., Lacaze, D. and Nurden, A.T. (1989): Studies on the platelets and megakaryocytes of a patient with type II Glanzmann's thrombasthenia. Thrombos. Haemostas. 62, 309 (abstr.).

Rosa, J.-P., Kieffer, N., Didry, D., Pidard, D., Kunicki, T.J. and Nurden, A.T. (1984): The human platelet membrane glycoprotein complex GP IIb-IIIa expresses antigenic sites not exposed on the dissociated glycoproteins. Blood 64, 1246-1253.

Sakariassen, K.S., Nievelstein, P.F.E.M., Coller, B.S. and Sixma J.J. (1986): The role of platelet membrane glycoproteins Ib and IIb-IIIa in platelet adherence to human artery subendothelium. Br. J. Haematol. 63, 681-691.

Shattil, S.J., Cunningham, M. and Hoxie, J.A. (1987): Detection of activated platelets in whole blood using activation-dependent monoclonal antibodies and flow cytometry. Blood 70, 307-315.

Sosnoskl, D.M., Emmanuel, B.S., Hawkins, A.L., van Tuinen, P., Ledbetter, D.H., Nussbaum, R.L., Kaos, F-T., Schwartz, E., Phillips, D.R., Bennett, J.S., Fitzgerald, L.A. and Ponz, M.A. (1988): Chromosomal localization of the genes for the vitronectin and fibronectin receptors α subunits and for platelet glycoproteins IIb and IIIa. J. Clin. Invest. 81, 1993-1998.

Taub, R., Gould, R.J., Garsky, V.M., Ciccarone, T.M., Hoxie, J., Friedman, P.A. and Shattil, S.J. (1989): A monoclonal antibody against the platelet fibrinogen receptor contains a sequence that mimics a receptor recognition domain in fibrinogen. J. Biol. Chem. 264, 259-265.

Weiss, H.J., Turitto, V.T. and Baumgartner, H.R. (1986): Platelet adhesion and thrombus formation on subendothelium in platelets deficient in glycoproteins IIb-IIIa, Ib, and storage granules. Blood 67, 322-330.

Woods, V.L., Wolff, L.E. and Keller, D.M. (1986): Resting platelets contain a substantial centrally located pool of glycoprotein IIb-IIIa complex which may be accessible to some but not other extracellular proteins. J. Biol. Chem. 261, 15242-14251.

Résumé

La thrombasthénie de Glanzmann est une pathologie héréditaire caractérisée par une absence d'agrégation plaquettaire induite par tous les inducteurs physiologiques. La conséquence en est la présence d'un syndrome hémorragique pouvant se manifester dès la naissance. La base moléculaire de cette maladie correspond à une absence, à un déficit, ou à une anomalie qualitative du complexe GP IIb-IIIa, le récepteur plaquettaire du fibrinogène et des autres protéines adhésives médiatrices de l'agrégation plaquettaire. On note également dans ce syndrome une absence ou une diminution de la rétraction du caillot et une diminution du taux de fibrinogène intraplaquettaire chez la plupart des patients. Dans ce chapitre nous avons décrit les principales anomalies fonctionnelles et moléculaires de la thrombasthénie de Glanzmann en illustrant notre texte par quelques cas étudiés personnellement. En particulier, nous avons fait référence aux études effectuées sur 64 malades à l'Hôpital Lariboisière à Paris pendant ces 15 dernières années. La très grande majorité de ces patients (75 %) présentent une anomalie de type I caractérisée par des taux de complexes en GP IIb-IIIa inférieurs à 5 %, une absence de rétraction du caillot et une diminution très importante du contenu intraplaquettaire en fibrinogène. Pour 16 % des patients ces mêmes anomalies sont plus modérées alors que l'absence d'agrégation est maintenue, suggérant que les taux de complexes GP IIb-IIIa nécessaires pour permettre une agrégation sont supérieurs à ceux qui assurent la rétraction du caillot. Ces patients sont classés dans le type II de la thrombasthénie de Glanzmann. Le troisième groupe plus rare (9%) correspond à des anomalies qualitatives des GP IIb ou IIIa avec comme résultat l'incapacité du complexe à fixer du fibrinogène suite à une activation plaquettaire. Malgré cette hétérogénéité dans la thrombasthénie de Glanzmann, le risque hémorragique s'est révélé être équivalent dans chacun des sous groupes. Les saignements sont toujours plus fréquents et plus graves pendant l'enfance. Le développement d'iso-anticorps dirigés contre les glycoprotéines affectées est un événement grave mais rare observé dans la plupart des cas chez des patients de type I polytransfusés. La présence de tels anticorps peut conduire à une inefficacité transfusionnelle. Dans un cas, un anticorps anti-GP IIIa s'est développé chez une femme enceinte avec comme conséquence le développement d'une thrombopénie néonatale. Les études des mégacaryocytes des patients avec la thrombasthénie de Glanzmann sont difficiles à réaliser. Chez les deux malades où cette étude a pu être effectuée, nous avons constaté un déficit comparable en GP IIb-IIIa à celui présent dans les plaquettes du même malade. L'absence de toute anomalie morphologique observée pour les mégacaryocytes d'un patient de type I suggère que ces GP ne sont pas impliquées dans le développement membranaire conduisant à la production plaquettaire.

En conclusion, l'étude d'un nombre important de patients a montré qu'il n'existait pas de relation stricte entre la sévérité du déficit en GP IIb-IIIa et les risques hémorragiques encourus par les patients. De telles constatations ont une importance pour l'évaluation de l'utilisation future de substances inhibant le fonctionnement des GP IIb-IIIa chez des adultes présentant des risques thrombotiques.

New cases of Glanzmann's thrombasthenia. Familial studies

N. Schlegel, M.-C. Morel*, T. Lecompte**, M.-F. Hurtaud and C. Kaplan*

Laboratoire d'Hématologie, Hôpital Robert Debré, 48, bd Sérurier, 75019 Paris, France
*Service d'Immunologie leuco-plaquettaire, INTS, 6, rue Alexandre Cabanel, 75015 Paris, France
**Laboratoire d'Hématologie, Hôpital Hôtel-Dieu, 1, place du Parvis-Notre-Dame, 75004 Paris, France

ABSTRACT

Nine new cases of Glanzmann's Thrombasthenia have been diagnosed, 8 in a gipsy population and 1 in an african family from Mali. Among these 9 cases, 4 could be extensively studied. They are characterized by the presence of residual amounts of GPIIIa on their platelets, a few binding sites for anti GP IIb IIIa monoclonal antibodies, and the existence of normal calcium changes (2 cases studied) after stimulation of aequorin loaded platelets, except in presence of ADP. Familial studies have shown that the 3 parents were heterozygous, as well as 1 brother and 1 sister. These results provide us the background for more extensive familial studies and further molecular biology investigations.

Characteristics of Glanzmann's Thrombasthenia (GT) have already been presented in this issue by different authors. The most flagrant data are the well established defect of GP IIb IIIa complexes. Generally, it is a quantitative defect, but, in a few cases, a qualitative one. As already highlighted by Caen (1972), GT appears to be very heterogeneous. Moreover, GT is strongly associated with consanguinity. Most cases of GT have been reported in France, in gipsy population, (George et al, 1990) in Israel and Jordan (Coller et al, 1986 ; Coller et al, 1987), and South India (Khanduri et al, 1981), populations where consanguinity is frequent.

The aim of this manuscript is to summarize the data obtained by studying new cases of GT from two different populations. These basic studies will provide us the background for further molecular biology studies on the GPIIb IIIa complexes and an approach for the understanding of the GT genetic defect.

PATIENTS AND METHODS

PATIENTS

The cases described here belong to a large gipsy population and to one african family.

Gipsy population

Since many years, we had the opportunity to study a very large gipsy population living in different parts of France. In this population, a high degree of consanguinity is observed.

Among 18 persons, 8 patients can be assumed to fulfill the clinical and platelet aggregation criteria of GT. Among these 8 patients, 3 could be more extensively studied. Patients 1 (P.F.) and 2 (C.F.) are brother and sister ; their maternal and paternal grand mothers are sisters. The grand mothers of these 2 patients and the maternal great grand mother of the patient 3 (E.R.) are also sisters. Moreover, the mother of P.F. and C.F. could also be studied. This mother and her husband (father of P.F. and C.F.) are first cousins.

The hemorrhagic manifestations observed in the 8 patients are frequent and classical. Furthermore, P.F. and E.R. underwent a surgical treatment. P.F., a young man who is now 20 years old, underwent a splenectomy after a traumatic splenic rupture, 2 years ago. He recovered after many platelet transfusions and developed an anti GPIIb IIIa antibody. E.R. a young woman who is now 21 years old, underwent a surgical treatment for gastro-intestinal hemorrhage. She also recovered after many platelet transfusions and developed an anti GPIIb IIIa antibody.

African family

This family is coming from Mali.

A case of GT was diagnosed in a 5 years old boy, who presented severe anemia due to gingivorragia. The hemorrhagic syndrome included epistaxis, hematomas and, at the age of 8 years, a very extensive and persistent hematoma of the thigh.

The two parents, the brother (11 years old) and the two sisters (6 years old and 4 years 6 months old) of the propositus could also be studied. No consanguinity could be assumed in this family, but the father and the mother are originated from the same village.

METHODS

Beside platelet numeration, clot retraction, and bleeding time, platelet functional studies included classical aggregation tests with various inducers : ADP, collagen, arachidonic acid and ristocetin.

Moreover, for P.F. and C.F. (gipsy population), calcium changes were studied by loading platelets with aequorin and stimulating them in an apparatus able to record simultaneous changes in light transmission and aequorin generated luminescence (Lecompte et al, in press).

Biochemical analysis included Sodium Dodecyl Sulphate - Polyacrylamide Gel Electrophoresis (SDS - PAGE), Western blot with lectins, and Crossed Immuno Electrophoresis (CIE) with an anti IIIa monoclonal antibody (Morel et al, this issue).

Binding sites for 2 monoclonal antibodies (MoAb) were also estimated. One antibody, PL2-49, is a murine monoclonal IgG1 antibody which binds GPIIb in a complex dependent manner (Morel et al, 1989). The other, PL2-73, is an anti GPIIb IIIa complex antibody (produced in the same laboratory than above).

RESULTS

PLATELET CLASSICAL STUDIES

These studies, i.e. platelet numeration, clot retraction, bleeding time, and aggregation tests have shown usual results observed in Type I GT for all the cases studied.

AEQUORIN DETECTED CALCIUM CHANGES IN STIMULATED THROMBASTHENIC PLATELETS

The patients P.F. and C.F. of the gipsy population could be studied on 3 and 2 separate occasions respectively. Aequorin loaded platelets of these 2 patients were stimulated with thrombin (1U/ml), calcium ionophore A23187 (1µM), Phorbol-Myristate Acetate (PMA) (0.1µM) and ADP (100µM). The results obtained are indicated on the Table 1. Estimated maximal calcium changes fall into the normal range in presence of calcium ionophore, thrombin and PMA, but tend to be lower than with normal platelets in presence of ADP.

Table 1 : Intra platelet calcium maximal levels (µM) in stimulated thrombasthenic platelets : Patients P.F. (1) and C.F. (2) of the gipsy population.

Patient	A23.187	Thrombin	ADP	PMA
1A	-	7.2	1.2	-
1B	9.5	5.6	1.4	2.8
1C	14.8	7.0	2.2	-
2A	17.8	8.0	2.2	3.9
2B	11.2	8.9	2.2	-
Normal range	7.9 31.9	4.0 20.0	2.0 4.0	2.5 4.5

Note : A, B, C : Different study occasions

BIOCHEMICAL AND IMMUNOLOGICAL RESULTS

Gipsy population

The results obtained by SDS-PAGE and Western blot with lectins are indicated on the Table 2. Similar profiles are obtained for the 3 patients : very low

Table 2 : Gipsy population. Platelet fibrinogen and GPIIb IIIa : SDS-PAGE and Western blot with lectins

Subjects	1	2	3	Mother
Fibrinogen (%)	<10	<10	<10	≈50
GPIIb IIIa PAS (%)	≈0	≈0	≈0	55
Lectins	residual amounts IIIa	residual amounts IIIa	ND*	id control

* ND = Not Determined

platelet fibrinogen, no detectable GPIIb IIIa by SDS-PAGE and PAS staining, but residual amounts of GPIIIa were detected with lectins. Concerning the mother we observed that platelet fibrinogen was decreased to fifty per cent, GPIIb IIIa was reduced to fifty five per cent after PAS staining, but no quantitative difference with the control could be evidenced with the lectins.

Crossed Immuno Electrophoresis (data not shown) with an anti IIIa monoclonal antibody could not detect any GPIIb IIIa complex peak in the platelets of the 3 patients. The peak observed with the mother's platelets was reduced to fifty per cent as compared to the control platelets.

The platelet binding sites for the 2 monoclonal antibodies PL2-49 and PL2-73 are indicated on the Table 3. They were markedly reduced on the platelets of the 3

Table 3 : Gipsy population. Platelet binding sites for monoclonal antibodies.

Subjects	1	2	3	Mother	Control
AntiIIb (PL2-49)	<1,000	<1,000	ND*	21,400	38,000 42,000
AntiIIb IIIa (PL2-73)	≈3,300	≈4,200	≈2,700	25,000	40,000

* ND = Not Determined

patients, the number of sites being lower with the MoAb anti IIb than with the MoAb anti IIb-IIIa. For the mother's platelets, the binding sites were estimated to be fifty per cent of the normal control with the same difference between the two MoAbs as for the children.

African family

The results obtained by SDS-PAGE and Western blot with lectins are indicated on the Table 4. The propositus (subject 1) has a profile similar to the gipsy

Table 4 : African family. Platelet Fibrinogen and GPIIb IIIa : SDS-PAGE and Western blot with lectins.

Subjects	Propositus	Brother	Sister	Sister	Father	Mother
Age (years-months)	9	11	6	4-6	46	31
Fibrinogen (%)	<10	100	75	100	70	100
GPIIb IIIa PAS (%)	≈0	50	50	≈N*	50	50
Lectins	residual amounts IIIa	---------------- id. control -------------				

N* = Normal

patients' one : very low platelet fibrinogen and residual amounts of GPIIIa.

The platelet fibrinogen is normal for 3 of 5 members of this family : the mother, the oldest brother and the youngest sister, and at the lower limit for 2 : the father and the other sister. After PAS staining, the GPIIb IIIa complex appeared to be reduced to fifty per cent of control for all members of the family except the youngest sister who exhibited a normal profil. No difference with control could be evidenced with the lectins.

The platelet binding sites for the 2 monoclonal antibodies PL2-49 and PL2-73 are indicated on the Table 5. They could be studied only on the 2 parents'

Table 5 : African family. Platelet binding sites for monoclonal antibodies.

Subjects	Father	Mother	Control
AntiIIb (PL2-49)	22,500	20,700	38,000 42,000
AntiIIb IIIa (PL2-73)	24,700	23,200	40,000

platelets. The results are similar for both of them : the binding sites are reduced to fifty per cent as compared to the control, but slightly lower with the anti IIb than with the anti IIb IIIa monoclonal antibody.

DISCUSSION

We have diagnosed 9 new cases of GT, 8 in a gipsy population, and 1 in an african family from Mali.

The recent publication of George et al (1990) remembers the high frequency of GT in gipsy population, due to the frequent intermarriages in this population. In contrast, the discovery of a GT case in an african family is unusual and more extensive studies of people from Mali or other neighbouring regions might have some interest to have a more complete view of GT in other human groups.

Classical hemorrhagic manifestations of GT occured in these 9 patients. Moreover, multiple platelets transfusions in two patients, P.F. and C.F., induced the synthesis of isoantibodies against GPIIb IIIa. It is interesting to notice that these antibodies appeared notwithstanding the patients had residual amounts of GP IIIa at the surface of their platelets. The mechanism(s) of production of such antibodies is (are) not elucidated yet, and several hypothesis are proposed in this issue (Nurden et al). More extensive studies regarding these antibodies are in progress.

Considering the 4 patients that have been more extensively studied, 3 from the gipsy population and 1 from the african family, the biological results are quite similar. The most flagrant data are the presence of residual amounts of GP IIIa, as it has been already published for Type I GT patients (Nurden et al, 1985) and as it is discussed by Nurden et al in this issue.

Moreover, we have demonstrated that aequorin loaded thrombasthenic platelets from 2 patients, P.F. and C.F., repeatedly studied, are able to induce luminescence signals corresponding to detectable calcium peaks, similar to those observed with normal platelets, except in presence of ADP (Lecompte et al, in press).

Familial studies have shown that the mother of P.F. and C.F. and the parents of the african child as one brother and one sister can be considered as heterozygous for GT. Three parameters are in favour of the heterozygous status in these 5 subjects : only fifty per cent of platelet fibrinogen, decrease to fifty per cent of the normal contain in GPIIb IIIa as estimated by PAS staining and platelet binding sites of two monoclonal antibodies directed against GPIIb and GPIIb IIIa complex. These results are in agreement with those of Coller et al (1986).

IN CONCLUSION, we have studied a large gipsy population and an african family in which we have diagnosed 9 cases of Type I GT and 5 heterozygous GT subjects. More extensive familial studies are now in progress in order to have more information on the GT transmission and genetic defects in these populations.

ACKNOWLEDGEMENTS

We would like to acknowledge the pediatricians who trust us to take care of their patients : Professor P. Narcy, Doctor J. Deffez, Professor M. Boureau, and Professor Y. Aujard, from Hopital Robert Debré in Paris, and Doctors Y. Kessler, M. Talon, M. Guesnu and Y. de St Martin from pediatric units near Paris and in Pau. We are also indebted to Doctor P. Besson, head of the blood bank at Hopital Robert Debré in Paris, for her helpful opinions about all the GT patients during many years. We are also grateful to Professor L. Drouet for his help in the study of the gipsy population, to Alan T Nurden for his participation to the study of two patients P.F. and C.F., and to J. Mac Gregor for his excellent advice.

REFERENCES

Caen, J.P. (1972) : Glanzmann's thrombasthenia Clin. Haematol. 1, 383-392.

Coller, B.S., Seligsohn, U., Zivelin, A., Zwang, E., Lusky, A., Modan, M. (1986) : Immunological and biochemical characterization of homozygous and heterozygous Glanzmann thrombasthenia in the Iraqi-Jewish and Arab populations of Israel : comparison of techniques for carrier detection. Br. J. Haematol. 62, 723-735.

Coller, B.S., Seligsohn, U., Little, P.A. (1987) : Type I Glanzmann Thrombasthenia patients from the Iraqi-Jewish and Arab populations in Israel can be differentiated by platelet glycoprotein IIIa immunoblot analysis. Blood 69, 1696-1703.

George, J.N., Caen, J.P., Nurden, A.T. (1990) : Glanzmann's Thrombasthenia : The spectrum of clinical disease. Blood 75, 1383-1395.

Khanduri, U., Pulimood, R., Sudarsanam, A., Carman, R.H. (1981) : Glanzmann's thrombasthenia. A review and report of 42 cases from South India. Thromb. Haemost. 46, 717-721.

Lecompte, T., Potevin, F., Champeix, P., Morel, M.C., Favier, R., Hurtaud, M.F., Schlegel, N., Samama, M., Kaplan, C. : Aequorin-detected calcium changes in stimulated thrombasthenic platelets. Aggregation-dependent calcium movement in response to ADP. Thromb. Res., in press.

Morel, M.C., Lecompte, T., Champeix, P., Favier, R., Potevin, F., Samama, M., Salmon, C., Kaplan, C. (1989) : PL2-49, a monoclonal antibody against glycoprotein IIb which is a platelet activator. Br. J. Haematol. 71, 57-63.

Nurden, A.T., Didry, D., Kieffer, N., Mc Ever, R.P. (1985) : Residual amounts of glycoproteins IIb and IIIa may be present in the platelets of most patients with Glanzmann's thrombasthenia. Blood 65, 1021-1024.

Résumé

Neuf nouveaux cas de Thrombasthénie de Glanzmann ont été diagnostiqués : 8 parmi une population gitane et 1 dans une famille africaine originaire du Mali. Parmi ces 9 cas, 4 ont pu être étudiés plus complètement. Ils sont caractérisés par la présence de faible quantité de GPIIIa sur les plaquettes, d'un faible nombre de sites de liaison pour des anticorps monoclonaux anti GPIIb IIIa, et l'apparition de changements calciques normaux (2 cas étudiés) après stimulation des plaquettes traitées par l'aequorine, sauf en présence d'ADP. Des études familiales ont montré que 3 parents étaient hétérozygotes, ainsi qu'1 frère et 1 soeur. Ces résultats constituent une base pour des études familiales plus approfondies ainsi que des investigations à l'aide de techniques de biologie moléculaire.

Use of murine monoclonal antibodies to study thrombopathies related to GPIIb-IIIa complexes

M.-C. Morel-Kopp*, T. Lecompte**, N. Schlegel***, P. Hivert****
and C. Kaplan*

* INTS, 6, rue Alexandre Cabanel, 75015 Paris, France
** Laboratoire central d'hémostase, Hôtel-Dieu, 1, place du Parvis-Notre-Dame, 75004 Paris, France
***Laboratoire d'hématologie, Hôpital Robert Debré, 48, bd Sérurier, 75019 Paris, France
****Laboratoire d'hématologie, CNTS, Hôpital Saint-Antoine, 184, rue Faubourg-Saint-Antoine, 75012 Paris, France

ABSTRACT

Glanzmann thrombasthenia is an autosomal recessive disorder of the platelet glycoproteins IIb-IIIa. In this work, extensive studies were performed on platelets of patients with different type of Glanzmann thrombasthenia: twenty one patients with type I thrombasthenia (platelets lack glycoproteins IIb and IIIa), one patient type II (platelet express 10% of the normal amount of glycoproteins IIb and IIIa) and two patients with a variant form of thrombasthenia (platelets show quantitative and qualitative abnormalities in GPIIb -GPIIIa). One of these variants has an unusual sensitivity to dissociation of the GPIIb-IIIa complexes in presence of calcium that may be related to abnormality of calcium binding sites. The second patient show a "new glycoprotein" of 118 kDa which could form a precipitation arc in crossed-immunoelectrophoresis recognized by anti-glycoprotein IIb and anti-glycoprotein IIIa monoclonal antibodies. As this pattern is seen in the patient's descendants, this case could represent a new constitutional hereditary disorder similar to Glanzmann thrombasthenia.These biochemical studies allow the characterization of the molecular abnormalities of our patients. In two type I Glanzmann thrombasthenia's patients, immunized against glycoproteic IIb-IIIa complex, crossed-immunoelectrophoresis showed the presence of residual complexes. With a very simple and sensitive western blotting method using monoclonal antibodies, we confirm that a considerable biochemical heterogeneity exist between all the patients classified as type I Glanzmann thrombasthenia.

This work was in part supported by the "Société d'Etudes et de Soins pour les Enfants Paralysés et Polymalformés" (S.E.S.E.P.).

INTRODUCTION

Glycoproteins (GP) IIb and IIIa, the major platelet membrane GP, are associated in a calcium-dependent heterodimer complex (Kunicki et al, 1981a). The complex integrity is crucial for adhesive proteins such as fibrinogen to bind (Caen, 1972; Ruggeri et al, 1983; Plow et al, 1986) and for platelet aggregation to occur. Glanzmann's thrombasthenia is a major hereditary platelet disease related to abnormalities in the GPIIb-IIIa complex, this hereditary platelet disease is characterized by a disorder of platelet functions producing a more or less lifelong bleeding tendency due to an absence of platelet aggregation. This autosomal recessive syndrome regroup qualitative and quantitative abnormalities of the GPIIb-IIIa complex. Patients are designated as type I : severe GPIIb-IIIa deficiency, type II : moderate GPIIb-IIIa deficiency . If the primary defect appears to be in the function of this complex rather than a quantitative deficiency, they are described as variants; absence of fibrinogen binding on activated platelets with normal amount of GP IIb/IIIa complexes, (Lightsey et al 1981); complex instability,(Nurden et al 1987); glycosylation defect, (Tanoue et al 1987); abnormal GP, (Jung et al 1988). It is of importance to characterize the biochemical defects and their relationships with functional abnormalities.

Monoclonal antibodies (MoAbs) are very useful to define each pathological case. They are epitope specific, and available in important quantities. The majority of these MoAbs against GPIIb-IIIa inhibit platelet aggregation by blocking adhesive protein binding sites (Bennett et al, 1983; Coller et al, 1983; Di Minno et al, 1983), but platelet activators against GPIIb or GPIIb-IIIa have been described (Bai et al, 1984; Morel et al, 1988, 1989; Modderman et al, 1988). Thus not only the structural but also the functional defects of the GPIIb-IIIa complex can be studied with the MoAbs.

MATERIAL AND METHODS

Unless otherwise specified, chemicals were purchased from Prolabo (France) and materials for sodium dodecyl sulfate polyacrylamide gel electrophoresis (SDS-PAGE) were from Bio-rad (Richmond, USA).

- *Patients*. All the patients we have studied showed absence or important decrease of ADP-induced platelet aggregation. They were referred to our laboratory for biochemical and immunological investigations.

- *Monoclonal antibodies*. The MoAb PL2-49 against GPIIb was from our laboratory and previously characterized (Morel et al, 1988,1989). XIIF9, MoAb anti GPIIIa was kindly supplied by Dr A. Nurden. P21 (= PL1-64, anti-GPIIb) and P22 (= PL2-73, anti-GPIIb-IIIa) were also from our laboratory and described during the IV International Workshop on Leucocyte Typing (Vienna, 1989) as P36 (anti- GPIIIa) and P63 (anti GPIIb).

- *SDS-PAGE and PAS staining*. The pellet of washed platelets was dissolved in 2% SDS, 10 mM Tris, 150 mM NaCl, 3 mM EDTA, 30 mM NEM, 1 mM PMSF buffer (pH 7,2). 300µg of proteins were electrophoresed by the Laemmli procedure (1970) and glycoproteins revealed after periodic-acid-schiff (PAS) staining (Fairbanks et al, 1971).

- *Crossed immunoelectrophoresis.* Washed platelets were prepared according to Mustard et al (1972) from ACD-PRP and solubilized in 1 % Triton X-100, 38 mM Tris, 100 mM Glycine buffer (pH 8.6) at a concentration of 6×10^9 platelets/ml. The method used was in first described by Laurell (1965) and modified by Bjerrum (1976, 1977). The second dimension electrophoresis was run against radiolabelled MoAbs in the intermediate gel and anti-human platelet polyclonal antibodies in the upper gel.

- *Western blotting.* After SDS-PAGE, separated proteins were transferred to nitrocellulose sheet according to Towbin et al (1979). Immunodetection was performed according to Blake et al (1984) with modification, antibody binding was revealed using luminescence (ECL, Amersham).

- *Binding assay.* Washed platelets prepared according to Mustard et al were resuspended in the same buffer containing 10^{-8}M Iloprost (2×10^8 platelets/ml). Platelet suspension was mixed with increasing concentrations of labelled PL2-49. Free radioactivity, percentage of bound radioactivity on platelets and non-specific binding were determined and used for Scatchard plot computerized analysis (1970).

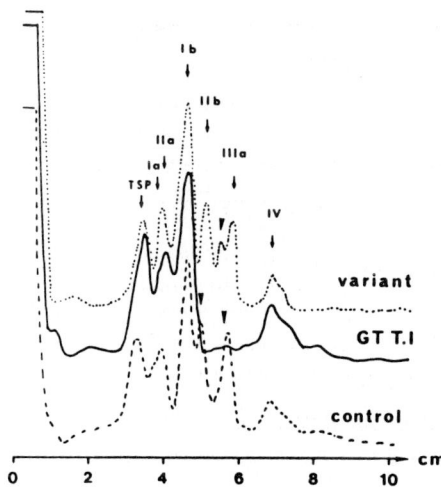

FIGURE 1 :

Densitometric scans of SDS-PAGE (6% acrylamide in non reducing condition) and PAS staining of control and Glanzmann's thrombasthenia platelet glycoproteins (300 µg of total platelet proteins were electrophoresed). The arrows show absence of peaks or presence of new extrapeak.

RESULTS

SDS-PAGE and PAS staining (figure 1).

Periodic-acid-schiff staining of electrophoresed type I Glanzmann's thrombasthenia platelet lysates showed in reduced condition a total absence of GPIIb and GPIIIa peaks; the same pattern was observed for the type II patient. Patient identified as variant A. has a moderate deficiency (50% reduction compared to the control) of GPIIb and GPIIIa. The second patient named variant L. has normal GPIIb and IIIa but presented an extra peak, identified between these two GP (figure 1), with a molecular weight estimated to 118 kDa.

Western-blot analysis.

The platelet lysates (150 µg) were separated by SDS-PAGE in non reduced conditions as described above and then electrophoretically transferred to a nitrocellulose membrane. After incubation with murine MoAbs P63 (anti-GPIIb) and P36 (anti-GPIIIa), the binding was then visualized by incubation with peroxidase-linked anti murine IgG and addition of the luminescence substrate. As shown on figure 2, the two bands corresponding to GPIIb and GPIIIa are detected for the normal control (lane 6). This figure illustrates the results obtained for our patients. Variable patterns were seen for the type I patients. The platelets of patients 2,5,6,7 demonstrated a GPIIIa band with a decreased intensity. The strongest one was observed for patients 2 and 7. A faint GPIIb was only observed for patient 2. The GPIIb and GPIIIa bands were present for patient 4 (type II subgroup) and patient 3 (variant A) as for the obligate heterozygous (lane 1). The relative proportions of these bands were similar to the control (lane 8). In only 3 cases variant A (lane 3), GT Type II(lane 4), GT Type I (lane 5)) another band, with a 160 kDa molecular weight, was observed analogous to the dimeric IIIa band as described elsewhere (Calvete et al, 1987).

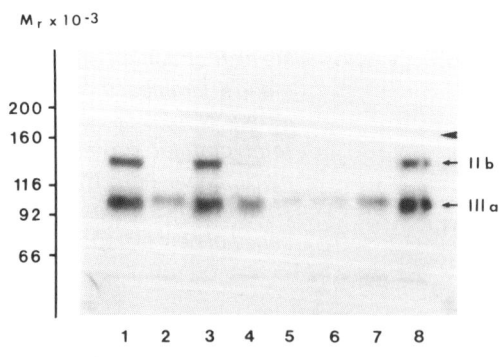

FIGURE 2:

Immunoblots of non-reduced SDS-solubilized platelets after SDS-PAGE (6% acrylamide, non-reduced condition) and transfer to nitrocellulose sheet, 150 µg of total platelet proteins were used. P36 anti-GPIIIa and P63 anti GPIIb (from the IV International Workshop on Leucocyte Typing) were used and horseradish-peroxidase conjugated secondary antibody. MoAb bindings were revealed using ECL procedure (Amersham). 1: heterozygous; 2, 5, 6, 7: type I; 3: variant; 4: type II; 8: normal platelets.

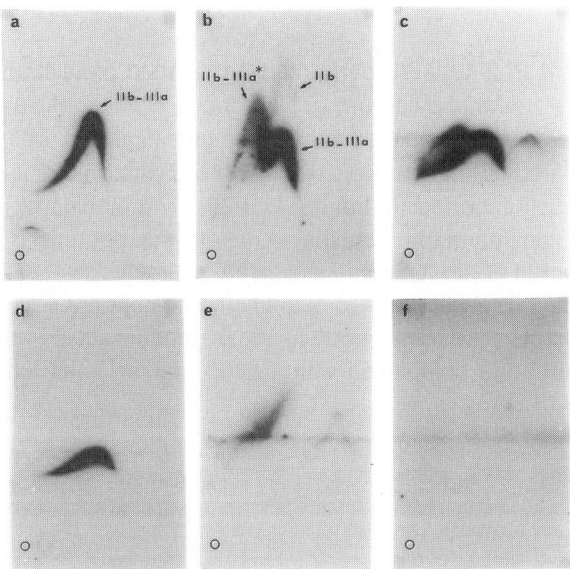

FIGURE 3 :

Autoradiograms of CIE analysis of platelet glycoproteins. Washed platelets (in the presence of 1 mM Ca++) were solubilized in 38 mM Glycine buffer (pH 8.6) containing 1% Triton X-100 and 100 µg used for analysis. The first dimension was electrophoresis at 10 V/cm for 90 minutes and the second dimension was 2 V/cm for 17 hours. The intermediate agarose section contained radiolabelled PL2-49, anti-GPIIb MoAb (a,b,d,f) or XIIF9, anti-GPIIIa MoAb (c,e), 200,000 cpm by gel and upper section contained rabbit antibodies to whole platelets. a: normal human platelets, b and c: variants of Glanzmann's thrombasthenia, d: type II, e and f: type I.

Crossed Immunoelectrophoresis.

Investigations were performed using triton X-100 extracts of platelets washed in presence of calcium and incorporation of ^{125}I labelled MoAbs in the intermediate gel. PL2-49 (anti-GPIIb) and XIIF9 (anti-GPIIIa) labelled only the GPIIb-IIIa complex when normal platelets were tested as shown on figure 3, platelets from patients were isolated in the same way. The results were variable depending of the patient's group. For type I group, two different patterns were observed : virtual absence of the GPIIb-IIIa complex or a faint print (figure 4e, 4f). Figure 4d illustrates the results obtained with type II platelets. Unusual profiles were observed for the two variants L. and A. A decrease in the size of GPIIb-IIIa precipitate was the feature of the two platelet patterns. But additional precipitates were clearly apparent. For variant L. an arc was observed in a position similar to that obtained for the free GPIIb after dissociating conditions of the complex as previously described (Kunicki et al, 1981b). Another extra peak in the cathodal position was equally recognized by the two MoAbs. The two MoAbs detected only 50 % of the normal contain of the GPIIb-IIIa complex for variant A. But XIIF9 (anti-GPIIIa) labelled a precipitate in the position of dissociated GPIIIa.

Binding assay.

Binding experiments of PL2-49 were performed on washed platelets in the presence of divalent cations (Ca++ 1 mM) and Iloprost 10^{-8} M (strong inhibitor of platelet activation and aggregation), this binding was completed after 20 minutes (figure 4). The saturation binding of PL2-49 to unstimulated normal platelets was achieved with 38,000 to 42,000 molecules per platelet as previously reported (Morel et al, 1989). The binding of PL2-49 to washed platelets from type I Glanzmann thrombasthenia patient was decreased to less than 2,000 molecules. The number of GPIIb-IIIa complexes were estimated to 4,100 +/ 300 copies per platelet for type II patient. We were able to quantify the number of GPIIb-IIIa complexes for obligate heterozygotes. It varied from 14,500 to 26,000 binding sites. Patient L. presented a slight decrease of GPIIb-IIIa complexes with 29,800 binding sites for PL2-49 (data not shown).

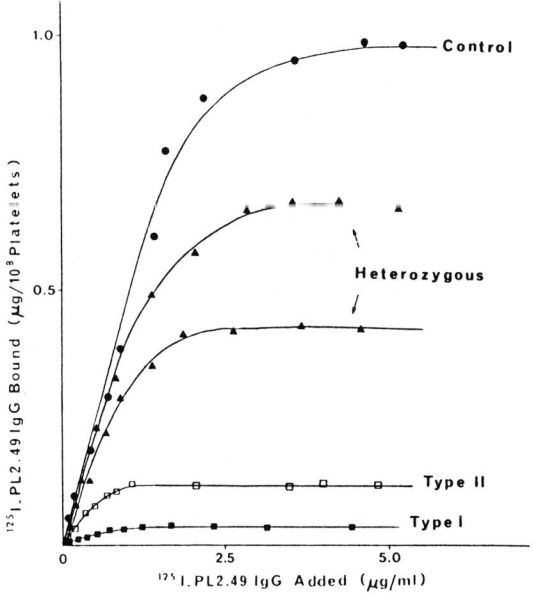

FIGURE 4 :

Specific binding of ^{125}I-PL2-49 to normal and Glanzmann's thrombasthenia platelets. Washed platelets ($2x10^8$/ml) were incubated under non-stirring conditions with increasing concentrations of ^{125}I-PL2-49 for 30 minutes at $20°C$. Platelet associated radioactivity was determined after centrifugation of the platelets through a layer of 20% sucrose and counting of the platelet pellet. Nonspecific binding value was subtracted from total binding to yield specific binding.

DISCUSSION

The major function of the activated GPIIb-IIIa complex is to be a receptor for adhesive proteins and to play a key role in the platelet aggregation (Bennett, 1985; Shattil et al, 1985). Glanzmann thrombasthenic platelets illustrate the crucial role of the GPIIb-IIIa complex in haemostasis (Caen et al, 1978). Monoclonal antibodies are useful tools to dissect the

GPIIb-IIIa structure, functions and regulations. We used MoAbs to better characterize the biochemical defects presented by patients referred to our unit, who showed a marked decrease of platelet aggregation. All but two patients were classified as Glanzmann thrombasthenia type I or type II according to the estimated amount of GPIIb and GPIIIa. We studied 21 patients with type I Glanzmann thrombasthenia. GPIIb and GPIIIa were not detected using PAS staining following SDS-PAGE. However, residual amounts of GPIIIa were detectable using monoclonal antibodies in a sensitive immunoblot technique, GPIIb was present only in two patients. In CIE we observed in two cases a residual amount of the GPIIb-IIIa complex. Binding methods using anti-GPIIb and anti-GPIIb-IIIa MoAbs (PL2-49, PL2-73) revealed no more than 2,000 binding sites per platelet. These results favoured an heterogeneity amoung the type I subgroup as it has been recently discussed (Coller et al, 1987; Seligsohn et al, 1989). Platelets of one patient classified as type II were evaluated to contain 10 % of the normal level of the complex by binding studies with MoAbs. The immunoblotting procedure showed the GPIIb and GPIIIa to be present in the same proportion as the normal control. In CIE a pattern similar to the control was observed with a diminution of the height of the precipitate arc. With the quantification of the monoclonal binding sites we can assess the GPIIb and GPIIIa platelet levels and thus allow the detection of Glanzmann heterozygotes. From a clinical point of view it is interesting to underline that in our series only type I patients were immunized following transfusions. If we consider the residual amounts of GPIIb-IIIa glycoproteins on the platelet surface, we therefore can assume that the formation of iso-antibody is related to the presence of less than 10 % of the normal level of these glycoproteins.

Concerning the variants of thrombasthenia, it has been shown that CIE analysis combined with ^{125}I labelled monoclonal antibody in the intermediate gel allowed the identification of GPIIb-IIIa abnormalities. The stability of the complex could be explored under exposure to variable conditions of pH, temperature, ionic concentration (Kunicki et al, 1981 ; Rosa, 1984b). The monoclonal antibody present in the intermediate gel binds only to its epitope and allow the identification of the immunoprecipitate after autoradiography (Pidard, 1989). Such an analysis, using four different monoclonal antibodies (PL2-49, P21, P22, XIIF9), was performed on patient L. and her family. The first analysis of the patient's platelet membrane showed no decrease of the GPIIb-IIIa but the presence of an extrapeak of 118 kDa after SDS-PAGE, in non reducing and reducing conditions. In immunoblotting this band was not recognized by the MoAbs we tested (anti-GPIb, anti-GPIIb, anti-GPIIIa). CIE in normal calcium concentration revealed the presence of normal GPIIb-IIIa complex as well as two other peaks, one free GPIIb and one of low mobility termed IIb-IIIa* recognized by three MoAbs, PL2-49, P21 (anti-GPIIb) and XIIF9 (anti-GPIIIa) but not with P22 (anti-GPIIb-IIIa). The presence of free GPIIb is unusual in these technical conditions (Rosa et al, 1984a) and implies an abnormal structure of the GPIIb-IIIa complex possibly due to the presence of the abnormal glycoprotein which could be structurally related to GPIIIa. The decrease number of MoAb binding sites which epitope is depending of the existence of normal GPIIb-IIIa complex (PL2-49) may imply abnormal structure of this complex or a lower accessibility of this epitope. Two children of this patient were examined and their platelets showed similar abnormalities. This case could represent a new case of constitutional hereditary disorder similar to Glanzmann thrombasthenia. The second patient, A., was studied in similar conditions. The CIE analysis showed that the normal GPIIb-IIIa complex was present but decreased and that in the presence of calcium a spontaneous moderate complex dissociation occurred with the presence of free GPIIIa. We may suppose that the calcium binding site on the GPIIb-IIIa complex is affected and this could be involved (this is currently under investigation); her haemostatic disorders reflect the necessity of the complex integrity.

PAS staining could not detect less than 15% of the normal amount of GP, neither western-blot nor CIE with MoAbs reveal structural heterogeneity due to abnormal glycosylation; the use of lectins allows going through this inhibitory factor in the qualitative approach.

In conclusion, the results we obtained in immunoblotting, binding analysis and CIE are relevant in several aspects. They provide evidence for residual amounts of GPIIb and GPIIIa and heterogeneity in the platelets of Glanzmann thrombasthenia patients. They allow the characterization of the molecular abnormalities and contribute to our knowledge of the pathology of the GPIIb-IIIa complex. They may provide insights into the role of crucial domains of the GPIIb-IIIa complex in the cellular interactions and lead to the better understanding of the relationship between molecular and gene defects.

BIBLIOGRAPHY

Bai, Y., Durbin, H. and Hogg, N. (1984): Monoclonal antibodies specific for platelet glycoproteins react with human monocytes. *Blood 64*:139-146.

Bennett, J.S., Hoxie, J.A., Leitman, S.F., Vilaire, G., Cines; D.B. (1983): Inhibition of fibrinogen binding to stimulated human platelets by a monoclonal antibody. *Proc. Natl. Acad. Sci. USA 80*:2417-2421.

Bennett, J.S. (1985): The platelet-fibrinogen interaction. *In Platelet Membrane Glycoproteins*. New York, Plenum, p196

Bjerrum, O.J., Bog-Hansen, T.C. (1976): Immunochemical gel precipitation techniques for analysis of membrane proteins. In : AH Maddy (ed.) : *Biochemical Analysis of Membranes*, Chapman and Hall, london, p363.

Bjerrum, O.J. (1977): Immunochemical investigation of membrane proteines. A methodological survey with emphasis placed on immunoprecipitation in gels. *Biochem. Biophys. Acta 472*:135.

Blake, M.S., Johnston, K.H., Russel-Jones, G.J., Gotschlich, E.C. (1984): A rapid, sensitive method for detection of alkaline phosphatase conjugated anti-antibody on Western blots. *Anal. Biochem. 136*:175-179.

Caen, J.P. (1972): Glanzmann thrombasthenia. *J. Clin. Haematol. 1*: 388-391.

Caen, J.P., Castaldi, P.A., Leclerc, J.C., Inceman, S., Larrieu, M-J., Probst, M., Bernard, J. (1978): Congenital bleeding disorders with long bleeding time and normal platelet count. I.Glanzmann's thrombasthenia (report of fifteen patients). *Am. J. Med. 41*:4

Calvete, J.J., Mac Gregor, J.L., Rivas, G., Gonzalez-Rodriguez, J. (1987): Identification of a glycoprotein IIIa dimer in polyacrylamide gel separations of human platelet membranes. *Thromb. Haemost. 58*:694-697.

Coller, B.S., Peerschke, E.I., Scudder, L.E., Sullivan, C.A. (1983): A murine monoclonal antibody that completely blocks the binding of fibrinogen to platelets produces a thrombasthenic-like state in normal platelets and bind to glycoproteins IIb/IIIa. *J. Cl. Invest. 72*:325-338.

Coller, B.S., Selighson, U., Little, P.A. (1987): Type I Glanzmann thrombasthenia patients from the Iraqui-Jewish and Arab populations in Israel can be differentiated by platelet glycoprotein IIIa immunoblot analysis. *Blood 69-6*:1696-1703.

Di Minno, G., Thiagarajan, P, Perussia, B., Martinez, J., Shapiro, S., Trinchieri, G., Murphy, S. (1983): Exposure of platelet fibrinogen-binding sites by collagen, arachidonic acid, and ADP: inhibition by a monoclonal antibody to the glycoprotein IIb-IIIa complex. *Blood 61*:140-148.

Fairbanks, G., Steck, T.L. and Wallach, D.F.H. (1971): Electrophoretic analysis of the major polypeptides of the human erythrocyte membrane. *Biochemistry 10* : 2606-2617.

Jung, S.M., Yoshida, N., Aoki, N., Tanoue, K., Yamazaki, H. and Moroi, M. (1988): Thrombasthenia with an abnormal platelet membrane glycoprotein IIb of different molecular weight. *Blood 71-4*: 915-922.

Kunicki, T.J., Nurden, A.T., Pidard, D., Russel, N.R. and Caen, J.P. (1981a): Characterization of human platelet glycoprotein antigens giving rise to individual immunoprecipitates in crossed-immunoelectrophoresis. *Blood 58*: 1190-1197.

Kunicki, T.J., Pidard, D., Rosa, J-P., Nurden, A.T. (1981b): The formation of Ca++ dependent complexes of platelet membrane glycoproteins IIb and IIIa in solution as determined by crossed immunoelectrophoresis. *Blood 58*:268-278.

Laemmli, U.K. (1970): Cleavage of structural proteins during the assembly of the head of the phage T4. *Nature 227*: 680-685.

Laurell, C.B. (1965): Antigen-antibody crossed electrophoresis. *Anal. Biochem. 10*:358.

Lightsey, A.L., Thomas, W.J., Plow, E.F., Mac Millan, R. and Ginsberg, M. (1981): Glanzmann's thrombasthenia in the absence of glycoprotein IIb and IIIa deficiency. *Blood 58 (suppl.):* 199a.

Modderman, P.W., Huisman, J.G., Van Mourik, J.A., Von Dem Borne, A.E.G.Kr. (1988): A monoclonal antibody to the human platelet glycoprotein IIb/IIIa complex induces platelet activation. *Thromb. Haemost. 60*:68-74.

Modderman, P.W., Van Mourik, J.A., Van Berkel, W., Cordell, J.L., Morel, M-C., Kaplan, C., Ouwehand, W.H., Huisman, J.G., Von Dem Borne, A.E.G.Kr. (1989): Decreased stability and structural heterogeneity of the residual platelet glycoprotein IIb/IIIa complex in a variant of Glanzmann's thrombasthenia. *Br. J. Haematol. 73*:514-521.

Morel, M-C., Favier, R., Champeix, P., Lecompte, T., Potevin F., Samama, M. and Kaplan, C. (1988): Characterization of an anti-IIb-IIIa monoclonal antibody which is a platelet activator. In:C. Kaplan-gouet, Ch. Salmon (Eds): *Platelet Immunology, Current Studies in Hematology and Blood Transfusion*, Karger, 53-63.

Morel, M-C., Lecompte, T., Champeix, P., Favier, R., Potevin, F., Samama, M., Salmon, C. and Kaplan, C. (1989): PL2-49, a monoclonal antibody against glycoprotein IIb which is a platelet activator. *Br. J. Haematol. 71*: 57-63.

Mustard, J.F., Perry, D.W., Ardlie, N.G. and Packam, M. (1972): Preparations of suspensions of washed platelets from humans. *Br. J. Haematol. 22*: 193-204.

Nurden, A.T., Rosa, J.P., Fournier, D., Legrand, C., Didry, D., Parquet, A. and Pidard, D. (1987): A variant of Glanzmann's thrombasthenia with abnormal IIb-IIIa complexes in the platelet membrane. *J. Clin. Invest. 79*: 962.

Pidard, D. (1989): The application of crossed-immunoelectrophoresis and related immunoassays to the characterization of glycoprotein structure and function. In Kunicki, George (eds): *Platelet immunobiology, molecular and clinical aspects*. Philadelphia, J.B. Lippincott Company, p193.

Plow, E.F., Ginsberg, M.H., Marguerie, G.A. (1986): Expression and function of adhesive proteins on the platelet surface. In Phillips, Shulman (eds): *Biochemistry of platelets*. San Diego, Academic Press, p226.

Rosa, J-P., Kieffer, N., Didry, D., Pidard, D., Kunicki, T.J., Nurden, A. (1984a): The human platelet membrane glycoprotein complex GP IIb-IIIa expresses antigenic sites not exposed on the dissociated glycoproteins. *Blood 64*:1246-1253.

Rosa, J-P (1984b): Etude d'un antigène plaquettaire membranaire impliqué dans les interactions plaquettes-plaquettes. Thèse de Doctorat de 3ème cycle.

Ruggeri, Z.M., De Marco, L., Gatti, L., Bader, R., Montgomery, R.R. (1983): Platelets have more than one binding site for von Willebrand factor. *J. Clin. Invest. 72*:1-12.

Scatchard, G. (1970): The attractions of proteins for small molecules and ions. *An. N.Y. Acad. Sci. 51*: 660-672.

Seligsohn, U., Coller, B.S., Zivelin, A., Plow, E.F., Ginsberg, M.H. (1989): Immunoblot analysis of platelet glycoprotein IIb in patients with Glanzmann thrombasthenia in Israel. *Br. J. Haematol. 72*:415-423.

Shattil, S.J., Brass, L.F., Bennett, J.S., Pandhi, P. (1985): Biochemical and functional consequences of dissociation of the platelet membrane glycoprotein IIb-IIIa complex. *Blood 66*:92-98.

Tanoue, K., Hasegawa, S., Yamaguchi, A., Yamamoto, N. and Yamazaki, H. (1987): A new variant of thrombasthenia with abnormally glycosylated GP IIb/IIIa. *Thromb. Res. 47*: 323-333.

Towbin, H., Staehelin, T., Gordon, J. (1979): Electrophoretic transfer of proteins from polyacrylamide gels to nitrocellulose sheets : procedure and some applications. *Proc. Natl. Acad. Sci. USA 76*:4350.

Résumé

Le complexe glycoproteique IIIb-IIIa plaquettaire est un hétérodimère Ca^{++} dépendant, qui change de forme après activation plaquettaire et devient le récepteur membranaire pour le fibrinogène plasmatique, permettant l'agrégation plaquettaire. La thrombasthénie de Glanzmann est une maladie autosomale récessive liée à une anomalie quantitative et/ou qualitative de ce complexe. Notre étude a porté sur 24 cas de thrombasthénie, 21 type I, 1 type II et 2 variants. L'utilisation d'anticorps monoclonaux associés à des techniques immunochimiques, comme le western-blot et l'immunoélectrophorèse croisée, nous a permis de confirmer l'existence d'une hétérogénéité biochimique entre les différents cas de type I, mais aussi de caractériser 2 variants. Les plaquettes de Mme L. présentent une "nouvelle" GP plaquettaire d'un poids moléculaire apparent de 118 kD, interférant avec le complexe GP IIb-IIIa et induisant une absence d'agrégation à l'ADP. Le patient A. présente un défaut à la fois quantitatif (50% de GP IIb et IIIa résiduelles) et qualitatif (complexe partiellement dissocié même en présence de Ca^{++}) du complexe GP IIb-IIIa.

Molecular aspects of Glanzmann's thrombasthenia

I. Djaffar, D. Vilette, J.-L. Wautier and J.-P. Rosa

INSERM U 150, Hôpital Lariboisière, 6, rue Guy Patin, 75475 Paris Cedex 10, France

Glanzmann's thrombasthenia is a congenital bleeding disorder characterized by a defect in platelet aggregation and binding of fibrinogen. The defect is due to quantitative or qualitative alterations in the platelet fibrinogen receptor GPIIb-IIIa, a member of the supergene family of integrins. Its 2 subunits, GPIIb and GPIIIa, are encoded by separate genes less than 200 kb apart on chromosome 17(q21-22). Processing and assembly of GPIIb-IIIa, as assessed in HEL cells, a human cell line with megakaryocytic features involve correct folding in the endoplasmic reticulum, of GPIIIa and preIIb (the uncleaved GPIIb precursor) which assemble just before or during transit to the Golgi. Then preIIb is clipped into the disulfide-linked 2-chain GPIIb and complex glycosylated, before GPIIb-IIIa is expressed at the cell surface. Unassembled preIIb does not transit to the plasma membrane. Given the colocalization of GPIIb and GPIIIa genes on chromosome 17, their large sizes, and their complex biosynthetic pathway, it is clear that multiple mechanisms will explain the molecular defects of thrombasthenia. In order to detect these mutations, we have developped the quantitative isolation of platelet RNA which allows Northern blot analysis of GPIIb and GPIIIa mRNAs to detect size anomalies, and PCR followed by sequencing to detect point mutations. To test our approach we have characterized the platelet GPIIb alloantigen Lek[a]/Lek[b], which leads to post-transfusion alloimmunisation. After PcR and sequencing of 60% of GPIIb mRNA, we found one single base substitution responsible of an Ile/Ser polymorphism in position 843. The same polymorphism was detected by Newman et al in the Bak[a]/Bak[b] system, which could therefore be identical. Definitive proof of the identity of the 2 systems will await further investigations. Thus these techniques when applied to patients should help characterize the mutations involved in Glanzmann's thrombasthenia, and in turn help understand better the regulation of expression as well as the structure-function relationship of GPIIb-IIIa.

A. INTRODUCTION.

Glanzmann's thrombasthenia is a congenital bleeding disorder characterized by the absence of platelet aggregation and fibrinogen binding (see reference 1 for review). The molecular anomaly was identified as a defect in membrane glycoproteins GPIIb and GPIIIa (2,

3). GPIIb and GPIIIa are respectively the α and β subunits of the heterodimer GPIIb-IIIa, the major platelet receptor for adhesive proteins such as fibrinogen, but also von Willebrand factor and fibronectin. Patients with undetectable or strongly reduced amounts of GPIIb and GPIIIa were termed type I thrombasthenics as opposed to patients in which quantitative amounts of functional glycoproteins could be detected (typically 10 to 15%) and who were termed type II thrombasthenics. A third category of patients was termed variants of thrombasthenia and is characterized by functionally deficient GPIIb-IIIa in normal or near normal amounts. In fact the heterogeneity of the disease is even greater than first suspected since a recent Western blotting analysis of platelet proteins from several type I thrombasthenics showed varying amounts of either GPIIb or GPIIIa among different patients (4).

The recent cloning and sequencing of cDNAs for GPIIb (5, 6, 7) and GPIIIa (8, 9, 10), has allowed access to the primary structure of both glycoproteins. In addition it was found that GPIIb and GPIIIa share strong sequence homology with respectively the α and β subunits of other adhesion receptors (11) defining the supergene family of Integrins (12). Integrins can be subdivided into subfamilies composed of receptors with different α subunits assembled with a common β subunit. GPIIIa is a β subunit common to platelet GPIIb-IIIa and endothelial vitronectin receptor. GPIIb is different from the α subunit of the endothelial vitronectin receptor.

The genes for GPIIb and GPIIIa were localized on chromosome 17. This was obtained by several methods including hybridization of [^{32}P]-labelled cDNAs for GPIIb and GPIIIa to the DNA of human chromosomes purified by dual laser chromosome sorting (6, 10), in situ chromosome hybridization and rodent-human somatic cell hybrids (10, 13, 14). The distance between the two genes was evaluated by pulse field electrophoresis at approximately 250 kb, the GPIIIa gene 5' to the GPIIb gene (14). However their respective orientation relative to the chromosome centromer has not been determined yet.

B. POSSIBLE MECHANISMS FOR GLANZMANN'S THROMBASTHENIA

Because Glanzmann's thrombasthenia is heterogeneous both clinically and biochemically, we expect that a broad spectrum of mutations will be detected. For example in type I Glanzmann's thrombasthenia, to account for the parallel deficit in GPIIb and GPIIIa, many mechanisms are possible. The simplest would be a large deletion encompassing both genes. Although such a gross genetic event is possible, it is not likely to represent a major mechanism because, 1) large deletions are rare events in human genetic diseases, and 2) most type I patients may have trace amounts of either or both polypeptides (4). Other mechanisms are possible including alteration of the expression of one gene affecting expression of the other gene. The abnormal gene would be affected by mutations already described in other genetic disorders, including large alterations, such as deletions, insertions, or rearrangements, or point mutations, which may affect correct mRNA maturation (mainly intron splicing, but also polyadenylation), transcription initiation, transcription regulation, translation (frame-shifts etc...).

Mutations more specific to GPIIb-IIIa may be expected. For example mutations affecting a coregulatory element may be found: the expression of GPIIb and GPIIIa genes may be coordinately regulated at the transcriptional level. Obviously the fact that GPIIb and GPIIIa genes are located at very close range from a genetic point of view (although 200 kb is a challenging distance from a molecular point of view), is intriguing and in contrast with several other members of the integrin supergene family of which α and β subunits genes are located on separate chromosomes (13). Indeed the 2 genes share virtually no homology and thus did not derive from each other or from a common ancestor gene by a duplication mechanism. Their physical association may therefore be fortuitous, or may have been positively selected for functional reasons: the close proximity of the GPIIb and GPIIIa genes may allow a common regulatory sequence to coordinately control expression of the two genes. This regulatory element could be megakaryocyte-specific, and mutations affecting its function may lead to altered expression of GPIIb-IIIa in platelets. Future studies, possibly including the study of the flanking regions of GPIIb and GPIIIa genes in thrombasthenic patients will be required to test this model.

Also mutations may affect the correct maturation and expression of GPIIb-IIIa at the cell surface. We have used a human leukemia cell line, HEL, to examine the biosynthesis, processing and assembly of GPIIb and GPIIIa. HEL cells exhibit megakaryocytic features (15), including the ability to synthesize platelet membrane glycoproteins GPIIb and GPIIIa. By means of pulse-chase experiments with [^{35}S]methionine Duperray et al. (16) and ourselves (17) showed that GPIIb and GPIIIa were synthesized from separate precursors first detected as high-mannose core glycosylated proteins in the endoplasmic reticulum (ER). The model that we propose for assembly and biogenesis of GPIIb-IIIa is summarized in Fig 1, and could be relevant to Glanzmann's thrombasthenia.

From our data we propose that thrombasthenia may be a consequence of mutations affecting such steps as the assembly of preIIb with GPIIIa (due to improper folding, or improper subunit association), or exit from ER to Golgi, or maturation in the Golgi (glycosylation or other post-translational modifications not yet defined), or correct targeting to the plasma membrane. We postulate, in case of improper assembly

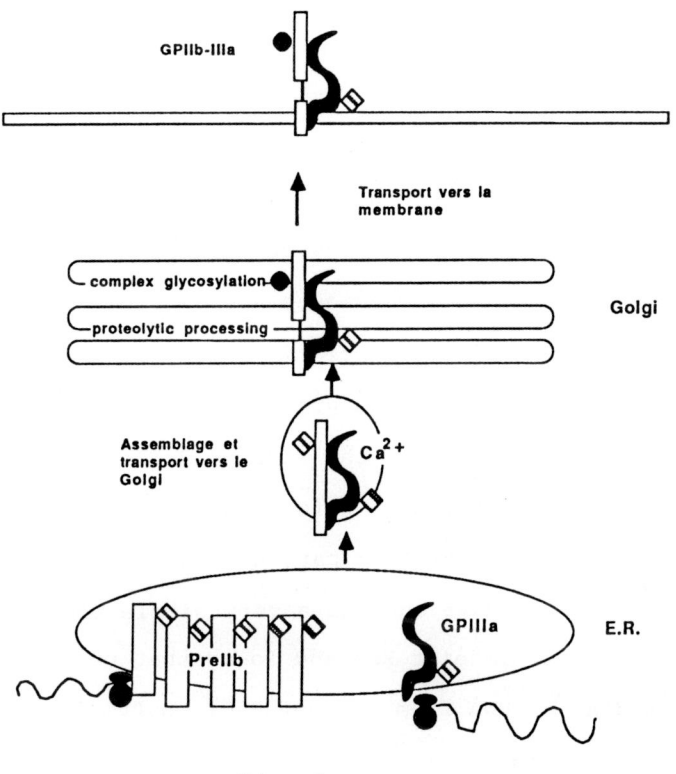

Fig. 1

that free subunits undergo rapid degradation. Turn-over rates of the 2 unassembled polypeptides in megakaryocytes of Glanzmann's patients are likely to be shorter than the half-life of circulating platelets (8 to 10 days), leading to the presence of only trace amounts of GPIIb (or preIIb) and GPIIIa in the platelets of thrombasthenics. Along the same lines, absence of synthesis of one of the 2 polypeptides, for example GPIIb, may lead to an apparent deficit in GPIIIa, at the platelet surface by rapid turn-over of the unassembled subunit in megakaryocytes.

C. MEANS OF DETECTING MUTATIONS IN GLANZMANN'S THROMBASTHENIA.

A major problem facing investigators in characterizing mutations involved in Glanzmann's thrombasthenia is that platelets are anucleated cells and presumably contain no or limited quantities of RNA. Although Southern blot analysis can provide some answers in some cases of large alterations, more refined techniques are usually required in most cases where more limited gene-tic alterations are encountered, e.g. point mutations. Access to RNA would greatly facilitate this task, allowing for Northern blot analysis of the size of GPIIb and GPIIIa transcripts, cDNA cloning and sequen-cing. Unfortunately, megakaryocytes from individuals, in particular from patients, are still very difficult to obtain. However, we have adapted a very simple technique of RNA extraction (18) to platelet RNA and found that one can recover approximately 1 to 3 µg of RNA from 1 ml of PRP. Sufficient material is usually obtained from 20 ml of whole blood to perform Northern blot analysis of GPIIb and GPIIIa mRNAs (19). Transcripts of 3.4 kb and 6.2 kb are detected for GPIIb and GPIIIa respectively. Thus anomalies in size and/or quantities of both messages can now be visualized in thrombasthenic patients and help orient investigations toward either or both genes.

In addition, µg quantities of platelet RNA can be subjected to enzymatic amplification by polymerase chain reaction or PcR, as was first described by Newman et al. (20) for GPIIIa. PcR consists in the in vitro amplification of a fragment of DNA or mRNA of known sequence by means of successive cycles of DNA polymerisation primed by two oligonucleotide primers flanking the region of interest (21). Tremendous amplification rates of 10^5 to 10^6 fold can be obtained yielding enough material to perform for example restriction mapping analysis or sequencing. We amplified GPIIb cDNA using 5 pairs of oligonucleotides, defining the 3' and 5' borders of 5 fragments encompassing 90% of the insert. DNA was first denatured by heating at 99°C for 7 min, and 2.5 U of Taq DNA polymerase (DNA polymerase from thermophilus aquaticus, which is resistant to high temperatures) was added. Consecutive cycles of primer annealing (1 min at 55°C), DNA extension (2 min at 70°C), and denaturation (45 s at 94°C) were performed using a programmable thermocycler (Hybaid). In Fig 2 is shown a gel of 5 overlapping fragments of the GPIIb cDNA amplified by PCR and covering the entire extracellular portion of GPIIb, i.e. 90% of the protein.

This technique was adapted so that the messenger RNA of GPIIb could be amplified from total RNA. The GPIIb fragments were then purified and sequenced either directly or after cloning into a vector such as M13. Such an approach could allow the determination of point mutations in the mRNA of GPIIb or GPIIIa, an otherwise extremely difficult task given the large size of the 2 genes.

In order to test our ability to determine point mutations, we decided to characterize the Lek^a platelet alloantigen which is defined by an alloantibody isolated from a patient who developed a lethal post-transfusion purpura (22). The Lek^a epitope is located on a 60 kDa chymotryptic fragment of GPIIbα as shown by Kieffer et al.(23).The 60 kDa fragment is the only extracellular part of GPIIbα which remains bound to the platelet membrane after chymotrypsin digestion of GPIIb-IIIa in whole platelets and presumably represents the C-terminal half of GPIIbα.

We amplified GPIIb mRNA from one Lek^b phenotype individual (i.e. whose platelets fail to bind the anti-Lek^a allo-antibody). After sequencing 80% of GPIIbα, and after eliminating several base differences apparently due to misincorporation of nucleotides by the Taq polymerase, we found a single substitution of a T into a G in position 2606. This substitution precisely corresponds to an aminoacid substi-

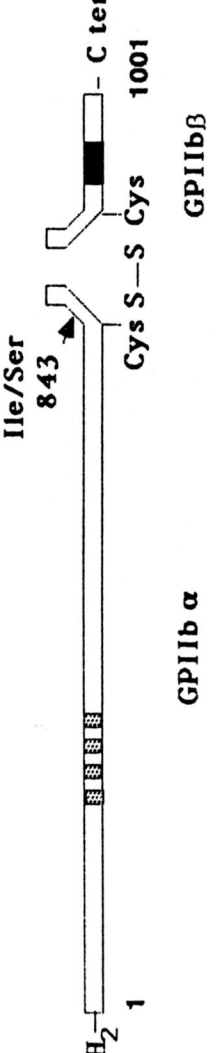

Fig. 2

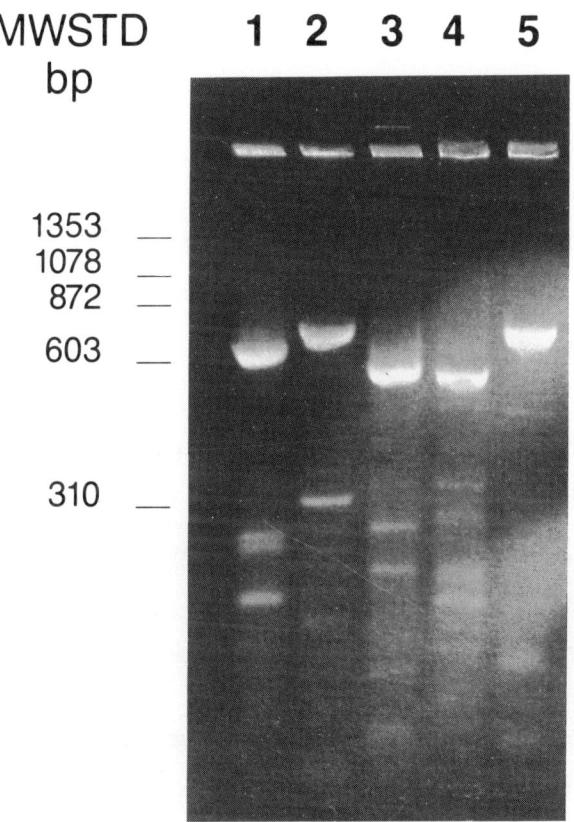

tution of Isoleucine into Serine in position 843, very close to the C-terminus of GPIIbα, shown in Fig. 3.

While our studies were in progress, the group of Peter Newman found the same isoleucine/serine 843 polymorphism associated with the Bak[a] / Bak[b] alloantigen system (24). This could indicate that Lek and Bak are identical. Studies are in progress to confirm this point.

In conclusion PcR of platelet RNA is a method of choice to determine single nucleotide substitutions in GPIIb and/or GPIIIa mRNAs and should turn out to be a very powerful means for determining the mutations responsible for Glanzmann's thrombasthenia.

REFERENCES

1 - Nurden AT (1989). In Kunicki TJ, George JN (eds): "Platelet Immunobiology. Molecular and Clinical Aspects," Philadelphia: J.B. Lippincott, pp.63-96.

2 - Nurden AT, Caen JP (1974). Br J Haematol 28:253-257

3 - Phillips DR, Agin PP (1977). J Clin Invest 60:535-545.

4 - Nurden AT, Didry D, Kieffer N, McEver RP (1985). Blood 65:1021-1024

5 - Poncz M, Eisman R, Heidenreich R, Silver SM, Vilaire G, Surrey S, Schwartz E, Bennett JS (1987). J Biol Chem 262:8476-8482.

6 - Bray PF, Rosa J-P, Johnston GI, Shiu DT, Cook RG, Lau C, Kan YW, McEver RP, Shuman MA (1987). J Clin Invest 80:1812-1817.

7 - Uzan G.,

8 - Fitzgerald LA, Steiner B, Rall SC, Jr, Lo S-S, Phillips DR (1987). J Biol Chem 262:3936-3939.

9 - Zimrin AB, Eisman R, Vilaire G, Schwartz E, Bennett JS, Poncz M (1988). J Clin Invest 81:1470-1475.

10 - Rosa J-P, Bray PF, Gayet O, Johnston GI, Cook RG, Jackson KW, Shuman MA, McEver RP (1988). Blood 72:593-600.

11 - Fitzgerald LA, Poncz M, Steiner B, Rall SC,Jr, Bennett JS, Phillips DR (1987). Biochemistry 26:8158-8163.

12 - Hynes, RO (1987). Cell 48:549-554.

13 - Sosnoski DM, Emmanuel BS, Hawkins AL, van Tuinen P Ledbetter DH, Nussbaum RL, Kaos FT, Schwartz E, Phillips DR, Fitzgerald LA, Poncz M (1988). J Clin Invest 81:1993-1998.

14 -Bray PF, Barsh G, Rosa J-P, Luo XY, Magenis E, Shuman MA (1988). Proc Natl Acad Sci USA 85:8683-8687.

15 - Tabilio A, Rosa J-P, Testa U, Kieffer N, Nurden AT, Del Canizo MZ, Breton-Gorius J, Vainchenker, W (1984). EMBO J 3:453-459.

16 - Duperray A, Berthier R, Chagnon E, Ryckwaert J-J, Ginsberg M, Plow E, Marguerie G (1987). J Cell Biol 104:1665-1673.

17 - Rosa J-P, McEver RP(1989). J Biol Chem 264:12596-12603.

18 - Chomczinsky P,and Sacchi N (1987). Anal Biochem 162:156-159.

19 - Djaffar I, Vilette D, Bray PF, and Rosa J-P (1990). Submitted for publication.

20 - Newman PJ, Gorski J, White GC, Gidwitz S, Cretney CJ, Aster RH (1988). J Clin Invest 82:739-743.

21 - Saiki RK, Scharf S, Faloona F, Mullis KB, Horn GT, Erlich HA, Arnheim N(1985). Science(Wash DC) 230:1350-1354.

22 - Boizard B. and Wautier J.-L., Vox Sang. : 46: 47, 1984

23 - Kieffer N., Didry D., Boizard B., Wautier J.-L., and Nurden A.T., Blood 64: 1212, 1984

24 - Newman et al, 1989, abstract.

Résumé

La thrombasthénie de Glanzmann est une maladie héréditaire hémorragique caractérisée par l'absence d'agrégation et de fixation du fibrinogène aux plaquettes. L'anomalie moléculaire est portée par le récepteur du fibrinogène, GPIIb-IIIa, un membre de la superfamille des intégrines. Ses 2 sous-unités, GPIIb et GPIIIa sont codées par 2 gènes séparés par moins de 200 kb sur le chromosome 17 (q21-22). La maturation et l'assemblage de GPIIb-IIIa, étudiés dans les cellules HEL, une lignée continue humaine aux caractéristiques mégacaryocytaires, comprennent le correct reploiement de GPIIIa et de préIIb (le précurseur non-clivé de GPIIb) dans le réticulum endoplasmique, suivi de leur assemblage juste avant ou au cours de leur transit vers le Golgi. Puis préIIb est clivé pour former les 2 chaînes liées par pont disulfure de GPIIb, puis est glycosylé par sucres complexes, avant que GPIIb-IIIa soit inséré dans la membrane plasmique. PréIIb non-assemblé ne transite pas jusqu'à la membrane. Etant donnés la colocalisation des 2 gènes sur le même chromosome, leurs grandes tailles, et la complexité de la biosynthèse, il est clair que de nombreux différents mécanismes seront trouvés à l' origine de la thrombasthénie. Pour les préciser, nous avons mis au point l'extraction d'ARNs de plaquettes permettant d'analyser les ARNms de GPIIb et GPIIIa par Northern blot pour déceler les anomalies de taille, PCR et séquence pour déterminer les mutations ponctuelles.
Pour tester notre approche nous avons décidé de caractériser l' alloantigène Lek^a/Lek^b porté par GPIIb, responsable d'alloimmunisation post-transfusion-nelle. Après amplification et séquence de 60% de l'ARNm de GPIIb, nous avons trouvé une substitution responsable d'un polymor-phisme Ilc/Ser près du C-terminus de la chaîne alpha de GPIIb. Ce même polymorphisme a aussi été trouvé par Newman et coll. pour le système Bak^a/Bak^b, qui pourrait donc être identique au système Lek. L'identité définitive des deux systèmes est en cours d'évaluation. Ces techniques, appliquées aux patients devraient aider considérablement à la caractérisation des mutations responsables de la maladie de Glanzmann, et par conséquent aider à mieux comprendre la régulation de l'expression ainsi que les relations structure-fonction de GPIIb-IIIa.

Clinical implications of platelet immunology

Implications cliniques de l'immunologie plaquettaire

Platelets, IgE and allergy

J.-P. Dessaint, A. Tsicopoulos, V. Pancré, M. Joseph, J.-C. Ameisen, A.-B. Tonnel and A. Capron

Centre d'immunologie et de biologie parasitaire, Unité mixte INSERM U 167-CNRS 624, Institut Pasteur, 1, rue du Pr A. Calmette, 59019 Lille Cedex, France

Platelet immunology has long been restricted to the study of platelets as targets of immune aggression, such as in auto or alloimmune thrombocytopenia, or of proinflammatory mediators such as platelet activating factor (PAF or PAF-acether). Yet, interaction of platelets with the immune system includes not only their well-known receptors for complement components and IgG, but also for other immunoglobulins and for various lymphokines or monokines such as gamma interferon (IFNγ) and tumor necrosis factor (TNF). Likewise, platelets generate besides factors that promote coagulation, cell growth, and tissue healing, several potent proinflammatory mediators including vasoactive amines (serotonine, histamine), and PAF itself. Extensive studies initiated in parasitic diseases have now established that IgE antibody can trigger platelets directly through a specific surface receptor designated Fc$_E$R$_{II}$ (Capron et al., 1986a). Thus, in the light of recent knowledge, platelets should now be considered not only as indirect or secondary effectors in immune pathways, but also as essential partners in some immune reactions such as defence against parasites and allergic disorders.

EVIDENCE FOR THE INVOLVEMENT OF PLATELETS IN ALLERGY

The involvement of platelets in allergic disorders, and particularly in asthma, is suggested by direct and indirect evidence (Day et al., 1975 ; Morley et al., 1984 ; Oxholm & Winther, 1986). The exposure of airways to allergen induces, in asthmatic patients or in sensitized rabbits and guinea pigs, bronchoconstriction as a primary effect, and platelet depletion of experimental animals suppresses the allergic respiratory syndrome (Pinckard et al., 1977). In this context, the role of PAF-acether in immediate response, although well-documented (Barnes et al., 1988), is far from being fully understood. Nevertheless, PAF-acether was shown to induce acute airway response after intravenous injection or intratracheal instillation (Denjean et al., 1983). Platelets seem to play a crucial role in this effect of PAF-acether. Thrombocytopenia has been associated with PAF-induced bronchoconstriction (Gateau et al., 1984). Platelet depletion, or platelet inhibition by prostacyclin, in rabbit or guinea-pig, suppressed the effects induced by PAF-acether on the lungs (Vargaftig & Benveniste, 1983). In vitro, PAF-acether contracted strongly surgical specimens of human bronchi, but only in the presence of platelets : neither PAF-acether nor platelets alone could induce bronchospasm (Schellenberg et al., 1983). Platelet activation mediated by PAF-acether is expressed by granule exocytosis. Compounds able to inhibit platelet degranulation also impaired the bronchoconstriction induced by antigen or PAF-acether (Vargaftig & Benveniste, 1983). In the rat, whose platelets have no demonstrable PAF-acether receptors, the intravenous injection of this phospholipid mediator was unable to provoke bronchoconstriction (Vargaftig & Benveniste, 1983). In the context of the eosinophil participation to bronchial hyperreactivity and tissue damage, it has been reported that platelet depletion reduced PAF-acether and allergen-mediated eosinophil infiltration into the lungs of normal and allergic animals respectively (Lellouch-Tubiana et al., 1988).

The participation of platelet degranulation is also suggested by experiments showing the release of platelet-derived mediators during allergic reactions. Both in animals and in man, allergic challenge or asthmatic shock - but not the non-allergic bronchoconstriction mediated by methacholine - has been shown to induce the release into plasma of platelet specific proteins, such as platelet factor 4 (Knauer et al., 1981) and ß-thromboglobulin (Gresele et al., 1982). These increases however vary widely from patients to patients and are not observed by all investigators (Greer et al., 1984 ; Durham et al., 1985). Yet in the bronchoalveolar lavage of asthmatics, significant elevations of ß-thromboglobulin and of fibrinopeptide-A were measured during the early and late phase response to allergen challenge (Metzger et al., 1985).

Although suggestive of the participation of platelets in the allergic drama, all the more so since platelets could be generated in the lung vasculature (Trowbrige et al., 1981), platelet activation was for long believed to occur indirectly through the effects of platelet activating factor. PAF is released by a variety of IgE-sensitized cells that express either the high affinity (Fc_ER_I) (mast cells, basophils) or lower affinity (Fc_ER_{II}) (macrophages, eosinophils), receptor for IgE, but PAF is also released by cells that do not bind IgE such as neutrophils and stimulated endothelial cells, and activated platelets themselves are known to generate PAF (Barnes et al., 1988).
The demonstration that platelets can damage parasite parasite targets <u>in vitro</u> in IgE antibody-dependent cytotoxicity reactions (Joseph et al., 1983 ; Haque et al., 1985) has opened the question of the direct participation of platelets in IgE-dependent allergic responses.

THE IgE Fc RECEPTOR OF PLATELETS

The binding of IgE to platelets is shown either by immunofluorescent flow cytometry with a monoclonal anti-IgE antibody or by using ^{125}I-labeled IgE myeloma protein, with approximately 6,000 sites on platelets and an average affinity constant of about 3.3×10^7 M^{-1} (Joseph et al., 1986). The binding of IgE is however restricted to a fraction of rat or human platelets, ranging from 10-20 % in controls, and up to 50 % in schistosome-infected rats or allergic patients (Joseph et al., 1986 ; Cines et al., 1986).

These findings, which indicate that the IgE Fc receptor on platelets differs from the classical, high affinity receptor of mast cells and basophils (Fc_ER_I), are however similar to the range of affinities reported for the binding of IgE to the corresponding receptors of monocytes/macrophages and eosinophils. The concept of similar receptors for IgE on platelet, eosinophil, and mononuclear phagocyte subsets is strenghtened by the demonstration of their common antigenicity, as shown by the use of polyclonal or monoclonal (BB10) antibodies. In particular, such anti-IgE receptor antibodies specifically inhibited the binding of radiolabeled IgE, but not of IgG (Joseph et al., 1986 ; Capron et al., 1986b). Purification and subsequent gel analysis of the platelet IgE receptor has provided evidence of two subunits of 43 kDa and 30 kDa, the latter differing from the smaller subunit in eosinophils and monocytes generally identified as a 23-25 kDa molecule (Capron et al., 1986b), and thought to be a breakdown product of the 43 kDa glycoprotein. Genes encoding for this class of IgE Fc receptors have been cloned and, although studies on molecular structure indicate a close homology between Fc_ER_{II} on inflammatory cells and Fc_ER_{II}/CD23 on B cells, there are now emerging indications of some degree of post-transcriptional heterogeneity among the second class of receptors for IgE (Dessaint et al., 1990).

An interesting finding has been the demonstration of the association of Fc_ER_{II} with adhesive molecules on the cell surface. In the case of platelets, those from patients with Glanzman's thrombasthenia, which partially (type II) or totally (type I) lack gp IIb/IIIa complexes, are also partially or totally deficient in Fc_ER_{II} and cannot be triggered into cytotoxic effectors by IgE. The same situation can be mimicked in normal platelets by using anti-IIb/IIIa polyclonal or monoclonal antibodies. The binding of radiolabelled IgE, but not of IgG, and the killing capacities are significantly inhibited by the preincubation of normal platelets with such antibodies (Ameisen et al., 1986). Besides the hypothesis of a sterical association or a molecular community between the gp IIb/IIIa complex, a receptor of the integrin superfamily, and the IgE Fc receptor, the possibility that the gpIIb/IIIa complex could work as a switch for platelet activation or deactivation deserves consideration, especially so since the presence of gpIIb/IIIa on other leukocyte populations has been suggested and is presently debated (Gogstad et al., 1984). Whereas platelets from patients with Glanzmann's thrombasthenia selectively fail to express both the gpIIb/IIIa complex and the IgE Fc receptor, the monocytes from the thrombasthenic patients however bind IgE normally and kill parasites efficiently. Similarly, anti-gpIIb/IIIa polyclonal and monoclonal antibodies, which inhibit both binding of IgE and IgE-mediated cytotoxicity in normal platelets, do not interfere with the capacity of normal monocytes to interact with IgE (Ameisen et al., 1986). However, inhibition of binding of anti-Fc_ER_{II} (BB10) monoclonal to eosinophils by peptides containing the tripeptide sequence Arg-Gly-Asp (RGD) common to a number of molecules that bind to the integrin family of receptors (Grangette et al., 1989) opens fascinating perspectives on the possible intersection between Fc_ER_{II} on inflammatory cells and the adhesive protein (integrin) superfamily.

The expression of Fc_ER_{II} by platelets, a property of a small subset of thrombocytes, is substantially increased in parasitic disease or allergic disorders, all situations associated with elevated IgE levels, and the "up-regulation" of the Fc_ER_{II} is generally attributed to slowering of receptor degradation consecutive to IgE binding. However, other extracellular factors than the ligand itself, appear to control Fc_ER_{II} expression. Several cytokines indeed directly or indirectly modify the size of the Fc_ER_{II}-positive cell pools. It has been shown that platelets exposed to recombinant human immune interferon increase their expression of Fc_ER_{II} (Pancré et al., 1988). This demonstration of the interrelationship between IFNγ and platelet function has to be related to the work of Molinas et al. (1987) who have demonstrated that human IFNγ binds to an estimate of 150-200 high-affinity specific receptors on human platelets with an apparent equilibrium dissociation constant (Kd) of 2×10^{-10} M. In fact, the control of Fc_ER_{II} on inflammatory cells seems to vary according to the cell population, and IFNγ does not increase Fc_ER_{II} expression by eosinophils contrary to its up-regulating effect on platelets and monocytes/macrophages (Dessaint et al., 1990).

IgE-DEPENDENT ACTIVATION OF PLATELETS THROUGH THEIR Fc_ER_{II}

The concept that platelets can participate directly in some IgE-mediated processes has arisen from the demonstration of the involvement of this cell population in IgE-dependent killing of parasites (Joseph et al., 1983 ; Haque et al., 1985). These effector functions were induced by the binding of parasite-specific IgE antibodies to their Fc_ER_{II}, and expressed by the excretion of cytocidal mediators as a consequence of the cross-linking of occupied receptors, through bound IgE antibodies by their interaction with their specific ligands (i.e. parasitic antigens, or, experimentally, anti-IgE antibody). In contrast with mononuclear phagocytes and eosinophils, which normally required a close contact with the target parasites, platelets could express their cytotoxic properties across filters by the release of soluble mediators (Joseph et al., 1985). Another parameter of platelet activation was associated with IgE-dependent activation : the generation of oxygen metabolites, expressed by a chemiluminescence in the presence of luminol, luciferin, and peroxidase. Platelet reactivity could be observed in the very conditions inducing parasite killing, i.e. with parasitic antigens on platelets collected from patients with schistosomiasis or filariasis. IgE-stimulated platelets induce significant catalase-inhibitable chemiluminescence, reaching its maximum between 3 and 5 minutes after the stimulus and decaying slowly ; spin trapping of hydroxyl radicals by reaction with stable nitroxyl radicals, and the generation of electron paramagnetic resonance (EPR) spectra have allowed the identification of °OH radicals after IgE-dependent activation (Cesbron et al., 1987).
This activation pathway appears strictly dependent on IgE and Fc_ER_{II} and is inhibited by the monoclonal antibody (BB10) to Fc_ER_{II} and, as mentioned previously, by antibodies to gpIIb or gpIIIa (Joseph et al., 1983 ; 1985 ; Ameisen et al., 1986). This IgE-dependent activation pathway appears to be selective, since no exocytose of serotonin nor platelet aggregation is elicited, when on the opposite IgG-dependent activation triggers these effects, but no parasite attrition nor oxygen radical production. However, both IgG and IgE-dependent signals can result in histamine release (M.M. Divry & J.P. Dessaint, unpublished).

EVIDENCE FOR IgE ANTIBODY-DEPENDENT PLATELET ACTIVATION IN ALLERGY

A first series of observations pointing to the cytophilic occupation of Fc_ER_{II} on platelets by IgE antibodies and the possibility to activate platelets through the IgE-dependent pathway is brought by *ex vivo* studies : platelets from allergic asthmatics, with mite or grass pollen-positive skin prick tests and high levels of specific IgE, generate cytotoxic mediators and reactive oxygen intermediates in the presence of the appropriate purified allergen. Alternatively, anti-human IgE antibodies induce the same response, whereas anti-IgG has no effect in this system. The IgE-dependence of these *ex vivo* studies is confirmed by the study of platelets from healthy controls incubated with the serum from the same allergic asthmatics ; subsequent addition of the relevant allergen, or of anti-IgE antibodies, induces the same platelet response as in platelets from allergic patients, and this is inhibited completely by previous immunoadsorption of IgE from the serum, or by preincubation of platelets with myeloma IgE, or with anti-Fc_ER_{II} polyclonal or monoclonal (BB10) antibodies (Joseph *et al.*, 1986).

Another example is provided by platelets from individuals sensitized to Hymenoptera venom, in whom platelets can be induced directly by the purified allergen (yellow-jacket or honey-bee venom) to produce cytocidal factors and oxygen metabolites, previously shown to be a characteristic feature of activation by IgE (Tsicopoulos *et al.*, 1988b). The allergen, anti-IgE or its F(ab')2 fragment could also trigger the release of histamine from platelets in such patients (Divry & Dessaint, unpublished observation).

A second series of evidence for the involvement of platelets in IgE-dependent reactions is provided by the demonstration that anti-allergic drugs formerly considered as mast cell stabilizers such as disodium cromoglycate (DSCG) also inhibit discharge of bioactive mediators by platelets (Tsicopoulos *et al.*, 1988a). Similar drugs such as nedocromil sodium (Joseph *et al.*, 1989) and cetirizine (De Vos *et al.*, 1989) also inhibit IgE-dependent platelet activation.

Finally, supportive evidence can be drawn from the studies of changes in platelet responses after specific desensitization of allergic patients. Indeed, after effective desensitization, the *ex vivo* reactivity of platelets to the allergen was significant decreased, which points to a close correlation between IgE-dependent activation of platelets and the clinical response of the patients to the allergen (Tsicopoulos *et al.*, 1988b).

This series of observations clearly indicates that platelets have the capacity to be activated, during local or systemic allergic reactions, by the interaction of membrane-bound IgE with the allergen. One therefore can consider that this strictly circulating Fc_ER_{II}-bearing cell subpopulation can be involved in the network of inflammatory cells which participate in the pathophysiology of allergic reactions. Although the contribution of platelets to systemic anaphylaxis is easy to postulate, the modalities of their interaction with the allergen during localized tissue anaphylactic reactions can only be hypothesized. This might be taking place in the vessels , with allergens leaking into the blood, or at the endothelium-tissue interface, through gaps forming between endothelial cells, particularly as a result of anaphylactic discharge of vasoactive amines by basophils or mast cells. In addition, platelet migration from the vessel into the bronchial musculature has been reported (Lellouch-Tubiana *et al.*, 1985).

CYTOKINE CONTROL OF IgE-DEPENDENT RESPONSE OF PLATELETS

The favourite hypothesis associated with desensitization mechanisms is the involvement of blocking IgG antibodies, produced in the course of the immunotherapy. In fact, an increase of the IgG antibodies could be observed in most of the patients studied. However, an alternative and interesting suggestion could be formulated, based on the observation of the control of platelet-dependent parasite killing and of the chemiluminescence response by lymphokines produced by mitogen- or antigen-stimulation of T lymphocytes. Indeed, IgE-dependent platelet cytotoxicity response was shown to be potentiated by IFNγ (Pancré *et al.*, 1987), TNFβ and to a lesser extend TNFα (Damonneville *et al.*, 1988). Contrariwise, ConA and antigen-stimulated CD4$^-$CD8$^+$ T lymphocytes release a factor able to inhibit the IgE-, IFNγ, and TNFβ-dependent platelet cytotoxcity toward the parasitic larvae. The production of oxygen metabolites by platelets in an IgE-antiIgE reaction was likewise strongly inhibited by the lymphokine (Pancré et al., 1986 ; 1989). This platelet activity suppressive lymphokine (PASL) is a 15-20 kDa acidic peptide which has recently been cloned. Taken together, these results demonstrates that in addition to IgE, antigen-specific T lymphocytes could activate platelets through IFNγ and TNFβ production, while a feedback regulation of the platelet immune functions is under the control of $CD4^-CD8^+$ stimulated T cells through PASL generation.

Accordingly, a follow-up study of hymenoptera venom-sensitive patients before and during rush-desensitization showed that, in parallel with abrogation of IgE antibody-dependent platelet responses, the treatment induces a switch in the lymphokine control of this response : before desensitization, T cell supernatants from in vitro cultures with the allergen could amplify IgE-dependent platelet activity, whereas 7 weeks after initiation of rush immunotherapy, allergen exposure led to release by T cells of inhibitory factors of platelet response to IgE (Ledru et al., 1988). A circulating suppressive factor with biological and chemical properties similar to PASL could be identified in the serum from patients receiving venom immunotherapy (Tsicopoulos et al., 1989). Thus, the acute changes in the immunophenotypes of circulating $CD4^+$ T cells (Tilmant et al., 1989) and increased proliferative response of $CD8^+$ cells to the allergen (Hsieh, 1984) induced by rush desensitization appear to be associated with a switch in the secretion of the lymphokines that control IgE-dependent platelet activation.

ASPIRIN-INDUCED ASTHMA

This common hypersensitivity does not appear to depend on IgE antibody to non-steroïdal anti-inflamatory drugs (NSAIDs). Yet, platelets from aspirin-sensitive asthmatics (ASA), exhibited anti-parasitic properties - and generated chemiluminescence - by the only addition of aspirin or other cyclooxygenase-inhibiting NSAIDs, such as indomethacin or flurbiprofen (Ameisen et al., 1985). The involvement of an IgE-dependent mechanism was ruled out by the absence of inhibitory effect of anti-Fc_ER_{II} antibody, and by the inability of serum from such patients to passively sensitize platelets from healthy donors. This abnormal responsiveness to NSAIDs was restricted, among inflammatory cells, to platelets : indeed, the patients' monocytes, which could kill parasites and generate chemiluminescence when triggered by IgE-dependent stimuli, did not express any cytocidal properties nor generate chemiluminescence in the presence of NSAIDs. It was shown that sodium salicylate and salicylamide, which are structurally related to aspirin but have no cyclooxygenase-inhibiting activity and do not induce adverse reactions, had no activating effect on platelets from ASA-patients. Furthermore, when platelets from patients with aspirin-induced asthma were incubated with salicylate before the addition of the NSAIDs, a highly significant inhibition of the activation induced by the drugs was observed. The preventive effect of salicylate was selective, since it did not affect the IgE-dependent triggering of the platelets. Thus, in aspirin-sensitive patients, NSAIDs abnormally trigger the specialized pathway normally dependent on IgE-dependent Fc_ER_{II} cross-linking that leads platelets to produce oxygen radicals. Interestingly, in aspirin-induced asthma, platelets lost their property to generate cytocidal factors after induction of a refractory period obtained by daily ingestion of high doses of aspirin. In this syndrome, platelets were deactivated at the very period when patients were unsensitive to the drug, and they recovered full reactivity as soon as the treatment with aspirin has been discontinued and patients were sensitive again (Ameisen et al., 1985).

CONCLUDING REMARKS

In the light of the observations reported here, it appears that if a definitive demonstration of a platelet involvement in allergic reactions and in their associated inflammatory effects is not acquired, the participation of these blood constituents in the physiopathological process is largely documented and can be considered now as more than an hypothesis. It should be unrealistic to stress only on platelets as responsible for such hypersensitivity reactions. Their reactivity has to be considered in the general concept of cellular networks, with the recruitement and IgE-antibody dependent activation of a large variety of Fc_ER_{II}-bearing cell populations, among which especially eosinophils, with the implication of endothelial cells, and, possibly cells from the peripheral nervous system. In this respect, it has been shown that the neuropeptide substance P could directly trigger platelet activation (Damonneville et al., 1988). Interestingly, the sequence of substance P actively involved in platelet activation is confined to the N-terminal region of the molecule, as for stimulation of T lymphocyte proliferation, whereas the C-terminal portion induces histamine release from mast cells. The construction of various synthetic peptides derived from the sequence of substance P has allowed the demonstration that the sequence 5-11 corresponded to the most active site of the molecule. In competition experiments, it has been also demonstrated that platelet activation by substance P can be inhibited by IgE itself and that the competitive inhibition observed might be related to the existence of limited but significant conformational homology between the primary structure of substance P and the binding domain of the E chain.

These examples, which do not represent an exhaustive list of the molecules potentially involved in platelet activation, provide evidence, in the framework of allergic disorders, that relevant stimuli such as IgE antibody, IgE-binding factors, or substance P can directly participate to platelet activation and to secretion of platelet-derived mediators. Similarly, in drug hypersensitivity, pseudoallergic reactions can be triggered at least in part by abnormal stimulation of platelets. Alltogether, such observations also focus to new therapeutical approaches in the control of allergic diseases and associated inflammatory disorders.

REFERENCES

Ameisen, J.C., Capron, A., Joseph, M., Maclouf, J., Vorng, H., Pancré, V., Fournier, E., Wallaert, B., and Tonnel, A.B. (1985): Aspirin-sensitive asthma: abnormal platelet response to drugs inducing asthmatic attacks. Int. Archs Allergy appl. Immunol. 78: 438-448.

Ameisen, J.C., Joseph, M., Caen, J.P., Kusnierz, J.P., Capron, M., Boizard, B., Wautier, J.L., Levy-Toledano, S., Vorng, H., and Capron, A. (1986): A role forglycoprotein IIb-IIIa complex in the binding of IgE to human platelets and platelet IgE-depenent cytotoxic functions. Brit. J. Haematol. 64: 21-32.

Barnes, P.J., Chung, K.F., and Page, C.P. (1988): Platelet-activating factor as a mediator of allergic disease. J. Allergy Clin. Immunol. 81: 919-934.

Capron, A., Dessaint, J.P., Capron, M., Joseph, M., Ameisen, J.C, and Tonnel, A.B. (1986a): From parasites to allergy: a second receptor for IgE. Immunology Today 7: 15-18.

Capron, M., Jouault, T., Prin, L., Joseph, M., Ameisen, J.C., Butterworth, A.E., Papin, J.P., Kusnierz, J.P., and Capron, A. (1986b): Functional study of a monoclonal antibody to IgE Fc receptor (Fc_ER_2) of eosinophils, platelets, and macrophages. J. Exp. Med. 164: 72-89.

Cesbron, J.Y., Capron, A., Vargaftig, B.B., Lagarde, M., Pincemail, J., Braquet, P., Taelman, H., and Joseph, M. (1987): Platelets mediate the action of diethylcarbamazine on microfilariae. Nature 325: 533-536.

Cines, D.B., van derKeyl, H., and Levinson, A.I. (1986): In vitro binding of an IgE protein to human platelets. J. Immunol. 136: 3433-3440.

Damonneville, M., Joseph, M., Auriault, C., Gras-Masse, H., Tartar, A., Joseph, M., and Capron, A. (1988): The neuropeptide substance P stimulates the effector functions of platelets. The neuropeptide substance P stimulates the effector functions of platelets. In Proc. 9th Eur. Immunol. Meeting Roma, Sept. 14-17, 1988 (Abstract).

Damonneville, M., Wietzerbin, J., Pancré, V., Joseph, M., Capron, A., and Auriault, C. (1988): Recombinant tumor necrosis factor mediate platelets cytotoxicity to Schistosoma mansoni larvae. J. Immunol. 140: 3962-3965.

Day, R.P., Behrmann, S., Dolovich, J., and Hargreave, F.E. (1975): Inflammatory effects of leukocytes and platelets. J. Allergy Clin. Immunol. 55: 87-92.

Denjean, A., Arnoux, B., Masse, R., Lockart, A., and Benveniste, J. (1983): Acute effects of intratracheal administration of platelet-activating factor in baboons. J. Appl. Physiol. 55: 799-804.

Dessaint, J.P., Capron, M., and Capron, A.: IgE antibody-mediated release of mediators by mononuclear phagocytes, eosinophils, and platelets. Fc Receptors and the Action of Antibodies (in press).

Devos, C., Joseph, M., Leprevost, C., Vorng, H., Tomassini, M., Capron, M., and Capron, A. (1989): Inhibition of human eosinophil chemotaxis and of the IgE-dependent stimulation of human blood platelets by Cetirizine. Int. Archs Allergy appl. Immunol. 88: 212-215.

Durham, S.R., Dawes, J., and Kay, A.B. (1985): Platelets in asthma. Lancet ii: 36.

Gateau, O., Arnoux, B., Deriaz, H., Viars, P., and Benveniste, J. (1984): Acute effects of intratracheal administration of PAF-acether in humans. Am. Rev. Resp. Dis. 133: 129A.

Gogstad, G., Heltland, O., Solum, N.O., and Prydz, H. (1983): Monocytes and platelets share the glycoproteins IIb and IIIb that are absent from both cells in Glanzmann's thrombasthenia type I. Biochem. J. 214: 331-337.

Grangette, C., Gruart, V., Ouaissi, M.A., Rizvi, F., Delespesse, G., Capron, A., and Capron, M. (1989): IgE receptor on human eosinophils (Fc$_E$R$_{II}$). Comparison with B cell CD23 and association with an adhesion molecule. J. Immunol. 143: 3580-3588.

Greer, I.A., Winter, J.H., Gaffney, D., McLoughlin, K., Belch, J.J.F., Boyd, G., and Forbes, C.D. (1984): Platelets in asthma. Lancet ii: 1479.

Gresele, P., Todisco, T., Merante, F., and Nenci, G.G. (1982): Platelet activation and allergic asthma. N. Engl. J. Med. 306: 549.

Haque, A., Cuna, W., Bonnel, B., Capron, A., and Joseph, M. (1985): Platelet-mediated killing of larvae from different filarial species in the presence of *Dipetalonema viteae* stimulated IgE antibodies. Parasite Immunol. 7: 517-526.

Hsieh, K.H. (1985): Altered interleukin-2 (IL-2) production and responsiveness after hyposensitization to house dust. J. Allergy Clin. Immunol. 76: 188-194.

Joseph, M., Auriault, C., Capron, A., Vorng, H., and Viens, P. (1983): A new function for platelets : IgE-dependent killing of schistosomes. Nature 303: 810-812.

Joseph, M., Auriault, C., Capron, M., Ameisen, J.C., Pancré, V., Torpier, G., Kusnierz, J.P., Ovlaque, G., and Capron, A. (1985): IgE-dependent platelet cytotoxicity against helminths. Adv. Exp. Med. Biol. 184: 23-31.

Joseph, M., Capron, A., Ameisen, J.C., Capron, M., Vorng, H., Pancré, V., Kusnierz, J.P., and Auriault, C. (1986): The receptor for IgE on blood platelets. Eur. J. Immunol. 16: 306-312.

Joseph, M., Thorel, T., Tsicopoulos, A., Tonnel, A.B., and Capron, A. (1989): Nedocromil sodium inhibition of IgE-mediated activation of human mononuclear phagocytes and platelets from asthmatics. Drugs 37: 32-36.

Knauer, K.A., Lichtenstein, L.M., Adkinson, N.F., and Fish, J.E. (1981): Platelet activation during antigen-induced airway reactions in asthmatic subjects. N. Engl. J. Med. 304: 1404-1407.

Ledru, E., Pestel, J., Tsicopoulos, A., Joseph, M., Wallaert, B., Tonnel, A.B., and Capron, A. (1988): Lymphocyte-mediated regulation of platelet activation during desensitization in patients with hymenoptera venom hypersensitivity. Clin. exp. Immunol. 73: 198-203.

Lellouch-Tubiana, A., Lefort, S., Pirotsky, E., Vargaftig, B., and Pfiser, A. (1985): Ultrastructural evidence for extravascular platelet recruitement in the lung upon intravenous injection of PAF to guinea pig. Brit. J. Exp. Pathol. 66: 345-355.

Lellouch-Tubiana, A., Lefort, J., Simon, M.T., Pfister, A., and Vargaftig, B.B. (1988): Eosinophil recruitment into guinea pig lungs after PAF-acether and allergen administration. Modulation by prostacyclin, platelet depletion, and selective antagonists. Am. Rev. Respir. Dis. 137: 948-953.

Metzger, W.J., Hunninghake, G.W., and Richerson, H.B. (1985): Late asthmatic response: inquiry into mechanisms and significance. Clin. Rev. Allergy 3: 145-165.

Molinas, F.C., Wietzerbin, J., and Falcoff, E. (1987) Human platelets possess receptors for a lymphokine : demonstration of high specific receptors for Hu IFNγ. J. Immunol. 138: 802-806.

Morley, J., Page, C.P., and Sanjar, S. (1984): The platelet in asthma. Lancet ii: 1142-1144.

Oxholm, P., and Winther, K. (1986) Thrombocyte involvement in immune inflammatory reactions. Allergy 41: 1-10.

Pancré, V., Auriault, C., Joseph, M., Cesbron, J.Y., Kusnierz, J.P., and Capron, A. (1986) A suppressive lymphokine of platelet cytotoxic functions. J. Immunol. 137: 585-591.

Pancré, V., Joseph, M., Capron, A., Delanoye, A., Vorng, H., and Auriault, C. (1989): Characterization of a suppressive factor of platelet cytotoxic functions in human and rat schistosomiasis *mansoni*. Clin. exp. Immunol. 76: 417-421.

Pancré, V., Joseph, M., Capron, A., Wietzerbin, J., Kusnierz, J.P., Vorng, H., and Auriault, C. (1988): Recombinant human immune interferon induces increased IgE receptor expression on human platelets. Eur. J. Immunol. 18: 829-832.

Pancré, V., Joseph, M., Mazingue, C., Wietzerbin, J., Capron, A., and Auriault, C. (1987): Induction of platelet cytotoxic functions by lymphokines : role of gamma interferon. J. Immunol. 138: 4490-4495.

Pinckard, R.N., Halonen, M., Palmer, J.D., Butler, C., Shaw, J.O., and Henson, P.M. (1977): Intravascular aggregation and pulmonary sequestration of platelets during IgE-induced systemic anaphylaxis in the rabbit: abrogation of lethal anaphylactic shock by platelet depletion. J. Immunol. 119: 2185-2193.

Schellenberg, R.R., Walker, B., and Snyder, F. (1983): Platelet-dependent contraction of human bronchi by platelet-activating factor. J. Allergy Clin. Immunol. 71: 145 (Abstract).

Tilmant, L., Dessaint, J.P., Tsicopoulos, A., Tonnel, A.B., and Capron, A. (1989): Concomittant augmentation of $CD24^+CD45^+$ suppressor inducer subset and diminution of $CD24^+CDw29^+$ diminution during hyposensitization. Clin. exp. Immunol. 767: 13-18.

Trowbridge, E.A., Martin, J.F., and Slater, D.N. (1982): Evidence for a theory of physical fragmentation of megakaryocytes, implying that all platelets are produced in the pulmonary circulation. Thromb. Res. 28: 461-463.

Tsicopoulos, A., Lassalle, P., Joseph, M., Tonnel, A.B., Thorel, T., Dessaint, J.P., and Capron, A. (1988a): Effect of disodium cromoglycate on inflammatory cells bearing the Fc epsilon receptor type II (Fc_ER_{II}). Int. J. Immunopharm. 10: 227-236.

Tsicopoulos, A., Tonnel, A.B., Wallaert, B., Joseph, M., Ameisen, J.C., Ramon, P.H., Dessaint, J.P., and Capron, A. (1988b): Decrease of IgE-dependent platelet activation in Hymenoptera hypersensitivity after specific rush desensitization. Clin. exp. Immunol. 71: 433-438.

Tsicopoulos, A., Tonnel, A.B., Wallaert, B., Joseph, M., Ramon, P.H., and Capron, A. (1989): A circulating suppressive factor of platelet cytotoxic functions after rush immunotherapy in *Hymenoptera* venom hypersensitivity. J. Immunol. 142: 2683-2688.

Vargaftig, B.B., and Benveniste, J. (1983): Platelet-activating factor today. Trends Pharmacol. Sci. 4: 341-350.

Résumé

L'étude des fonctions plaquettaires dans les modèles d'immunité anti-parasitaire a révélé la participation des thrombocytes comme effecteurs dans des réactions de cytotoxicité dépendant d'anticorps anti-parasite de classe IgE. Ces observations ont conduit à la caractérisation sur une fraction des plaquettes sanguines d'un récepteur pour le Fc de cette immunoglobuline (Fc_ER_{II}), avec des propriétés communes aux récepteurs portés par les monocytes/macrophages et les éosinophiles. Sous stimulation IgE dépendante, les plaquettes génèrent non seulement des molécules cytotoxiques mais aussi des radicaux libres et libèrent l'histamine. Chez les patients allergiques, on peut mettre en évidence des réponses significatives des plaquettes à la stimulation IgE-dépendante, qui décroissent lors de la désensibilisation spécifique. Les fonctions plaquettaires IgE-dépendantes sont soumises à une modulation par diverses lymphokines, activatrices (IFN-gamma, TNF-ß) et inhibitrice (PASL : Lymphokine Suppressive de l'Activation Plaquettaire). Ainsi, les modifications de l'équilibre des sous-populations lymphocytaires T induites par la désensibilisation spécifique pourraient contribuer à l'inhibition progressive des réponses des plaquettes à l'IgE chez l'allergique.

Thrombospondin binding by human osteosarcoma cells : relationship to platelet-aggregating activity of osteosarcoma cells

P. Clezardin, E. Alfaro*, J. Grange**, C. Desgranges**, C. Kaplan***, P. Delmas**** and M. Dechavanne

*INSERM U 331-Laboratoire d'Hémobiologie, Faculté de Médecine Alexis Carrel ; INSERM U234, Pavillon F, Hôpital Edouard Herriot****; INSERM U271, cours Albert-Thomas**; Laboratoire d'Immunologie, Centre Régional de Transfusion Sanguine de Gerland*, Lyon et Service d'Immunologie Leuco-Plaquettaire, Institut National de Transfusion Sanguine***, Paris, France*

INTRODUCTION

Thrombospondin is a high molecular mass (450 kDa) glycoprotein composed of three equivalent disulfide-linked chains of 150-160 kDa (Lawler et al., 1982). Each thrombospondin chain is made up of several protease-resistant domains, which bind specifically to heparin, sulfated glycolipids, fibrinogen, fibronectin, collagen, laminin, histidine-rich glycoprotein, plasminogen (reviewed by Lawler, 1986) and osteonectin (Clezardin et al., 1988a). Thrombospondin is a major component of platelet α-granules and thus is secreted when platelets are stimulated with thrombin (Baenziger et al., 1972). The secreted thrombospondin binds to the surface of activated platelets (Wolff et al., 1986) and is involved in platelet aggregation (Leung, 1984; Tuszynski et al., 1988). This glycoprotein is also synthesized by a wide range of cultured cells including fibroblasts (Raugi et al., 1982; Jaffe et al., 1983), monocytes and macrophages (Jaffe et al., 1985), osteoblasts (Gehron-Robey et al., 1989; Clezardin et al., 1989), endothelial (McPherson et al., 1981; Mosher et al., 1982), osteosarcoma (Clezardin et al., 1989), squamous carcinoma (Varani et al., 1986), melanoma (Apelgren et al., 1989) and smooth muscle cells (Raugi et al., 1982). The exact physiological function(s) of thrombospondin in these cells is unknown; however, there is growing evidence that it is involved in cell adhesion (Roberts et al., 1988a; Clezardin et al., 1988b).

Since Gasic et al. (1973) demonstrated that cells from a variety of tumors can induce platelet aggregation in vitro, several different mechanisms have been proposed for the activation of platelets by tumor cells including mechanisms that are dependent on ADP secretion and thrombin generation (Bastida et al., 1981; Bastida et al., 1982) as well as mechanisms involving the presence of a trypsin-sensitive membrane tumor cell protein (Hara et al., 1980;

Lerner *et al.*, 1983) or the formation of a sialolipoprotein complex (Pearlstein *et al.*, 1979). In addition, recent studies have implicated several cell-surface molecules as adhesion receptors during platelet-tumor cell interaction. Among these molecules involved in platelet tumor interaction are membrane glycoproteins Ib (Kitawaga *et al.*, 1989) and IIb/IIIa (Karpatkin *et al.*, 1988; Chopra *et al.*, 1988; Grossi *et al.*, 1989; Kitawaga *et al.*, 1989; Boukerche *et al.*, 1989), von Willebrand factor (Karpatkin *et al.*, 1988), fibronectin (Karpatkin *et al.*, 1988) and laminin (Terranova *et al.*, 1982; Iwamoto *et al.*, 1987). Moreover, thrombospondin has recently been shown to potentiate T241 sarcoma cell lung colonization in mice (Tuszynski *et al.*, 1987). These findings, taken together with the fact that thrombospondin is secreted by osteosarcoma cells, prompted us to examine whether or not it is involved in the platelet-aggregating activity of osteosarcoma cells.

In this study we report that cell surface expression of thrombospondin by osteosarcoma cells directly correlates with the ability of thrombospondin to mediate platelet-tumor cell interaction.

MATERIALS AND METHODS

Materials

Medium 199 was from Eurobio. Pansorbin, a 10% suspension *Staphylococcus aureus* cell preparation, was purchased from Calbiochem. Bovine serum albumin was purchased from Miles Laboratories Inc. (Elkhart). Iodo-Beads were from Pierce Chemical Co. Carrier-free sodium ^{125}I, [^{35}S]Methionine and [^{14}C]methylated proteins used as molecular mass markers were purchased from Amersham. Apyrase (Grade 1) was from Sigma Chemical Co. D-phenylalanyl-L-prolyl-L-arginine chloromethylketone (PPACK) was purchased from Calbiochem.

Cell cultures

Human osteosarcoma cells designated MG-63 and TE-85 were obtained from the American Type Culture Collection. Osteosarcoma cells to be used in aggregation studies were harvested from culture dishes with Ca^{2+}, Mg^{2+}-free Hanks' solution containing 10 mM EGTA. Alternatively osteosarcoma cells were harvested with brief trypsin treatment (0.5 mg/ml). After incubation, EGTA-treated and trypsin-treated cells were diluted with a 5-fold excess of Hanks' solution or M199 medium containing 10% (vol./vol.) fetal calf serum, respectively. Cell suspensions were then centrifuged at 160 x g for 4 min, the supernatants were removed and the cell pellets resuspended in Hanks' solution containing 0.2% (mass/vol.) bovine serum albumin. Cell suspensions had viabilities of approximatively 80 to 90% by trypan blue exclusion.

However, cell viability of osteosarcoma cells decreased rapidly after 60 min. Tumor cells were therefore used as quickly as possible after isolation.

Metabolic labelling of cultured cells

Prior to labelling, cultures of osteosarcoma cells were incubated for 30 min in methionine-free M199 medium. Incorporation was then initiated with fresh methionine-free M199 medium containing [^{35}S]methionine (50 µCi/ml). After an 18-h incubation, the labelled medium was harvested and centrifuged at 10 000 x g to remove cellular debris. The labelled cells were washed once with phosphate-buffered saline then solubilized with lysis buffer (1% Triton X-100, 1% sodium deoxycholate, 1 mM phenylmethylsulfonylfluoride, 17 U aprotinin/ml and 1 mM EDTA in phosphate-buffered saline, pH 7.4) for 1h at 4°C. After solubilization, the lysate was clarified by centrifugation at 10 000 x g.

Immunoprecipitation

The procedure was essentially as previously described (Clezardin *et al.*, 1986). Briefly, the cell lysate and the medium were adsorbed with an equal volume of a 10% suspension (mass/vol.) of *S. aureus* and regularly agitated at room temperature for 30 min. The *S. aureus* was then pelleted by centrifugation and the recovered cell lysate and medium were incubated for 2 h at room temperature with 20 µl of anti-thrombospondin or non-immune serum. After incubation, a 10% suspension of *S. aureus* was added and the mixture was continuously agitated for 30 min at room temperature. The immune complexes were then pelleted by centrifugation (6000 x g) in an Eppendorf microfuge for 3 min, washed once in a buffer (50 mM Tris, 150 mM NaCl, 1 mM EDTA, 1% Triton X-100, 1% sodium deoxycholate, 0.1% SDS, 2 mM phenylmethylsulfonyl fluoride, 17 U aprotinin/ml) containing 0.5% (mass/vol.) bovine serum albumin and twice with the buffer alone. The pellet was then resuspended in sample buffer for gel electrophoresis and heated at 100°C for 5 min.

Gel electrophoresis of immunoprecipitates and fluorography

Immunoprecipitates were electrophoresed on a 6% SDS/polyacrylamide gel by the method of Laemmli. The gels were then processed for fluorography.

Purification and radiolabelling of thrombospondin

Human platelet thrombospondin was purified by Mono Q anion-exchange chromatography (Clezardin *et al.*,1984) and iodinated using immobilized chloramine T on nonporous polystyrene beads (Iodobeads). Free iodine was removed by filtration on a Sephadex G-25 column. [^{125}I]thrombospondin was then repurified on a heparin affinity colum in the presence of 2 mM calcium chloride. The labelled protein appeared intact on a 7.5% SDS/polyacrylamide gel analyzed by autoradiography (results not shown).

Thrombospondin binding assays

Binding assays were performed on confluent monolayers in 24-wells culture dishes as follows. Monolayers were rinsed twice with M199 medium supplemented with 0.2% (mass/vol.) bovine serum albumin. A third wash with serum-free M199 medium containing 0.2% (mass/vol.) bovine serum albumin was left for 30 min at room temperature. After the incubation period, 0.25 ml of fresh M199 medium containing 0.2% (mass/vol.) bovine serum albumin, appropriate amounts of [^{125}I]thrombospondin, with or without 100-fold excess of unlabelled thrombospondin, was added and cells were incubated for the appropriate time (normally 60 min at room temperature). At the end of the incubation, cell layers were washed four times with cold M199 medium containing 0.2% (mass/vol.) bovine serum albumin and solubilized overnight with 1 ml 1 N sodium hydroxide. Solubilized material was removed, and plates were washed with an additional 1 ml of 1 N sodium hydroxide. The radioactivity in the pooled extracts was then determined in a γ-counter. All samples were run in triplicate with parallel cultures used to determine cell numbers. Specific binding was defined as the total radioactivity bound minus the amount bound in the presence of 100-fold excess unlabelled thrombospondin and was adjusted in each experiment to a standard cell number. Each experiment was performed at least three times.

Platelet Aggregation

Platelet-rich plasma was obtained by centrifugation of freshly drawn blood of healthy donors [collected in heparin (10U/ml)] at room temperature for 20 min at 160 x g. The remaining blood was centrifuged at 1500 x g for 15 min to obtain platelet-poor plasma. Platelet-poor plasma was used to calibrate light transmission at 100%. The platelet count in platelet-rich plasma was adjusted to 2×10^8 platelets/ml for each experiment. EDTA- or trypsin-treated osteosarcoma cells (0.5 to 2×10^6 cells/ml) were either preincubated with a anti-thrombospondin polyclonal antibody or directly added to the platelet-rich plasma. The aggregation pattern was then recorded in a Chrono-Log Dual Channel aggregometer at 37°C under continuous stirring.

To study the development of procoagulant activity by osteosarcoma cells, PPACK (10^{-4}M), a synthetic peptide which specifically inhibits thrombin, was incubated with the platelet-rich plasma 2 min. prior to the addition of osteosarcoma cells. Apyrase (130 μg/ml), an ADP scavenger, was added to the platelet-rich plasma immediately prior to the addition of tumor cells.

RESULTS

Immunoprecipitation

To demonstrate the presence of thrombospondin in human MG-63 osteosarcoma cells, immunoprecipitation of the cell lysate and the culture medium were performed using an anti-thrombospondin rabbit polyclonal antibody (Fig. 1). The polyclonal antibody immunoisolated from the cell lysate a single protein band with a molecular mass of 450 kDa under nonreducing conditions (Fig. 1A, lane 1) and of 160 kDa under reducing conditions (Fig. 1B, lane 1). No band corresponding to thrombospondin was seen from precipitates employing nonimmune serum (Fig. 1A and B, lane 2). Immunoprecipitation of thrombospondin from the culture

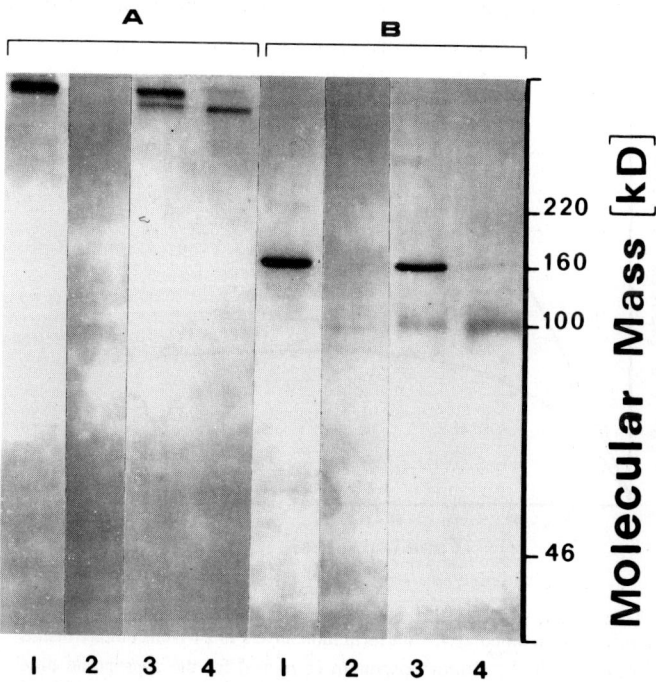

Fig. 1. SDS/polyacrylamide gel electrophoresis analysis of thrombospondin immunoprecipitated from biosynthetically labelled human MG-63 osteosarcoma cells. MG-63 were cultured in the presence of [^{35}S]methionine. After an 18-h incubation thrombospondin was immunoprecipitated from the cells and the culture medium. The immunoprecipitates were analysed by SDS/polyacrylamide gel electrophoresis under nonreducing (A) and reducing (B) conditions and fluorography. Lanes 1 and 2, immunoprecipitation of the cells using an anti-thrombospondin polyclonal antibody and a nonimmune serum, respectively; lanes 3 and 4, immunoprecipitation of the medium using an anti-thrombospondin polyclonal antibody and a nonimmune serum, respectively. (Reproduced from Clezardin et al., 1989).

medium showed that there was no difference in the mobility of cellular and secreted thrombospondin under nonreducing and reducing conditions (Fig. 1A and B, lane 3). In addition to the thrombospondin band immunoisolated from the culture medium, there was another band with a molecular mass of approximately 440 kDa under nonreducing conditions (Fig. 1A, lane 4) and 100 kDa under reducing conditions (Fig. 1B, lane 4). This precipitation is nonspecific as it is present in the precipitates employing nonimmune serum (Fig. 1A and B, lane 4).

Saturation of binding of thrombospondin to MG-63 and TE-85 osteosarcoma cells

Time course binding of [^{125}I]thrombospondin to MG-63 and TE-85 cells in monolayer indicated that binding was time dependent and that there was a plateau after 60 minutes regardless of the osteosarcoma cell line used (Fig. 2). Therefore in all subsequent binding assays [^{125}I]thrombospondin was incubated for 60 minutes.

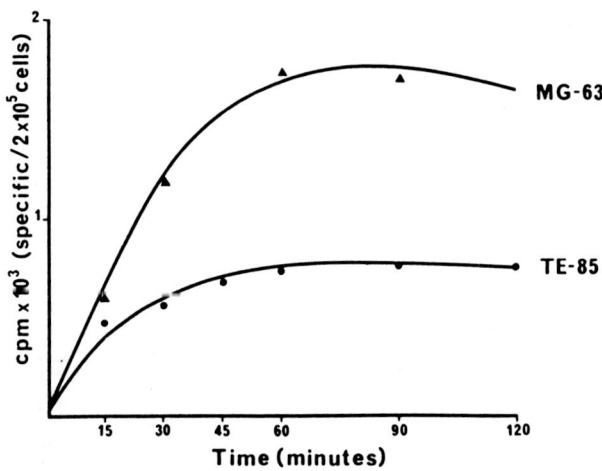

Fig. 2. Time course of [^{125}I]thrombospondin binding to MG-63 and TE-85 osteosarcoma cells in monolayer. Confluent monolayers in 24-wells culture dishes were incubated with [^{125}I]thrombospondin (1 µg/ml) for the appropriate time (from 15 to 120 minutes). At the end of the incubation, cell layers were washed and solubilized with sodium hydroxide. The radioactivity in the extracts was then determined in a γ-counter. Specific binding was defined as the total radioactivity bound minus the amount bound in the presence of 100-fold excess unlabelled thrombospondin and was adjusted to a standard cell number (2×10^5 cells).

[^{125}I]thrombospondin bound to both MG63 and TE-85 osteosarcoma cells in a saturable manner (Fig. 3). In the presence of 100-fold excess unlabelled thrombospondin, binding to MG-63 and TE-85 cells was reduced by 65 to 85%. Analysis of the binding data shown in Fig. 3 by the Scatchard method was consistent with a single class of binding sites (results not shown). However, MG-63 cells had eightfold more thrombospondin binding sites than TE-85 cells (Fig. 3).

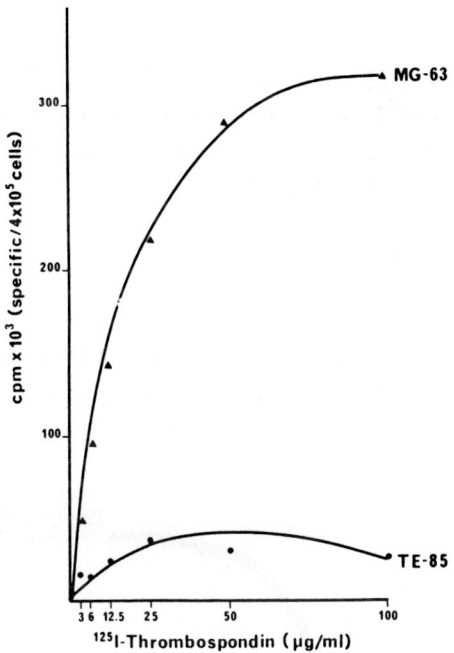

Fig. 3. Saturation of binding of [^{125}I]thrombospondin to MG-63 and TE-85 osteosarcoma cells in monolayer. The experimental procedure was essentially as described in the legend of Fig. 2 except that cell monolayers were incubated with increasing amounts of [^{125}I]thrombospondin (ranged from 3 to 100 µg/ml) for 60 minutes at room temperature. Specific binding was adjusted to 4×10^5 cells.

Platelet aggregation

MG-63 and TE-85 osteosarcoma cells were found to dose dependently induce aggregation of platelets. Increasing the number of tumor cells (0.5 to 2×10^6 cells/ml) caused a progressive increase in platelet aggregation with a maximum effect at 2×10^6 cells/ml (Table 1).

Table 1.

Effect of Osteosarcoma Cell Concentrations on Platelet Aggregation

Cells/ml	Platelet Aggregation (%)	
	MG-63	TE-85
0.5×10^6	13	9
1×10^6	38	24
2×10^6	80	75

MG-63 and TE-85 cells were added to platelet-rich plasma at various cell concentrations, and platelet aggregation response was measured as the peak height of the aggregation curve. Platelet-poor plasma was used to calibrate light transmission at 100%. No increase in aggregation occurred at cell concentrations greater than 2×10^6 cells/ml.

Presence of apyrase (130 μg/ml) or PPACK (10^{-4}M) in platelet-rich plasma had no effect on platelet responses to MG-63 and TE-85 osteosarcoma cells (results not shown). On the other hand, pretreatment of MG-63 cells (1×10^6 cells/ml) with trypsin (0.5 mg/ml) inhibited the subsequent aggregation response to osteosarcoma cells (Fig. 4).

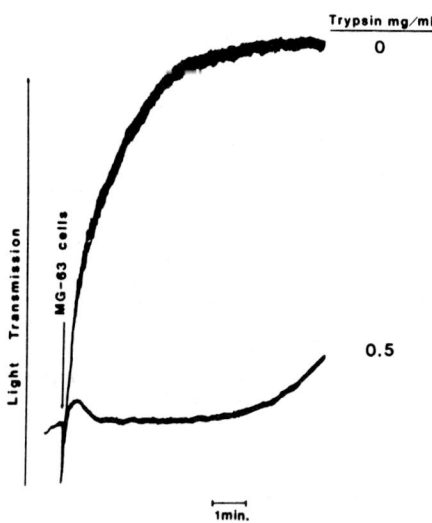

Fig. 4. Effect of trypsin on the platelet-aggregating activity of MG-63 osteosarcoma cells. MG-63 cells in monolayer were harvested from culture dishes with brief trypsin (0.5 mg/ml) or EGTA treatment (10 mM). Trypsin- or EGTA-treated MG-63 cells (1×10^6/ml) were then added to the platelet-rich plasma (2×10^8 cells/ml) and the aggregation pattern recorded.

This inhibition occurred only temporarily as trypsin increased the lag time (between 3 and 10 min.) prior to the onset of aggregation. Supernatants of cell suspensions had no platelet-aggregating activity (results not shown). Similar results were obtained with trypsin-treated TE-85 osteosarcoma cells (results not shown).

Preincubation of MG-63 osteosarcoma cells (1×10^6/ml) with an anti-thrombospondin polyclonal antibody (100 µg/ml) significantly inhibited platelet aggregation (Fig. 5). Similar results were obtained with anti-thrombospondin monoclonal antibody P10 (100 µg/ml) (results not shown).

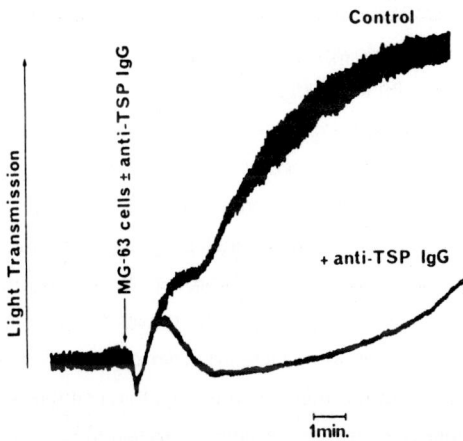

Fig. 5. Platelet-aggregating activity of MG-63 osteosarcoma cells in the presence or absence of an anti-thrombospondin polyclonal antibody (anti-TSP IgG). EGTA-treated MG-63 cells (1×10^6 cells/ml) preincubated with an anti-thrombospondin polyclonal antibody (100 µg/ml) were directly added to the platelet-rich plasma (2×10^8 cells/ml) and the aggregation pattern recorded. Hanks' buffer instead of the anti-thrombospondin antibody was used as control.

In contrast, the anti-thrombospondin polyclonal antibody had no effect on platelet aggregation induced by TE-85 osteosarcoma cells at concentrations which did inhibit the platelet-aggregating activity of MG-63 cells (results not shown). The inhibitory effect of the anti-thrombospondin antibodies was specifically directed toward the platelet-aggregating activity of MG-63 osteosarcoma cells since these antibodies did not affect platelet aggregation induced by collagen or ADP (results not shown).

DISCUSSION

In a recent study we showed by immunoprecipitation techniques that human osteosarcoma cells synthesize and secrete thrombospondin (Clezardin *et al.*, 1989). The present study indicates that osteosarcoma cells bind thrombospondin in a receptor-like fashion. Using [^{125}I]thrombospondin as the ligand, binding to cell monolayers is time- and concentration-dependent, saturable and inhibitable with excess cold thrombospondin. However, we have observed significant variability between the two osteosarcoma cell lines in binding thrombospondin: MG-63 cells has eightfold more thrombospondin binding sites than TE-85 cells. It was recently shown that the capacity of human squamous carcinoma and melanoma cells to synthesize thrombospondin was directly correlated with their ability to bind this glycoprotein (Varani *et al.*, 1986; Riser *et al.*, 1988). It is therefore conceivable that MG-63 osteosarcoma cells synthesized much more thrombospondin than TE-85 osteosarcoma cells.

It has been previously reported that human MG-63 osteosarcoma cells induce aggregation of platelets (Mehta *et al.*, 1987). However, the mechanism(s) by which osteosarcoma cells do induce platelet aggregation as well as the ligand(s) mediating platelet-osteosarcoma interaction are unknown. We find that the platelet-aggregating activity of human MG-63 and TE-85 osteosarcoma cells is closely related to the cell surface, as the supernatants of cell suspensions had no activity and preincubation of osteosarcoma cells with trypsin abolished the aggregating activity of these tumor cells. The activation of platelets by osteosarcoma cells seems therefore to occur via a trypsin-sensitive membrane tumor cell protein. Such a requirement of a trypsin-sensitive surface protein for platelet-aggregating activity was also reported for B16F10 and HM29 melanoma, and for CT26 carcinoma cells (Lerner *et al.*, 1983). Preincubation of MG-63 osteosarcoma cells with an anti-thrombospondin polyclonal antibody inhibits the tumor-platelet interaction as demonstrated by aggregometry. On the other hand, such an antibody does not affect the platelet aggregating activity of TE-85 osteosarcoma cells. Taken together, these results suggest therefore that human osteosarcoma cells which express thrombospondin at their surface do induce platelet-osteosarcoma interaction at least in part by this ligand. Whether the expression of receptors for thrombospondin occurs primarily to allow interaction of osteosarcoma cells with platelets remains to be determined. MG-63 osteosarcoma cells have been shown to express the vitronectin receptor (CD51) (Suzuki *et al.*, 1987) which functions as a thrombospondin receptor on the surface of platelets, endothelial, smooth muscle (Lawler *et al.*, 1988; Lawler & Hynes, 1989) and melanoma cells (Tuszynski *et al.*, 1989). Thrombospondin also binds specifically to proteoglycans (Murphy-Ullrich *et al.*, 1988; Roberts, 1988b), sulfated glycolipids (Roberts, 1988b) and membrane glycoprotein IV (CD36) (Asch *et al.*, 1987; McGregor *et al.*, 1989). Further studies are being undertaken to identify the thrombospondin receptor(s) involved in mediating platelet-osteosarcoma interaction.

This study was supported in part by Grant from the Fondation de France and by Grant 6840 from the Association pour la Recherche contre le Cancer.

REFERENCES

Asch, A.S., Barnwell, J., Silverstein, R.L. & Nachman, R.L. (1987): Isolation of the thrombospondin membrane receptor. *J. Clin. Invest.*, 79, 1054-1061.

Baenziger, N.L., Brodie, G.N. & Majerus, P.W. (1972): Isolation and properties of a thrombin-sensitive protein of human platelets. *J. Biol. Chem.*, 247, 2723-2729.

Bastida, E., Ordinas, A & Jamieson, G.A. (1981): Differing platelet-aggregating effects by two tumor cell lines: absence of role for platelet-derived ADP. *Am. J. Haematol.*, 11, 367-378.

Bastida, E., Ordinas, A., Giardina, S.L. & Jamieson, G.A. (1982): Differentiation of platelet-aggregating effects of human tumor cell lines based on inhibition studies with apyrase, hirudin and phospholipase. *Cancer Res.*, 42, 4348-4352.

Boukerche, H., Berthier-Vergnes, O., Tabone, E., Doré, J.F., Leung, L.L.K. & McGregor, J.L. (1989): Platelet-melanoma cell interaction is mediated by the glycoprotein IIb-IIIa complex. *Blood*, 74, 658-663.

Chopra, H., Hatfield, J.S., Chang, Y.S., Grossi, I.M., Fitzgerald, L.A., O'Gara, C.Y., Marnett, L.J., Diglio, C.A., Taylor, J.D. & Honn, K.V. (1988): Role of tumor cell cytoskeleton and membrane glycoprotein IRGpIIb/IIIa in platelet adhesion to tumor cell membrane and tumor cell-induced platelet aggregation. *Cancer Res.*, 48, 3787-3800.

Clezardin, P., McGregor, J.L., Manach, M., Robert, F., Dechavanne, M. & Clemetson, K.J. (1984): Isolation of thrombospondin released from thrombin-stimulated human platelets by fast protein liquid chromatography on an anion-exchange Mono Q column. *J. Chromatogr.*, 296, 249-256.

Clezardin, P., McGregor, J.L., Lyon, M., Clemetson, K.J. & Huppert, J. (1986): Characterization of two murine monoclonal antibodies (P10,P12) directed against different determinants on human blood platelet thrombospondin. *Eur. J. Biochem.*, 154, 95-102.

Clezardin, P., Malaval, L., Ehrensperger, A.S., Delmas, P., Dechavanne, M. & McGregor, J.L. (1988a): Complex formation of human thrombospondin with osteonectin. *Eur. J. Biochem.*, 175, 275-284.

Clezardin, P., Bourdillon, M.C., Hunter, N.R. & McGregor, J.L. (1988b): Cell attachment and fibrinogen binding properties of platelet and endothelial cell thrombospondin are not affected by structural differences in the 70 and 18 kDa protease-resistant domains. *FEBS Lett.*, 228, 215-218.

Clezardin, P., Jouishomme, H., Chavassieux, P. & Marie, P.J. (1989): Thrombospondin is synthesized and secreted by human osteoblasts and osteosarcoma cells. A model to study the different effects of thrombospondin in cell adhesion. *Eur. J. Biochem.*, 181, 721-726.

Gasic, G.J., Gasic, T.B., Galanti, N., Johnson, T. & Murphy, S. (1973): Platelet-tumor cell interactions in mice: the role of platelets in the spread of malignant disease. *Int. J. Cancer*, 11, 704-718.

Gehron-Robey, P., Young, M.F., Fisher, L.W. & McLain, T.D. (1989): Thrombospondin is an osteoblast-derived component of mineralized extracellular matrix. *J. Cell Biol.*, 108, 719-727.

Grossi, I.M., Fitzgerald, L.A., Umbarger, L.A., Nelson, K.K., Diglio, C.A., Taylor, J.D. & Honn, K.V. (1989): Bidirectional control of membrane expression and/or activation of the tumor cell IRGpIIb/IIIa receptor and tumor cell adhesion by lipoxygenase products of arachidonic acid and linoleic acid. *Cancer Res.*, 49, 1029-1037.

Hara, Y., Steiner, M. & Baldini, M.G. (1980): Characterization of the platelet-aggregating activity of tumor cells. *Cancer Res.*, 40, 1217-1222.

Iwamoto, Y., Robey, F.A., Graf, J., Sasaki, M., Kleinman, H.K., Yamada, Y. & Martin, G.R. (1987): YIGSR, a synthetic laminin pentapeptide, inhibits experimental metastasis formation. *Science*, 238, 1132-1134.

Jaffe, E.A., Ruggiero, J.T., Leung, L.L.K., Doyle, M.J., McKeown-Longo, P.J. & Mosher, D.F. (1983): Cultured human fibroblasts synthesize and secrete thrombospondin and incorporate it into extracellular matrix. *Proc. Natl. Acad. Sci.USA*, 80, 998-1002.

Jaffe, E.A., Ruggiero, J.T. & Falcone, D.J. (1985): Monocyte and macrophages synthesize and secrete thrombospondin. *Blood*, 65, 79-84.

Karpatkin, S., Pearlstein, E., Ambrogio, C. & Coller, B.S. (1988) Role of adhesive proteins in platelet tumor interaction in vitro and metastasis formation in vivo. *J. Clin. Invest.*, 81, 1012-1019.

Kitawaga, H., Yamamoto, N., Yamamoto, K., Tanoue, K., Kosaki, K. & Yamazaki, H. (1989): Involvement of platelet membrane glycoprotein Ib and glycoprotein IIb/IIIa complex in thrombin-dependent and -independent platelet aggregations induced by tumor cells. *Cancer Res.*, 49, 537-541.

Lawler, J.W., Chao, F.C. & Cohen, C.M. (1982): Evidence for calcium-sensitive structure in platelet thrombospondin. Isolation and partial characterization of thrombospondin in the presence of calcium. *J. Biol. Chem.*, 257, 12257-12265.

Lawler, J.W. (1986): The structural and functional properties of thrombospondin. *Blood*, 67, 1197-1209.

Lawler, J., Weinstein, R. & Hynes, R.O. (1988): Cell attachment to thrombospondin: the role of Arg-Gly-Asp, calcium and integrin receptors. *J. Cell Biol.*, 107, 2351-2361.

Lawler, J. & Hynes, R.O. (1989): An integrin receptor on normal and thrombasthenic platelets that binds thrombospondin. *Blood*, 74, 2022-2027.

Lerner, W.A., Pearlstein, E., Ambrogio & C., Karpatkin, S. (1983): A new mechanism for tumor-induced platelet aggregation. Comparison with mechanisms shared by other tumors with possible pharmacological strategy toward prevention of metastases. *Int. J. Cancer*, 31, 463-469.

Leung, L.L.K. (1984): Role of thrombospondin in platelet aggregation. *J. Clin. Invest.*, 74, 1764-1772.

McGregor, J.L., Catimel, B., Parmentier, S., Clezardin, P., Dechavanne, M. & Leung, L.L.K. (1989): Rapid purification and partial characterization of human platelet glycoprotein IIIb. Interaction with thrombospondin and its role in platelet aggregation. *J. Biol. Chem.*, 264, 501-506.

McPherson, J., Sage, H. & Bornstein, P. (1981): Isolation and characterization of a glycoprotein secreted by aortic endothelial cells in culture. Apparent identity with platelet thrombospondin. *J. Biol. Chem.*, 256, 11330-11336.

Metha, P., Lawson, D., Ward, M.B., Kimura, A. & Gee, A. (1987): Effect of human tumor cells on platelet aggregation: Potential relevance to pattern metastasis. *Cancer Res.*, 47, 3115-3117.

Mosher, D.F., Doyle, M.J. & Jaffe, E.A. (1982): Synthesis and secretion of thrombospondin by cultured human endothelial cells. *J. Biol. Chem.*, 93, 343-348.

Murphy-Ullrich, J.E., Westrick, L.G., Esko, J.D. & Mosher, D.F. (1988): Altered metabolism of thrombospondin by chinese hamster ovary cells defective in glycosaminoglycan synthesis. *J. Biol. Chem.*, 263, 6400-6406.

Pearlstein, E., Cooper, L. & Karpatkin, S. (1979): Extraction and characterization of a platelet-aggregating material from SV-40-transformed mouse 3T3 fibroblasts. *J. Lab. Clin. Med.*, 93, 332-344.

Raugi, G.J., Mumby, S.M., Abbott-Brown, D. & Bornstein, P. (1982): Thrombospondin: synthesis and secretion by cells in culture. *J. Cell Biol.*, 95, 351-354.

Riser, B.L., Varani, J., O'Rourke, K. & Dixit, V.M. (1988): Thrombospondin binding by human squamous carcinoma and melanoma cells: Relationship to biological activity. *Exp. Cell Res.*, 174, 319-329.

Roberts, D.D. & Ginsburg, V. (1988a): Sulfated glycolipids and cell adhesion. *Arch. Biochem. Biophys.*, 267, 405-415.

Roberts, D.D. (1988b): Interactions of thrombospondin with sulfated glycolipids and proteoglycans of human melanoma cells. *Cancer Res.*, 48, 6785-6793.

Suzuki, S., Argraves, S., Arai, H., Languino, L.R., Pierschbacher, M.D. & Ruoshlati, E. (1987): Amino acid sequence of the vitronectin receptor alpha subunit and comparative expression of adhesion receptor mRNAs. *J. Biol. Chem.*, 262, 14080-14085.

Terranova, V.P., Liotta, L.A., Russo, R.G. & Martin, G.R. (1982): Role of laminin in the attachment and metastasis of murine tumor cells. *Cancer Res.*, 42, 2265-2269.

Tuszynski, G.P., Gasic, T.B., Rothman, V.L., Knudsen, K.A. & Gasic, G.J. (1987): Thrombospondin, a potentiator of tumor cell metastasis. *Cancer Res.*, 47, 4130-4133.

Tuszynski, G.P., Rothman, V.L., Murphy, A., Siegler, K. & Knudsen, K.A. (1988): Thrombospondin promotes platelet aggregation. *Blood*, 72, 109-115.

Tuszynski, G.P., Karczewski, J., Smith, L., Murphy, A., Rothman, V.L. & Knudsen, K.A. (1989): The GPIIb-IIIa-like complex may function as a human melanoma cell adhesion receptor for thrombospondin. *Exp. Cell Res.*, 182, 473-481.

Varani, J., Dixit, V.M., Fligiel, S.E.G., McKeever, P.E. & Carey, T.E. (1986): Thrombospondin-induced attachment and spreading of human squamous carcinoma cells. *Exp. Cell Res.*, 167, 376-390.

Wolff, R., Plow, E.F. & Ginsberg, M.H. (1986): Interaction of thrombospondin with resting and stimulated human platelets. *J. Biol. Chem.*, 261, 6840-6846.

SUMMARY

Thrombospondin (TSP) is a 450 kDa glycoprotein synthesized and secreted by MG-63 osteosarcoma cells (P.Clezardin et al., Eur.J.Biochem., 1989). In this study, we have explored the expression of TSP to the surface of MG-63 cells and investigated the involvement of TSP in the platelet-aggregating activity of these tumor cells. Binding of (^{125}I) TSP to MG-63 cells in monolayer was time and concentration-dependent, saturable and inhibitable with excess cold TSP. MG-63 cells induced aggregation of platelets in a dose-dependent fashion. Preincubation of MG-63 cells with an anti-TSP polyclonal antibody inhibited by 80 % the plateletaggregating activity of these tumor cells. Another human osteosarcoma cell line, TE-85, induced platelet aggregation to the same extent as MG-63 cells. However, TE-85 cells had few TSP binding sites and the platelet-aggregating activity of these tumor cells was not inhibited by an anti-TSP antibody. In conclusion, these results demonstrate that osteosarcoma cells which express high amounts of TSP at their surface induce platelet aggregation via this ligand.

Résumé

La thrombospondine (TSP) est une glycoprotéine de 450 kDa synthétisée et sécrétée par les cellules d'une lignée humaine d'ostéosarcome appelée MG-63 (P.Clezardin et al., Eur.J.Biochem., 1989). Dans cette étude nous avons étudié l'expression de la TSP à la surface des MG-63 ainsi que le rôle de cette glycoprotéine dans l'agrégation plaquettaire induite par ces cellules tumorales. La fixation de (^{125}I) TSP à la surface des cellules MG-63 cultivées en monocouche se fait en fonction du temps et de la concentration : elle est saturable et est inhibée par un excès de TSP "froide". Les cellules tumorales MG-63 induisent l'agrégation des plaquettes entre elles. Cependant, l'activité proagrégante de ces cellules est inhibée à 80 % en présence d'un anticorps polyclonal anti-TSP. Une deuxième lignée humaine d'ostéosarcome (TE-85) induit également l'agrégation plaquettaire dans des proportions équivalentes aux cellules MG-63. Toutefois, les cellules TE-85 ont peu de sites de fixation pour la TSP et l'agrégation plaquettaire induite par ces TE-85 n'est pas inhibée par un anticorps anti-TSP. En conclusion, ces résultats indiquent que lorsque la TSP est fortement exprimée à la surface des cellules d'une lignée d'ostéosarcome, celles-ci exercent un effet proagrégant par le biais de la TSP.

Platelet immunology : fundamental and clinical aspects. Ed. C. Kaplan-Gouet, N. Schlegel, Ch. Salmon, J. McGregor. Colloque INSERM/John Libbey Eurotext Ltd © 1991. Vol. 206, pp. 209-217.

The role of cytoadhesins in mediating platelet-melanoma cell interaction and *in vivo* melanoma tumor growth

H. Boukerche*, O. Berthier-Vergnes**, E. Tabone***, and J.L. McGregor*

*INSERM U 331, Laboratoire d'hémobiolgie, **Faculté de médecine Alexis Carrel, INSERM U 218, ***Centre Léon Bérard, Unité de morphologie cellulaire et tissulaire, Lyon, France

Abstract :

Platelet-tumor cell interactions are believed to be a major mechanism in promoting metastasis. Human or animal tumor cell lines are known to aggregate human blood platelets, under in vitro conditions, by secreting ADP, or generating thrombin. However, the identity of membrane binding sites, present on platelets or tumor cells, that are involved on the formation of platelet-tumor cell aggregates remains to be elucidated. Evidence is presented in this review to indicate that glycoprotein (GP) IIb-IIIa-like protein (vitronectin receptor) is present on melanoma cells and that it may serve as the binding site through which tumors cells interact with the GPIIb-IIIa platelet membrane glycoprotein complex. Moreover, the GPIIb-IIIa-like complex may play also an important role in the growth of tumor metastasis. These results give additional support to the involvement of this receptor in the adhesive and migratory behavior of malignant cells.

Introduction :

Metastasis is a complex multistep process initiated by the detachement of tumor cells from the primary tumor mass, invasion into the circulation, arrest in the cappillary bed, extravasation and the formation of secondary metastatic colonies (Roos, 1979). Extensive evidence suggest that platelet-tumor cell interactions may play a crucial role in the dissemination of cancer cells. Human or animal tumor cell lines can aggregate human blood platelets, under in vitro conditions, by secreting ADP, or generating thrombin (Gasic et al., 1973; Bastida et al., 1981; 1982). Such platelet-tumor cell agregates show an increased tendancy to induce the formation of lung metastasis in vivo (Sindelar et al., 1975). Tumor cells infused intraveneously into mice cause a significant thrombocytopenia which is accompanied by an accumulation of platelet-tumor cell aggregates in the vessel of the lungs (Hilgard et al., 1973; 1974; Gasic et al., 1978). Pretreatment of animals with anticoagulants or antiplatelet polyclonal antibodies reduces the metastatic spread of lung tumors (Gasic et al., 1968; Pearlstein et al., 1984). However, the identity of membrane binding sites, present on platelets or tumor cells, that are involved on the formation of platelet-tumor cell aggregates remains to be elucidated. This review summarizes the importance of cytoadhesins present on platelets and tumors cells in mediating tumor-platelet interactions. Evidence is also presented to show that cytoadhesins play also a crucial role in metastasis formation and tumor growth in vivo.

The cytoadhesins family

The cytoadhesins are members of a recently recognized superfamily of proteins, the "integrins", which bind adhesive proteins (fibrinogen, fibronectin, and vitronectin) bearing an Arg-Gly-Asp (R-G-D) peptide recognition sequence (Buck & Howitz, 1987; Ginsberg et al., 1988). Many of these integrins are well characterized, consisting of two non convalently associated α and β subunits that are expressed as a complex form on the cell surface on various species from drosophila to mammals. The cytoadhesins subfamily consists of the platelet glycoprotein IIb-IIIa ($\alpha IIb/\beta_3$) and the vitronectin receptor (VNR) ($\alpha v \beta_3$) expressed by endothelial (Cheresh, 1987), melanoma cells (Cheresh & Spiro, 1987), and other cell types (Pytela et al., 1986). VNR like GPIIb-IIIa promote adhesion to a number of extracellular matrix proteins including vitronectin, fibrinogen, fibronectin and thrombospondin (Cheresh, 1987; Cheresh & Spiro, 1987; Knudsen et al., 1988; Tuszynski et al., 1989). New members of the cytoadhesins subfamily have been recently described in which the α subunit can associate with more than one β subunit : $\alpha v \beta_1$ identified as a predominant VNR in human embryonic kidney cell line (Bodary & McLean, 1990), $\alpha v \beta_5$ identified in carcinoma cells (Cheresh et al., 1989), and an αv subunit associated with a novel β_S subunit ($\alpha v \beta_S$) in osteosarcoma cells (Freed et al., 1990). Unlike the $\alpha v \beta_5$ and $\alpha v \beta_S$ which promote attachment to vitronectin, fibronectin and other ligands (Cheresh et al., 1989; Freed et al., 1990), $\alpha v \beta_S$ appears to bind only to vitronectin (Bodary & McLean, 1990).

Involvement of the glycoprotein IIb-IIIa-like complex (vitronectin receptor) in platelet-tumor cell interaction :

As stated above, a number of tumor cell lines induce platelet aggregation in vitro in heparinized platelet-rich plasma (PRP) via the release of ADP by tumor cells or the generation of thrombin (Bastida et al., 1981; 1982; Mehta, 1984). In our laboratory, a human cell line derived from an achromic skin metastasis of a patient with malignant melanoma (Berthier-Vergnes et al., 1986) has been shown to aggregate platelets in heparinized PRP (Boukerche et al., 1989a). This aggregation appeared to be ADP-dependant since it was inhibited by apyrase. A clear proof showing interacting platelets-tumor cells was provided by electron microscopy. Platelets in contact with tumor cell surface were almost all degranulated as compared with platelets at the periphery of the tumor platelet aggregates, suggesting that the latter had undergone aggregation but no complete release. At the site of their interaction with platelets, tumor cells formed extrusions or processes which penetrated into the platelet aggregates. The significance of these processes is not known but may prevent dissociation of emboli once they are formed (Menter et al., 1987). These phenomenon have also been observed in vivo by Crissman and colleagues (1985; 1988).

Several lines of evidence strongly suggest that platelet GPIIb-IIIa complex is involved in the interaction between platelets and tumors cells. Platelets from patients with Glanzmann thrombasthenia, lacking GPIIb and GPIIIa, were not aggregated by tumor cells (Boukerche et al., 1989a). Incubation of platelets with anti-GPIIb-IIIa monoclonal (10E5, LYP18) or polyclonal antibodies inhibited platelet aggregation induced by tumor cells (Yamamoto et al., 1986; Grossi et al., 1988; Boukerche et al., 1989a, Kitagawa et al., 1989). Thus, the deficiency of GPIIb and GPIIIa in Glanzmann's thrombasthenic platelets associated with no binding of fibrinogen, accounts for the defective platelet aggregation induced by melanoma cells. Interestingly, melanoma cells pretreated with LYP18 Fab fragments did not aggregate platelets (Boukerche et al., 1989a). The lack of inhibition of platelet aggregation induced by melanoma cells pretreated with MoAb LYP18 was not due to LYP18 released from melanoma cells onto the medium and its subsequent binding to platelets since less than 4% of the total melanoma cell bound labelled LYP18 was recovered in the supernate of the aggregation studies. Ultrastructural studies showed no platelet-platelet or platelet-melanoma interactions. Moreover, the tumor cell surface did not show cytoplasmic extrusions or processes.

A number of tumor cell lines (e.g., human melanoma, human colon carcinoma, human cervical carcinoma, rat walker 256 carcinosarcoma) synthesize and express on their surface two proteins with the characteristic changes similar in mobility to that observed with platelet GPIIb-IIIa and the vitronectin receptor member of the cytoadhesins family (Pytela et al., 1985; Knudsen et al., 1988; Chopra et al., 1988; Boukerche et al., 1989a). Recent results from our laboratory indicate that our monoclonal antibody to GPIIb-IIIa (LYP18) and polyclonal antibodies to the human vitronectin receptor immunoprecipitate from surface labelled melanoma cells the same complex (H. Boukerche et al., unpublished results). Moreover, in agreement with others (Ginsberg et al., 1988, Knudsen et al. 1988), we showed that the alpha subunit of the IIb-IIIa-like GPs is different from platelet GPIIb since it was not recognized by either an anti-platelet GPIIb polyclonal or monoclonal antibody. In contrast, the IIIa-like GP immunocross-react with either a polyclonal or a monoclonal antibody to platelet GPIIIa. Cheresh and Harper (1987) and others (Knudsen et al., 1988) have recently reported that a M21 or a C32 human melanoma cell lines express on their surface an glycoprotein complex recognized by Arg-Gly-

Asp peptide recognition sequence which shares biochemical and immunological similarities with the vitronectin receptor. These data suggest that the IIb-IIIa-like complex and the vitronectin receptor are the same and that we are most likely studying the same receptor reported by Cheresh and Harper (1987) and others (Knudsen et al., 1988; Chopra et al., 1988). While the GPIIb-IIIa-like complex present on tumor cells have been shown to be critically involved in the tumor cell-aggregation process, it appears to be insufficient by itself in the initial attachement of platelets to tumor cells. Initial interactions between platelets and tumor cells may result in a reorganization of tumor cell cytoskueleton (e.g., microfilaments and/or intermediate filaments) leading to the redistribution and clustering of the GPIIb-IIIa-like complex. Such areas of high concentration of this receptor may represent focal points through which platelets interact with tumor cells (Chopra et al., 1988).

In vivo function of the GPIIb-IIIa-like complex (vitronectin receptor) :

The in vivo function of the GPIIb-IIIa-like complex was demonstrated by the ability of a synthetic peptide containing Arg-Gly-Asp sequence to drastically decrease the formation of lung tumor colonies of murine melanoma cells (Humphries et al., 1986). Similarly, preincubation of human platelets with an anti-GPIIb-IIIa monoclonal antibody before infusion into mice inhibited by 77% the reconstitution with human platelets of pulmonary metastases induced by CT26 colon carcinoma cells (Karpatkin et al., 1988). Recent results from our laboratory indicate that coinjection in mice of M3Da. human melanoma cells with an anti-platelet GPIIb-IIIa MoAb (LYP18) that cross-reacts with the IIb/IIIa-like GPs on melanoma cells dramatically decreased the growth of tumor in mice (Boukerche et al., 1989b). This effect was not due to complement-dependant cytotoxicity or a direct cytotoxic effect of monoclonal antibody LYP18. These new results supply evidence that this particular integrin plays a crucial role in the control of tumor growth. Tumor cell growth is the first step of a complex interaction between tumor cells and their surrouding stromacal matrices leading to metastasis. Two possible explanations may account for the observation reported in this paper. The first explanation is based on the idea the IIb/IIIa-like GPs may bind to adhesive proteins present in the stroma (eg., vWF, fibronectin and fibrin) and, in so doing, may allow the stroma matrix to regulate tumor growth and differenciation in vivo (Ruoslahti & Pierschbacher, 1987). Another explanation is that MoAb by binding to the IIb/IIIa-like GPs may prevent macrophage access and activation leading to rapid destruction of the melanoma cells in vivo (Dvorak, 1986). In postransplant times studies, we showed that MoAb LYP18 have no effect if injected after tumor cell grafting, suggesting that LYP18 may interfere with one or more of the early steps in the establishement of tumor (Boukerche et al., 1989b).

Conclusions :

The integrins superfamily, in particular, the members of the cytoadhesin subfamily form a class of cell surface receptors that play an important role in tumor cell metastasis. Evidence is presented in this review to show that the GPIIb-IIIa-like proteins (vitronectin receptor) present on tumor cells may serve as the binding site through which tumor cells interact with the IIb-IIIa platelet membrane glycoprotein complex. The observed inhibition of platelet-tumor cell interactions is probably due to an inhibition of fibrinogen binding or other ligands (e.g., vWF, fibronectin, vitronectin, thrombospondin) to platelet membrane GPIIb-IIIa and subsequent platelet-platelet and platelet-tumor cell interactions. The use of MoAbs raised against cytoadhesive receptors present on melanoma cells and others malignant cells or anti-adhesive peptides (RGDS series) provide attractive concept for possible application as therapeutical approach in tumor treatment.

Acknoweldgements :

This work was carried out with the help of the Association pour la Recherche sur le Cancer (ARC, subvention 6586), of la Ligue contre la Cancer.

References :

Bastida, E., Ordinas, A., Giardina, S.L., and Jamieson, G.A. (1981). Differing platelet aggrgating effects by two tumor cell lines : absence of role of platelet-derived ADP. Am. J. Haematol. 11, 367-378.

Bastida, E., Ordinas, A., and Jamieson, G.A. (1982) : Differenciation of platelet aggregating effects of human tumor cell lines bases on inhibition studies with apyrase, hirudin, and phospholipase. Cancer Res. 42, 4348-4352.

Berthier-Vergnes, O., Reano, A., and J-F., Doré. (1986) : Lectin binding glycoproteins in human melanoma cell lines with high or low tumorigenicity. Int. J. Cancer 37, 747-751.

Bodary, S., and McLean, J.W. (1990) : The integrin β_1 subunit associates with the vitronectin receptor α_V subunit to form a novel vitronectin receptor in a human embryonic kidney cell line. J. Biol. Chem. 11, 5938-5941.

Boukerche, H., Berthier-Vergnes, O., Tabone, E., Doré, J-F., Leung, L.L.K., and J.L. McGregor. (1989a). Platelet-melanoma interaction is mediated by the glycoprotein IIb-IIIa complex. Blood 74, 658-663.

Boukerche, H., O. Berthier-Vergnes, M. Bailly, J-F Doré, L.L.K. Leung, and J.L. McGregor. (1989b) : A monoclonal antibody (LYP18) directed against the blood platelet glycoprotein IIb-IIIa complex inhibits human melanoma growth in vivo. Blood 74, 909-912.

Buck, C.A., and Howitz, A.F. (1987) : Cell surface receptors for extracellular matrix molecules. Ann. Rev. Cell Biol. 3, 179-205.

Cheresh, D.A. (1987) : Human endothelial cells synthesize and express an Arg-Gly-Asp -directed adhesion receptor involved in attachment to fibrinogen and von Willebrandt factor. Proc. Natl. ACad. Sci. USA 84, 6471-6475.

Cheresh, D.A. & Harper, J.R. (1987) : Arg-Gly-Asp. recognition by a cell adhesion receptor requires its 130-kDa subunit. J. Biol. Chem., 267, 1434-1437.

Cheresh, D.A. & Spiro, R.C. (1987) : Biosynthesis and functional properties of an Arg-Gly-Asp-directed receptor involved in human melanoma cell attachment to vitronectin, fibrinogen, and von willebrandt factor. J. Biol. Chem. 36, 17703-17771.

Cheresh, D.A., Smith, J.W., Cooper, H.M., and Quaranta, V. (1989) : A novel vitronectin receptor integrin ($\alpha v \beta_x$) is responsible for distinct adhesive properties of carcinoma cells. Cell 57, 59-69.

Chopra, H., Hatfield, J., Chang Y.S., Grossi, I.M., Fitzgerald, L.A., O'Gara, C.Y., Marnett, L.J., Diglio, C.A., Taylor, J.D., and Honn, K.V. (1988) : Role of tumor cell cytosqueleton and membrane glycoprotein IRGpIIb/IIIa in platelet adhesion to tumor cell membrane and tumor cell-induced platelet aggregation. Cancer Res. 48, 3787-3800.

Crissman, J., Hatfield, J.S., Schaldenbrand, M., Sloane, B., and Honn, K.V. (1985) : Arrest and extravasation of B16 amelanotic melanoma in murine lungs. A light and electron microscopic study. Lab. Invest. 53, 470-478.

Crissman, J., Hatfield, J.S., Menter, D.G., Sloane, B.F., and K.V. Honn. (1988) : Morphological study of interaction of intravascular tumor cells with endothelial cells and subendothelial matrix. Cancer Res. 48, 4065-4072.

Dvorak, H.F. (1986) : Tumors : Wounds that not heal. N. Engl. J. Med. 315, 1650-1652.

Freed, E., Gailit, J., van der Geer, P., Ruoslahti, E., and Hunter T. (1990) : A novel integrin β subunit is associated with the vitronectin receptor α subunit (αv) in a human osteosrcoma cell line and is a substrate for protein kinase C. EMBO 8, 2955-2965.

Gasic, G.J., Gasic T.B., and Stewart, C.C. (1968) : Antimetastatic effect associated with platelet reduction. Proc. Natl. Acad. Sci. USA 61, 46-52.

Gasic, G.J., Gasic, T.B., Galanti, N., Johnson, T., and Murphy, S. (1973) : Platelet-tumor cell interactions in mice. The role of platelets in the spread of malignant disease. Int. J. Cancer 11, 704-718.

Gasic, G.J., Boettiger, D., Catalfamo, J.L., Gasic, T.B., and Stewart, G.J. (1978). Aggregation of platelets and cell membrane vesiculation by rat cells transformed in vitro by roux sarcoma virus. Cancer Res. 38, 2950-2955.

Ginsberg, M.H., Loftus, J.C., and Plow, E.F. (1988) : Cytoadhesins, integrins and platelets. Thromb. Haemost. 59, 1-6.

Grossi, I.M., Hatfield, J.S., Fitzgerald, L.A., Newcombe, M., Taylor, D., and Honn, K.V. (1988) : Role of tumor cell glycoprotein immunologically related to glycoprotein Ib and IIb/IIIa in tumor cell-platelet and tumor-matrix interactions. FASEB J. 2, 2385-2395.

Hilgard, P. (1973) : The role of blood platelets in experimental matastases. Br. J. Cancer 28, 429-435.

Hilgard, P., and Gordon-Smith, E.C. (1974) : Microangiopathic haemolytic anaemia and experimental tumor-cell emboli. Br. J. Haematol. 26, 651-659.

Humphries, M.J., Olden, K., and Yamada, K.M. (1986) : A synthetic peptide from fibronectin inhibits experimental metastasis of murine melanoma cells. Science 233, 467-470.

Karpatkin, S., Pearlstein, E., Ambrogio, C., and B.S. Coller. (1988) : Role of adhesive proteins in platelet tumor interaction in vitro and metastasis formation in vivo. J. Clin. Invest. 81, 1012-1019.

Knudsen, K.A., Smith, L., Smith, S., Karczeski, J. and Tuszynski, P. (1988). Role of IIb-IIIa-like glycoproteins in cell substratum adhesion of human melanoma cells. J. Cell. physiol. 136, 471-478.

Kitagawa, H., Yamamoto, N., Yamamoto, K., Tanoue, K., Kosaki, G., and Yamasaki, H. (1989) : Involvement of platelet membrane glycoprotein Ib and glycoprotein IIb/IIIa complex in thrombin-dependant and independant platelet aggregations induced by tumor cells. Cancer Res. 49, 537-541.

Mehta, P. (1984). Potential role of platelets in the pathogenesis of tumor metastasis. Blood 63, 55-63.

Menter, D.G., Hatfield, J.S., Harkins, C., Sloane, B.F., Taylor, J.D., Crissmn, J.D., and Honn, K.V. (1987) : Tumor cell-platelet interaction in vitro and their relationship to in vivo arrest of hematogenously circulating tumor cells. Clin. Exp. Metastasis 5, 65-78.

Pearlstein, E., Ambrogio, C., and Karpatkin, S. (1984) : Effect of antiplatelet antibody on the development of pulmonary metastases following injection of CT26 colon adenocarcinoma, Lewis lung carcinoma and B16 amelanotic melanoma tumor cells into mice. Cancer Res. 44, 3884-3887.

Pytela, R. Pierschbacher, M.D., Ginsberg, M.H., Plow, E.F., and Ruoslahti, E. (1986) : Platelet membrane glycoprotein IIb-IIIa : member of a family of Arg-Gly-Asp-specific adhesion receptors. Science 231, 1559-1562.

Roos, E., and Dingemans, K.P. (1979). Mechanisms of metastasis. Biochim. Biophys. Acta 560, 135-166.

Ruoslahti, E. & Pierschbacher, M.D. (1987) : New perspectives in cell adhesion : RGD and integrins. Science 238, 491-497.

Sindelar, W.F., Tralka, T.S., and Ketcham, A.S. (1975) : Electron microscopic observations on formation of pulmonary metastases. J. Surg. Res. 18, 137-161.

Tuszynski, G.P., Karczewski, J., Smith, L., Murphy, A., Rothman, V.L., and Knudsen, K.A. (1989) : The GPIIb IIIa like complex may function as a human melanoma cell adhesion receptor for thrombospondin. Exp. Cell Res. 182, 473-481.

Yamamoto, K., Kitagawa, H., Tanoue, K., Tsuruo, T., Yamamoto, N., and Yamasaki, H. (1986) : Role of heparin in tumor cell-induced platelet aggregation. Thromb. Haemost. 56, 90-94.

Résumé

Les interactions entre les plaquettes et les cellules tumorales sont un des mécanismes mis en jeu au cours de la formation des métastases. Il est bien reconnu aujourd'hui que les cellules tumorales d'origine humaine ou animale agrègent les plaquettes sanguines humaines, in vitro, selon un mécanisme mettant en jeu soit l'ADP soit la génération de la thrombine. Cependant, l'identité des récepteurs, présents sur la plaquette ou la cellule tumorale, mis en jeu au cours de ces interactions restait encore à déterminer. Les arguments présentés dans cette revue montrent que les interactions entre les plaquettes et les cellules tumorales apparaissent être dues à un mécanisme mettant en jeu le complexe de glycoproteines GP (IIb-IIIa) de la plaquette et un complexe de GPs apparenté (GPIIb-IIIa-like ou récepteur de la vitronectine) présent sur la cellule tumorale. De plus, ce pseudo-complexe joue aussi un rôle clef dans la croissance d'une tumeur métastatique (in vivo). Ce qui constitue autant d'arguments en faveur du rôle de ce récepteur dans le comportement migratoire et adhésif des cellules malignes.

Platelet antigens, new aspects

A.E.G. Kr. von dem Borne and R.W.A.M. Kuijpers

Department of Immunologic Haematology, Central Laboratory of the Netherlands Red Cross Blood Transfusion Service, Department of Experimental and Clinical Immunology, University of Amsterdam and Department of Haematology, Academic Medical Centre, CLB, Plesmanlaan 125, 1066 CX Amsterdam, The Netherlands

SUMMARY

From the different types of platelet antigens the socalled platelet specific allo-antigens are discussed in detail. These antigens play an important role in neonatal alloimmune thrombocytopenia and posttransfusion purpura. Xenoantigens detected by murine monoclonal antibodies (also known as CD antigens of platelets) are only briefly mentioned. The description of many new platelet specific alloantigens in recent years has made it necessary to develop a new nomenclature system. This HPA nomenclature system is discussed in detail. Many new data have become available concerning the glycoprotein location of platelet antigens. HPA-1 and HPA-4 antigens are on GPIIIa, HPA-3 on GPIIb, HPA-5 on GPIa, and Nak^a on GPIV. We found that the HPA-2 (Ko) antigens are probably localized on GPIb , notably on its N-terminal part. Many of the platelet GP's which carry these antigen belong to the adhesion molecules of the integrin superfamily. This explains why they may be expressed not only on platelets, but on other cells (endothelial cells, smooth muscle cells, fibroblasts, activated T-cells) as well. Thus, they are not always as platelet specific as previously thought. Studies on the molecular genetics of HPA-antigens have recently started. By applying PCR on cDNA prepared by reversed transcriptase from platelet RNA Newman and coworkers unravelled the molecular basis of HPA-1 and HPA-3 antigens. HPA-1 (Zw) antigens are due to a leucine/proline polymorphism of aminoacid 33 of the mature GPIIIa chain. HPA-3 antigens are caused by a isoleucine/serine polymporphism of aminoacid 843 of mature GPIIb. However, there are indications that the actual HPA-epitopes are not these aminoacids. Probably the epitopes result from differences in the secundary and/or tertiary structure of the glycopeptide chains induced by the different amino acids.

Introduction

In the last decade platelet immunology has experienced a rapid evolution. New methods to define and measure platelet antigens and antibodies have been deviced. This has led not only to the recognition of new antigen systems, but also to new insights into the pathophysiology of immune mediated platelet disorders. Moreover, and most importantly, the study of platelet antigens at a molecular level has intensified, providing the necessary fundamental knowledge for a further expansion of our field.

Therefore, the emphasis of this review will be on this latter aspect and notably on the molecular nature of platelet alloantigens, allthough some new serological, genetical and clinical data of interest will be discussed as well. Also in the field of platelet xenoantigens rapid progress has occurred, especially of those antigens recognized by monoclonal antibodies (Mab's). Mab's against platelets have been studied in detail during the last Workshop on Human Leukocyte Differentiation antigens (Vienna 1989) from which a voluminous report has recently appeared (1). Therefore, this new aspect will not be discussed here. Suffice it to say that Mab's are most outstanding tools in the study of platelet membrane glycoproteins and are very helpful in serological analyses. At present there are already 26 different Mab specificities available for such studies, of which 24 assigned in clusters (CD's) or subclusters. From the glycoproteins recognised by these antibody groups already 20 have been cloned and characterised by sequencing (table 1).

Platelet Specific Alloantigen Systems

Apart from antigens shared with other blood cells and tissues (such as glycoconjugate antigens of the blood group ABH, Le, I, P systems and the HLA class I glycoprotein antigens) platelets carry an apparently unique set of so-called platelet specific antigens. As will be discussed later, many of these antigens appear not to be as platelet-specific as previously thought.

The platelet specific antigens or antigen systems described so far, are listed in table 2, together with their frequency of occurrence. Many have been and/or are still published under different names. A historical record in this respect

Table 1

Monoclonal Antibody Clusters and Subclusters Reactive with Platelets

Clusters	Platelet Membrane Component	Synonyms	Cloned
CD9	p24	-	y
CDw17	lactosyl ceramide	-	-
CD23	gp50-45	FcεR-II	y
CD29	GPIIa	VLAβ-chain	y
CD31	GPIIa'	PE-CAM	y
CDw32	gp40	FcγR-II	y
CD36	GPIV=IIIb	TRSP-R	y
CD41	GPIIb(IIb/IIIa)	$CA\alpha^{IIb}$-chain	y
CD42a	GPIX	} vWF-R	y
CD42b	GPIb		y
CD45(CD45RA,RO)	gp220/180	LCA(T200)	y
CD46	gp66/56	MCP	y
CD47	gp47-52	Rh-associated gp	n
CD49b	GPIa	$VLA\alpha_2$-chain	y
CD49d	gp150	$VLA\alpha_4$-chain	y
(CD49e)	GPIc'	$VLA\alpha_5$-chain	y
CD49f	GPIc	$VLA\alpha_6$-chain	n
CD51	gp140	$CA\alpha^v$-chain (VNRα chain)	y
CD55	gp75	DAF	y
CD58	gp40-65	LFA-3 (CD2-R)	y
CD59	gp18-20	MIRL	y
CDw60	$(NeuAc)_2$-Gal	-	-
CD61	GPIIIa	CAβ-chain	y
CD62	GMP-140	PADGEM	y
CD63	gp53	-	n
CD69	gp32/28	AIM	n
u.c.	GPV	TSP	n
u.c.	gp180	-	n

Abbreviations: FcεR=IgE Fc receptor; VLA=very late antigen; PE-CAM= platelet--endothelial cell adhesion molecule, FcγR=IgG Fc receptor; TRSP= thrombospondin; CA= cytoadhesin; vWF= von Willebrand factor; LCA= leucocyte common antigen; MCP= membrane cofactor protein; VNR= vitronectin receptor; DAF= decay accelerating factor; LFA= leucocyte function antigen; MIRL= membrane inhibitor of reactive lysis; PADGEM= platelet activation dependent granule external membrane protein; AIM= activation inducer molecule; TSP= thrombin sensitive protein

Table 2

Platelet Specific Antigen Systems Described Sofar

System	Antigens	Frequency (%)*	Reference
Duzo	$Duzo^a$	22.0	2
$Zw=Pl^A$	$Zw^a=Pl^{A1}$	97.9	3,4,5
	$Zw^b=Pl^{A2}$	26.5	
Ko= Sib	$Ko^a=Sib^a$	14.9	4,6,7,8
	Ko^b	99.3	
Pl^E	Pl^{E1}	> 99.9	5
	Pl^{E2}	5.0	
Bak=Lek	$Bak^a=Lek^a$	87.7	9,10,11,12
	Bak^b	64.1	
Pen=Yuk	$Pen^a=Yuk^b$	> 99.9	13,14
	Yuk^a	< 0.2	
Br=Hc=Zav	$Br^a=Hc^a=Zav$	20.6	15,16,17,18
	$Br^b=Zw^b$	99.2	
Pl^T	Pl^{T1}	> 98.1	19
Nak	Nak^a	96.00**	20
Sr	Sr^a	< 0.1	21
Gov	Gov^a	78.1	22
	Gov^b	71.7	

*   in Caucasians
** in Japanese

is the Zw system, the first platelet specific antigen system described which is still persistingly called the Pl^A system by authors from North America. Another more recent record is the Br system, also described under the names Hc and Zav.

It is clear that a new nomenclature system for such antigen systems will be helpful to avoid further confusion. Recently, a group of platelet serologists all members of the International Working Party on Platelet Serology of the ISBT and ISH has tackled the nomenclature problem. This has led to the proposal depicted in table 3. Platelet-specific alloantigen system will be called HPA (for Human Platelet Antigen). The different systems will be numbered chronologically in order of the date of description in the literature. A high frequency allele of a system will be indicated with the letter a, its low frequency counterpart with a letter b. New antigen systems will be included only if they

Table 3

A New Nomenclature of Platelet-specific Allo-antigens

System	Original name(s)	Antigens	Original name(s)
HPA-1	Zw, Pl^A	HPA-1a	Zw^a, Pl^{A1}
		HPA-1b	Zw^b, Pl^{A2}
HPA-2	Ko, Sib	HPA-2a	Ko^b
		HPA-2b	Ko^a, Sib^a
HPA-3	Bak, Lek	HPA-3a	Bak^a, Lek^a
		HPA-3b	Bak^b
HPA-4	Pen, Yuk	HPA-4a	Pen^a, Yuk^b
		HPA-4b	Pen^b, Yuk^a
HPA-5	Br, Hc, Zav	HPA-5a	Br^b, Zav^b
		HPA-5b	Br^a, Zav^a, Hc^a

have been accepted officially as such by the Working Party. This is not yet the case for Pl^T, Nak, Sr and Gov. Note that neither Duzo nor PL^E were included in the new nomenclature. This is because Duzo and Pl^{E2} antisera are not available anymore. Moreover, Pl^{E1} antiserum was probably from a Bernard Soulier syndrome patient immunized by blood transfusion i.e. the serum may contain isoantibodies instead of alloantibodies. Indeed, up till now no normal donors have been found whose platelets did not react with anti PL^{E1}.

Note that all HPA systems described so far appear to be biallelic systems. In recently performed population studies it appeared that the phenotype and genotype frequencies may vary considerably between different ethnic groups (8,23, 24,25). For example, HPA-1a (Zw^a) is (nearly) ubiquitous in Japanese, Koreans and Blacks, whereas HPA-1b (Zw^b) seems to be rare. HPA-4b ($Yuk^a=Pen^b$) is found only in Japanese and Koreans, although quite infrequently. This antigen is rare or absent in Caucasians (and has not yet been studied in Black people). South American Indians (Mapuches) have also (nearly) all HPA-1a (Zw^a), have HPA-4b (Yuk^a) in a low frequency as well and HPA-5b (Br^a) in a lower frequency in comparison to Caucasians (see also table 4).

Table 4

Phenotype frequency (%) in different populations

System	Antigens	Caucasians	Blacks	Japanese	Koreans	Indians
Zw=HPA-1	Zw^a=1a	97.9	99.6	> 99.9	100	99.9
	Zw^b=1b	26.5	-	3.7	11.5	-
Ko=HPA-2	Ko^b=2a	99.3	-	-	-	-
	Ko^a=2b	14.9	-	25.4	-	-
Bak=HPA-3	Bak^a=3a	87.7	-	78.9	87.3	89.3
	Bak^b=3b	64.1	-	70.7	-	-
Pen=HPA-4	Pen^a=4a	> 99.9	-	99.9	100	99.9
	Pen^b=4b	< 0.2	-	1.7	1.6	0.9
Br=HPA-5	Br^b=5a	99.2	-	-	-	-
	Br^a=5b	20.6	-	-	-	4.9

The biallelism of platelet antigens and the marked differences between different ethnic groups suggest that single evolutionary events have been responsible for their diversifaction and that these events are of a late date, probably occurring during postspecies evolution.

Clinical Importance of Platelet Specific Alloantigens

The $Duzo^a$ antibodies came from the blood of a mother with a newborn suffering from neonatal alloimmune thrombocytopenia (NAIT) while anti HPA-1a (Zw^a) antibodies were from the blood of a patient with post transfusion purpura (PTP).

Since these early descriptions of platelet specific alloantibodies as causes of a specific platelet disease sera from such cases have been the main source for further studies. This has led to the discovery of many more new antibody specificities and antigens. Only recently the study of platelet transfusion refractoriness has also contributed. The involvement of the different platelet antigen systems in specific clinical situations is summarized in table 5. The diversity of antibody specificities involved in NAIT appears to be far greater than of those involved in PTP. In fact, with the possible exception of anti-Gov-antibodies, the antibodies in PTP are all directed against antigens present on the glycoprotein IIb/IIIa complex of platelets. This intriguing association is still unexplained.

Refractoriness to platelet transfusion (PTR) therapy is mostly due to allo-antibodies directed against HLA class I antigens and sometimes anti A and/or anti B. Recent publications indicate that sometimes PTR also may be due to platelet specific alloantibodies, although this has been shown only in a few patients. Notably, these are mostly patients who became refractory for transfusions of HLA matched platelets.

Glycoprotein localisation of Platelet Specific Antigens

Mainly due to modern methods such as immunoprecipitation and SDS poly-acrylamide gel electrophoresis, immunoblotting and recently monoclonal antibody capture immuno assays most platelet specific antigens have been definitely localized on specific platelet membrane glycoproteins.

This is depicted in table 6. Most of the data on glycoprotein location have been published in detail in the literature (see the references). However, those on HPA-2 (Ko=Sib), Sr, Pl^T and Gov are still from preliminary reports. The data on Nak have not yet been reported (Ikeda, personal communication). The localization studies on HPA-2 were performed in our laboratory. With a panel of anti HPA-2a (Ko^b) and anti HPA-2b (Ko^a) sera we found that (chloro-

Table 5

Clinical importance of Platelet Alloantigens Involved in	References
Neonatal alloimmune thrombocytopenia: Duzo, Zw, Ko, Bak, Pen, Br, Pl^E, Pl^T, Sr	2,5,9,13,14,15,19,21,26 27,28,29,30
Posttransfusion purpura: Zw, Bak, Pen, Gov	3,5,10,11,12,22,31,32, 33,34
Transfusion refractoriness: HLA-ABC, bloodgroup ABO, Zw, Ko, Bak, Br, Nak, Gov	8,20,22,35,36,37

Table 6

Glycoprotein localization of platelet alloantigens

System	Original names	Glycoprotein location	Reference
HPA-1	Zw, Pl^A	GPIIIa	38,39
HPA-2	Ko, Sib	GPIbα	40
HPA-3	Bak, Lek	GPIIb	39,41
HPA-4	Pen, Yuk	GPIIIa	42,43,44
HPA-5	Br, Hc, Zav	GPIa	17,18,45
-	Pl^E	GPIbα	46
-	Sr	GPIIIa	21
-	Nak	GPIV?	-
-	Pl^T	GPV	19
-	Gov	gp175/150	22
-	Cr-related	gp75	47

Figure 1:

Amino-acid Sequence Difference Related to Zw Polymorphism in the NH2 terminal part of GPIIIa

```
        1                   11                  21
Zwa:  G P N I C T T R G V S S C Q Q C L A V S P M C A W C S D E A . . . .

Zwb:  . . . . . . . . . . . . . . . . . . . . . . . . . . . . . . . . .

        31        *        41                  51
      L P L G S P R C D L K E N L L K D N C A P E S I E F P V S E . . . .

      . . P . . . . . . . . . . . . . . . . . . . . . . . . . . . .
```

Figure 2:

Amino Acid Sequence Difference in GPIIb Related to Bak Polymorphism

```
        820                     30                    40
Baka:   P Q G G L Q C F P Q P P V N P L K V D W G L P I P
Bakb:   . . . . . . . . . . . . . . . . . . . . . . . * S .

                50                    60
        S P S P I H P A H H K R D R R Q I F L P E P E Q P
        . . . . . . . . . . . . . . . . . . . . E . . . .

        70                    80                    90
        S R L Q D P V L V S C D S A P C T V V Q C D L Q E
        . . . . . . . . . . . . . . . . . . . . . . . . .

            900                               10
        M A R G Q R A M V T V L A F L W L P S L Y Q R P L
        . . . . . . . . . . . . . . . . . . . . . . . . .

                            30                          40
        D Q F V L Q S H A W F N V S S L P Y A V P P L S L
        . . . . . . . . . . . . . . . . . . . . . . . . .

            50                    60
        D R G E A Q V W T Q L L R A L E E R A I P I W W V
        . . . . . . . . . . . . . . . . . . . . . . . . .
```

LIBS-1 (PMI-1 site)   IIbα-IIbβ cut   transmembrane part

quine stripped) platelets from two patients with Bernard Soulier syndrome and platelets from normal donors treated with elastase were not expressing the respective antigens. 'Bernard Soulier' platelets are deficient in the GP Ib/IX/V complex. Elastase treatment removes the N-terminal 45-75 kDa part of GP Ibα leaving GP Ibβ and GP IX intact. Then, we found that HPA-2 antibodies were captured in the MAIPA (48) only by Mab's against GP Ib (CD42b) and GP IX (CD42a) but not by a anti GP V Mab or Mab's directed against other glycoproteins or glycoprotein complexes such as GP IIb/IIIa, GP Ia/IIa, GP Ic/IIa, GP IIa' and GPIV. Finally, we could show that some HPA-2 antibody containing sera were able to block ristocetin induced aggregation of platelets (also after formalin fixation), but not aggregation by other agonists. All together these data strongly suggest that the HPA-2 system is due to a genetically determined polymorphism of the N-terminal part of GP Ibα. However, we are not yet able to definitely prove this location by immunoprecipitation or immunoblotting.

To the list in table 5 the Cr-related antigens have been added. Recently, it has been found that this family of red cell antigens (Cr^a, Tc^a, Tc^b, Tc^c, Dr^a, WES^a, WES^b, Es^a, UMC and IFC) is located on the decay accelerating factor (DAF or CD55 antigen) (for review see 47). Because DAF is also present on platelets (as well as on all white cells of the blood, endothelial cells and on most so not all tissue cells) this polymorphic structure is of interest to platelet immunologists as well.

The molecular nature of platelet specific antigens

Studies into the molecular nature of platelet antigens have only just started. It was shown that the Zw^a and Zw^b antigens (HPA-1a,b) are detectable on a small peptide fragment of 17-23 kDa (140-190 amino acid) obtained by trypsin digestion of GP IIIa (39, 49). The HPA-1 (Zw)-antigens are destroyed by reduction (50,51) indicating that they are dependent on the secondary structure of the protein with intact disulfide bridges. Recently, Newman et al. (52) used reverse transcriptase and the polymerase chain reaction (PCR) to study platelet-RNA from donors with different HPA-1 (Zw) phenotypes. They found that a C → T polymorphism at base 196 of the GP IIIa DNA sequence (53) may form the basis of HPA-1 (Zw) polymorphism. The C → T polymorphism leads to a unique Nci I restriction enzyme cleavage site in HPA-Ib (Zw^b)-DNA. The single base change results in a leucine/proline polymorphism at aminoacid postion 33 from the NH2-terminal part of GP IIIa (figure 1). This region of GP IIIa is rich in cysteines (7 in the first 50 N-terminal amino-acids) and extensive disulfide pairing will probably occur around amino acid 33. Thus, because HPA-1 (Zw) antigens are sensitive to reduction it is likely that the aminoacids leucine and proline are probably not part of the actual HPA-1 (Zw) epitopes but induce the epitopes in the folded GP IIIa chain at another site.

The localization of the HPA-1 (Zw) epitopes on the NH2-terminal part of GP IIIa explains the old finding that anti-HPA-1a (Zw^a) antibodies inhibit platelet aggregation via the inhibition of fibrinogen binding. This part of the molecule is thought to be involved in the formation of a fibrinogen binding site.

In an even more recent study by the group of Newman the PCR method was also applied to study the nature of Bak = HPA-3 polymorphism (54). In this latter study they found again a single base substitution and showed with allele specific oligonucleotide probes that this substitution was linked with the Bak-phenotype in normal donors. The base pair substitution results in an isoleucine-serine polymorphism of residue 843 of the mature GP IIb heavy chain (figure 2). Interestingly, this polymorphism is very close to the binding site of the monoclonal antibody PMI-1, a functionally important region of GP IIb regulated by divalent cation and ligand binding, and involved in platelet adhesion to collagen (55).

Platelet specificity of platelet-specific alloantigens

An important recent finding is that platelet specific alloantigens may be expressed on other cells and tissues as well.

Antigens of the HPA-1 (Zw) and HPA-4 (Pen=Yuk) system have been detected on endothelial cells, smooth muscle cells and fibroblasts (56,57,58). Antigens of the HPA-5 (Br) system have been found on activated T-lymphocyte and endothelial cells (59,60). HPA-2 (Ko) and HPA-3 (Bak) antigens, however, appear to be expresssed on platelets only.

These findings are not at all unexpected. Many antigen-carrying glycoproteins of platelets are present in the surface membrane as hetero-dimeric or hetero-trimeric complexes. The complexes have important functions as receptor molecules for ligand binding in platelet aggregation and adhesion. Similar or related receptors may be present on other cells and are involved in cell-cell or cell-matrix interactions in general. In fact, these glycoprotein complexes often belong to a large superfamily of adhesion molecules, named the integrins (61). Integrins are heterodimers of a noncovalently linked α- and β-chain. The superfamily consists of at least three (sub)families: the VLA (very late antigen) family, the LFA (leukocyte function antigen or leukocyte adhesion molecule (Leu-CAM) family) and the cytoadhesin family. Each family shares a common β-chain ($β_1$, $β_2$ and $β_3$, respectively). The members of a family have different α-chains and show different ligand-binding capacity. The different family β-chains have homologous amino-acid sequences, as have the different inter- and intra-family α-chains.

Platelet GP IIb and GP IIIa form a complex (also denoted as $α^{IIb}β_3$), which belongs to the cytoadhesin family. The complex has as ligands fibrinogen, fibronectin, von Willebrand factor (vWF) and vitronectin (S protein). All these adhesive proteins share the short peptide stretch RGDS (arg-gly-asp-ser) involved in binding to the receptor (62). On endothelial cells, fibroblasts, smooth muscle cells and osteoclasts (and in low amounts also on platelets) a related cytoadhesin is expressed, vitronectin receptor (VNR). This receptor has the ability to bind vitronectin, fibrinogen and vWF. VNR has the same β_3 chain (GP IIIa) which as discussed carries HPA-1 (Zw) and HPA-4 (Yuk=Pen) antigens. However, the α-chain (α^v) is different and appears not to carry HPA-3 (Bak) antigens, which are therefore unique for platelets. The VNR is also denoted as $\alpha^v\beta_3$.

Patients with Glanzmann's disease (GD) have platelets deficient in the membrane GP IIb/IIIa complex or $\alpha^{IIb}\beta_3$. However, their endothelial cells may express the VNR or $\alpha^v\beta_3$ normally (63). Thus, the endothelial cells in GD patients (as well as the smooth muscle cells) are expected to express HPA-1 (Zw) and HPA-4 (Pen) antigens normally. This was indeed found to be so for HPA-1 (58). Platelets express three members of the VLA family e.g. VLA-2 ($\alpha_2\beta_1$) or GP Ia/IIa complex, VLA-5 ($\alpha_5\beta_1$) and VLA-6 ($\alpha_6\beta_1$) both known as GP Ic/IIa complex (and possibly also some VLA-4=$\alpha_4\beta_1$). They are receptors for collagen, fibronectin and laminin, respectively (64,65). The VLA family encompasses at least six different members (VLA1-6) which are expressed on nearly every cell of the body, albeit in a different composition (and with different ligand binding capacity). All cells which carry VLA-2 or GP Ia/IIa will therefore also carry HPA-5 (Br) antigens including activated T cells and endothelial cells.

On platelets GP Ib (itself a heterodimer of GP Ibα and GP Ibβ) is complexed to GP IX. The complex is the major vWF receptor of platelets. So far, it has been found to be a unique adhesion structure, confined to platelets and megakaryocytes only. Thus Pl^E and HPA-2 (Ko) antigens are probably unique for this cell lineage. GP V may also be complexed to GP Ib/IX because as discussed together with GP Ib and GP IX this protein is not expressed on the platelet surface membrane of patients with Bernard Soulier syndrome. GP V seems to be present on endothelial cells (PW Modderman et al., unpublished). Thus, it is possible that Pl^T antigens are also present on the latter cell type.

The broad tissue expression of some platelet-antigen system is of more than basic interest. It suggests that antibodies directed against such antigens may not only attack and destroy platelets but other cells as well, including cells which form an integral part of vessel walls. More specifically, it is possible that purpura, which form such a characteristic sign of immune mediated thrombocytopenias may (also) result from direct vessel wall damage by the antibodies. Moreover, it is possible that an alloimmune response against these antigens may follow not only blood tranfusion, bone marrow transplantation and pregnancy, but also organ transplantation. Perhaps graft rejection may sometimes results from such an immune response.

Conclusion

Remarkable progress has been made in platelet immunology in the last decade and in all fields covered by it, including diagnosis and treatment of immune mediated platelet disorders. But, most remarkable has been the description of six new platelet specific antigens or antigen systems within 5 years, the detailed glycoprotein localization of all the antigens and last but not least the elucidation of the molecular basis of platelet antigen polymorphism in case of two antigen systems.

Thus, in the coming years platelet immunology is expected to become a science not only dealing with interesting and clinically important platelet disorders but also with the molecular basis of antigens (and immune response).

References

1. Leucocyte Typing IV. White cell differentiation antigens
   W. Knapp, B. Dörken, W.R. Gilks, E.P. Rieber, R.E. Schmidt, H. Stein,

   A.E.G. Kr. von dem Borne, editors. Oxford University Press, 1989
2. J. Moulinier
   Iso-immunisation maternelle antiplaquettaire et purpura néo-natal. Le système de groupe plaquettaire "duzo".
   Proc. 6th Congress Europ. Soc. Haematol., Copenhagen 1957:236;817-820. Karger, Basel

3. J.J. van Loghem, H. Dorfmeyer, M. van der Hart
   Serological and genetical studies on a platelet antigen (Zw)
   Vox Sang. 4;161-169 (1959)
4. Ch.M. van der Weerdt, L.E. Veenhoven-von Riesz, L.E. Nijenhuis, J.J. van Loghem
   The Zw blood group system in platelets
   Vox Sang. 8;513-530 (1963)
5. N.R. Shulman, V.J. Marder, M.C. Hiller, E.M. Collier
   Platelet and leucocyte isoantigens and their antibodies: serologic, physiologic and clinical studies
   Progress in Haematology 4;222-304 (1964)
6. C.M. van der Weerdt, H. van de Wiel-Dorfmeyer, C.P. Engelfriet, J.J. van Loghem
   A new platelet antigen
   Proc. 8th Congress Europ. Soc. Haematol. Vienna 1961:379. Karger, Basel
7. C.M. van der Weerdt
   The platelet agglutination test in platelet grouping. Histocompatibility testing 1965:161-166. Munksgaard, Kopenhagen
8. H. Saji, E. Maruya, H. Fujii, T. Maekawa, Y. Akiyama, T. Matsura, T. Hosoi
   New platelet antigen, Sib[a], involved in platelet transfusion refractoriness in a Japanese Man
   Vox Sang. 56;283-287 (1989)
9. A.E.G. Kr. von dem Borne, E. von Riesz, F.W.A. Verheugt, J.W. ten Cate, J.G. Koppe, C.P. Engelfriet, L.E. Nijenhuis
   Bak[a], a new platelet-specific-antigen involved in neonatal allo-immune thrombocytopenia
   Vox Sang. 39;113-120 (1980)
10. B. Boizard, J.W. Wautier
    Lek[a], a new platelet antigen absent in Glanzmann's thrombasthenia
    Vox Sang. 46;47-54 (1984)
11. T.S. Kickler, J.H. Herman, K. Furihata, T.J. Kunicki, R.H. Aster
    Identification of Bak[b], a new platelet-specific antigen associated with post-transfusion purpura
    Blood 71;894-898 (1988)
12. V. Kiefel, S. Santoso, W.M. Glöckner, B. Katzmann, W. Mayer, C. Mueller-Eckhardt
    Post-transfusion purpura associated with an antibody against an allele of the Bak[a] antigen
    Vox Sang. 56;93-97 (1989)

13. J.M. Friedman, R.H. Aster
    Neonatal alloimmune thrombocytopenic purpura and congenital porencephaly in two siblings associated with a 'new' maternal antiplatelet antibody
    Blood 66;1412-1415 (1985)
14. Y. Shibata, T. Miyayi, Y. Ichikawa, I. Matsuda
    A new platelet antigen system, Yuk^a/Yuk^b
    Vox Sang. 51;334-336 (1986)
15. V. Kiefel, S. Santoso, B. Katzmann, C. Mueller-Eckhardt
    A new platelet-specific alloantigen Br^a. Report of 4 cases with neonatal alloimmune thrombocytopenia
    Vox Sang. 54;101-106 (1988)
16. V. Kiefel, S. Santoso, B. Katzman, C. Mueller-Eckhardt
    The Br^a/Br^b alloantigen system on human platelets
    Blood 73;2219-2223 (1989)
17. V.L. Woods, K.D. Pischel, E.D. Avery, H.G. Bluestein
    Antigenic polymorphism of human very late activation protein-2 (platelet glycoprotein Ia-IIa). Platelet alloantigen Hc^a
    J. Clin. Invest 83;978-985 (1989)
18. J.W. Smith, J.G. Kelton, P. Horsewood, C. Brown, A. Giles, R. Meyer, V. Woods, R. Burrows
    Platelet specific alloantigens on the platelet glycoprotein Ia/IIa complex
    Brit. J. Haemat. 72;534-538 (1989)
19. D.S. Beardsley, J.S. Ho, T. Moulton
    Pl^T: a new platelet antigen on glycoprotein V
    Blood 70; suppl. 1, 347a,1244 (1987)
20. H. Ikeda, T. Mitani, M. Ohnuma, H. Haga, S. Ohtzuka, T. Kato, T. Nakase, S. Sekiguchi
    A new platelet-specific antigen, Nak^a, involved in the refractoriness of HLA-matched platelet transfusion
    Vox Sang. 57;213-217 (1989)
21. C. Mueller-Eckhardt, V. Kiefel, H. Kroll, S. Santoso
    A new low-frequency ("private") platelet alloantigen [Sr(a)] on glycoprotein IIIa associated with neonatal alloimmune thrombocytopenia (NAIT)
    Blood 74; suppl. 1, 188a,706 (1989)
22. J.W. Smith, J.G. Kelton, P. Horsewood, J.R. Humber, T.E. Warhentin
    A novel platelet alloantigen system, Gov^a/Gov^b, on a protein of 175 kDa
    Blood 74; suppl. 1, 69a,248 (1989)

23. G. Ramsey, D.J. Salamon
    Frequency of Pl^{A1} in blacks
    Transfusion 26;531-532 (1986)
24. J. Inostroza, V. Kiefel, C. Mueller-Eckhardt
    Frequency of platelet-specific antigens Pl^{A1}, Bak^a, Yuk^a, Yuk^b and Br^a in South American (Mapuches) Indians
    Transfusion 28;586-587 (1988)
25. K.S. Han, H.I. Cho, S.I. Kim
    Frequency of platelet-specific antigens among Koreans determined by a simplified immunofluorescence test
    Transfusion 29;708-710 (1989)
26. A.E.G. Kr. von dem Borne, E.F. van Leeuwen, L.E. von Riesz, C.J. van Boxtel, C.P. Engelfriet
    Neonatal alloimmune thrombocytopenia; detection and characterization of the responsible antibodies by the platelet immunofluorescent test
    Blood 57;649-656 (1980)
27. C. Mueller-Eckhardt, T. Bleker, M. Weisheit, C. Wirtz, S. Santoso
    Neonatal alloimmune-thrombocytopenia due to fetomaternal Zw^b incompatiblity
    Vox Sang 50;94-96 (1986)
28. N. Bizzaro, G. Dianese
    Neonatal alloimmune amegakaryocytosis
    Vox Sang. 54;112-114 (1988)
29. K. McGrath, R. Minchinton, I. Cunningham, H. Ayberk
    Platelet anti-Bak^b antibody associated with neonatal alloimmune thrombocytopenia
    Vox Sang. 57;182-184 (1989)
30. C. Mueller-Eckhardt, V. Kiefel, A. Grubert, H. Kroll, M. Weisheit, S. Schmidt, G. Mueller-Eckhardt, S. Santoso
    348 cases of suspected neonatal alloimmune thrombocytopenia
    Lancet I;363-366 (1989)
31. N.R. Shulman, R.H. Aster, A. Leitner, M.C. Hiller
    Immunoreactions involving platelets. V. Post-transfusion purpura due to a complement-fixing antibody against a genetically controled platelet antigen. A proposed mechanism for thrombocytopenia and its relevance in autoimmunity.
    J. Clin. Invest. 40;1597-1620 (1961)
32. E. Taaning, N. Morling, H. Ovesen, A. Svejgaard
    Posttransfusion purpura and anti-Zw^b(-Pl^{A2})
    Tissue Antigens 26;143-146 (1985)

33. R.M. Keimowitz, J. Collins, K. Davis, R.H. Aster
    Posttransfusion purpura associated with alloimmunization against the platelet-specific antigen, Bak^a
    Am. J. Haematol. 21;79-88 (1986)
34. T.L. Simon, J. Collins, T.J. Kunicki, K. Furihata, K.J. Smith, R.H. Aster
    Posttransfusion purpura associated with alloantibody specific for the platelet antigen Pen^a
    Am. J. Haemat. 29;38-40 (1988)
35. A.E.G. Kr. von dem Borne, W.H. Ouwehand, R.W.A.M. Kuijpers
    Theoretical and practical aspects of platelet cross matching
    Transf. Med. Rev. in press (1990)
36. F. Langerscheidt, V. Kiefel, S. Santoso, C. Mueller-Echardt
    Platelet transfusion refractoriness associated with two rare platelet-specific alloantibodies (anti-Bak^a and anti-Pl^{A2}) and multiple HLA antibodies
    Transfusion 28;597-600 (1988)
37. P. Bierling, P. Fromont, A. Bettaieb, N. Duedari
    Anti-Br^a antibodies in the French population
    Brit. J. Haemat. 73;428-429 (1989)
38. T.J. Kunicki, R.H. Aster
    Isolation and immunologic characterization of the human platelet alloantigen Pl^{A1}
    Molecular Immunology 16;353-360 (1979)
39. C.E. van der Schoot, M. Wester, A.E.G. Kr. von dem Borne, J.G. Huisman
    Characterization of platelet-specific alloantigens by immunoblotting: localization of Zw and Bak antigens
    Brit J. Haemat. 64;715-723 (1986)
40. R.W.A.M. Kuijpers, P.W. Modderman, P.M.M. Bleeker, W.H. Ouwehand, A.E.G. Kr. von dem Borne
    Localization of the platelet specific Ko system antigens Ko^a/Ko^b on GP Ib/IX
    Blood 74; suppl 1, 226a,842 (1989)
41 N. Kieffer, B. Boizard, D. Didry, J.L. Wautier, A.T. Nurden
    Immunochemical characterization of the platelet-specific alloantigen Lek^a: a comparative study with the Pl^{A1} alloantigen
    Blood 64;1212-1219 (1984)

42. Y. Shibata, H. Mori
   A new platelet-specific alloantigen system, Yuk^a/Yuk^b, is located on platelet membrane glycoprotein IIIa
   Proc. Japan Academy 63; ser B, no 1,36-38 (1987)
43. K. Furihata, D.J. Nuyent, A. Bissonette, R.H. Aster, T.J. Kunicki
   On the association of the platelet-specific alloantigen, Pen^a, with glycoprotein IIIa. Evidence for heterogeneity of glycoprotein IIIa
   J. Clin. Invest. 80;1624-1630 (1987)
44. S. Santoso, Y. Shibata, V. Kiefel, C. Mueller-Eckhardt
   Identification of the Yuk^b alloantigen on platelet glycoprotein IIIa
   Vox Sang. 53;48-51 (1987)
45. S. Santoso, V. Kiefel, C. Mueller-Eckhardt
   Immunochemical characterization of the new alloantigen system Br^a/Br^b
   Brit. J. Haemat. 72;191-198 (1989)
46. K. Furihata, J. Hunter, R.H. Aster, G.R. Koewing, N.R. Shulman, T.J. Kunicki
   Human anti-Pl^{E1} antibody recognizes epitopes associated with the alpha subunit of platelet glycoprotein Ib
   Brit. J. Haemat. 68;103-110 (1988)
47. G. Daniels
   Cromer-related antigens-bloodgroup determinants on decay-accelerating factor
   Vox Sang. 56;205-211 (1989)
48. V. Kiefel, S. Santoso, M. Weisheit, C. Mueller-Eckhardt
   Monoclonal antibody specific immobilization of platelet antigens (MAIPA): a new tool for the identification of platelet reactive antibodies
   Blood 70;1722-1726 (1987)
49. P.J. Newman, L.S. Martin, M.A. Knipp, R.A. Kahn
   Studies on the nature of the human platelet alloantigen, Pl^{A1}
   Mol. Immunol. 22;719-729 (1985)
50. R. McMillan, D. Mason, P. Tani, M. Schmidt
   Evaluation of platelet surface antigen: localization of the Pl^{A1} alloantigen
   Brit. J. Haemat. 51;297-304 (1982)
51. J.G. Huisman
   Immunoblotting: an emerging technique in immunohaematology
   Vox Sang. 50;129-136 (1986)

52. P.J. Newman, R.S. Derbes, R.H. Aster
    The human platelet alloantigens, Pl^{A1} and Pl^{A2}, are associated with a leucine^{33}/proline^{33} aminoacid polymorphism in membrane glycoprotein IIIa, and are distinguishable by DNA typing
    J. Clin. Invest. 83;1778-1781 (1989)
53. L.A. Fitzgerald, B. Steiner, S.C. Rall, S.S. Lo, D.R. Philips
    Protein sequence of endothelial glycoprotein IIIa derived from a cDNA clone
    J. Biol. Chem. 262;3936-3939 (1987)
54. S. Lyman, R.H. Aster, P.J. Newman
    Polymorphism of human platelet membrane glycoprotein IIb associated with the Bak^a/Bak^b alloantigen system
    Blood 74; suppl. 1, 58a,205 (1989)
55. J.C. Loftus, E.F. Plow, A.L. Felinger III, S.E. D'Souza, D. Dixon, L. Lacy, J. Sorge, M.H. Grinsberg
    Molecular cloning and chemical synthesis of a region of platelet glycoprotein IIb involved in adhesive function
    Proc. Nat. Acad. Science 84;7114-7118 (1987)
56. O.C. Leeksma, J.C. Giltay, J. Zandbergen-Spaargaren, P.W. Modderman, J.A. van Mourik, A.E.G. Kr. von dem Borne
    The platelet alloantigen Zw^a or Pl^{A1} is expressed by cultured endothelial cells
    Brit. J. Haemat. 66;369-373 (1987)
57. J.C. Giltay, O.C. Leeksma, A.E.G. Kr. von dem Borne, J.A. van Mourik
    Alloantigenic composition of the endothelial vitronectin receptor
    Blood 72;230-233 (1988)
58. J.C. Giltay, H.J.M. Brinkman, A.E.G. Kr. von dem Borne, J.A. van Mourik
    Expression of Zw^a (or Pl^{A1}) on human vascular smooth muscle cells and foreskin fibroblasts: a study on normal individuals and a patient with Glanzmann's thrombosthenia
    Blood 74;965-970 (1989)
59. S. Santoso, V. Kiefel, C. Mueller-Eckhardt
    Human platelet alloantigens Br^a/Br^b are expressed on the very late activation antigen 2 (VLA-2) of T-lymphocytes
    Human Immunology 25;237-346 (1989)

60. J.C. Giltay, H.J.M. Brinkman, A. Vlekke, V. Kiefel, J.A. van Mourik, A.E.G. Kr. von dem Borne
    The platelet glycoprotein Ia-IIa associated Br-alloantigen system is expressed by cultured endothelial cells
    Submitted for publication (1989)
61. R.C. Hynes
    Integrins: a family of cell surface receptors
    Cell 48;549-554 (1987)
62. M.H. Ginsberg, J.C. Loftus, E.F. Plow
    Cytoadhesins, integrins and platelets
    Thrombosis and haemostasis 59;1-6 (1989)
63. J.C. Giltay, O.C. Leeksma, C. Breederveld, J.A. van Mourik
    Normal synthesis and expression of endothelial IIb/IIIa in Glanzmann's Thrombasthenia
    Blood 69;809-812 (1987)
64. A. Sonnenberg, P.W. Modderman, F. Hogervorst
    Laminin receptor on platelets is the integrin VLA-6
    Nature 336;487-489 (1988)
65. M.E. Hemler
    Adhesive protein receptors on haematopoietic cells
    Immunology Today 9;109-113 (1988)

Résumé

Des différentes classes d'antigènes plaquettaires celle des alloantigènes "spécifiques" jouant un rôle fondamental dans les TNN et les PPT est décrite en détail. Les xénoantigènes mis en évidence par les monoclonaux murins sont brièvement cités. Ces dernières années plusieurs nouveaux alloantigènes plaquettaires ont été décrits nécessitant la création d'un nouveau système de nomenclature (HPA = human platelet antigen). La localisation de certains antigènes plaquettaire sur une glycoprotéine a été possible par l'apport de nouveaux outils. Les antigènes des systèmes HPA-1 et HPA-4 sont portés par la GPIIIa, HPA-3 sur la GPIIb, HPA-5 sur la GPIa et l'antigène Nak^a sur la GPIV ; les antigènes HPA-2 (Ko) étant probablement porté par la chaine alpha de la GPIb (extrémité N-terminale). La plupart de ces glycoprotéines fait partie de la superfamille des récepteurs de protéines adhésives (intégrines), ce qui explique leur expression non seulement sur les plaquettes mais aussi sur d'autres types cellulaires (cellules endothéliales, fibres musculaires lisses, fibroblastes, lymphocytes T activés...); elles ne sont donc plus strictement plaquettaires. Des études en biologie moléculaire ont récemment commencé permettant de mettre en évidence des polymorphismes au niveau des acides aminés pour certains antigènes. Le polymorphisme épitopique résulte des différences entre les structures secondaires et/ou tertiaires dues aux changements en acides aminés (structure primaire).

Platelet glycoproteins IIa, IIIa and Ib carry blood group A and B determinants

S. Santoso, V. Kiefel and C. Mueller-Eckhardt

Institute of Clinical Immunology and Transfusion Medicine, Justus Liebig University, Langhansstrasse 7, D-6300 Giessen, Germany

ABSTRACT

We report the localization of A, B blood group determinants on intrinsic platelet glycoproteins using anti-A, B IgG antibodies. By radioimmunoprecipitation and subsequent analysis in two dimensional gel electrophoresis (isoelectric focussing/SDS-PAGE) anti-A precipitated six spots with identical mobilities as platelet glycoprotein (GP) complexes Ia/IIa, Ic'/IIa, Ib/IX and IIb/IIIa. The results were confirmed by data obtained by an assay employing monoclonal antibody-specific immobilization of platelet antigens (MAIPA). By this technique, blood group A, B determinants were shown to be immobilized by monoclonal antibodies (mabs) specific for GP Ia, Ic', IX, IIb/IIIa and strongly by mab specific for GP IIa, but not by mab specific for HLA class I molecules.
The more precise localization on platelet glycoproteins was achieved by immunoblotting technique by which blood group A determinants could be assigned to GPs IIa, IIIa and Ib.

INTRODUCTION

Although ABH blood group determinants have been recognized on platelets for many years (Moreaux & Andre, 1954), there is little information regarding their localization on platelet membranes. Dunstan et al. (1985a) demonstrated that ABH determinants on platelets, like on erythrocytes, consisted of intrinsic type 2 chains and passively absorbed type 1 chains in approximately equal amounts. The intrinsic determinants are believed to be borne by glycolipids rather than by glycoproteins (Dunstan et al., 1985b).
More recently, Mollicone et al. (1988) have shown that a variety of platelet glycoproteins do carry intrinsic ABH determinants. Since the major glycoprotein comigrated with GP Ibα, the authors suggested that glycocalicin, a highly O-glycosylated fragment of this glycoprotein, contributes to the major part of the glycoprotein-borne ABH determinants of platelets.
In this study, we have identified at least three different platelet glycoproteins, i.e. GP IIa, IIIa, Ib containing A, B determinants of which GP IIa appears to be the most prominent.

MATERIALS AND METHODS

Human antisera
Anti-A serum with high-titer of IgG antibodies was obtained from a polytransfused patient who developed refractoriness to platelet transfusions (Santoso et al., 1990a). Anti-B serum was from a healthy mother who delivered a child with neonatal alloimmune thrombocytopenia (Mueller-Eckhardt et al., 1989). The control serum was collected from a non-transfused male blood donor of blood group AB. All sera were stored at -25°C until use.

Monoclonal antibodies (mabs)
The specificities of the mabs used in this study are listed in Table 1.

Table 1: Specificities of the monoclonal antibodies used in the MAIPA assay for immobilization of platelet glycoproteins.
VLA: Very Late Activation Antigen

Mab	Specific for an epitope on	References
FMC 25	GP IX	Berndt et al, 1985
Gi3	GP IIb/IIIa	Santoso et al, 1989
A-1A5	GP IIa (VLAß)	Hemler et al, 1983
Gi 14	GP Ia (VLAα2)	Santoso et al, 1989
GoH3	GP Ic' (VLAα6)	Sonnenberg et al, 1987
w6/32	HLA class I	Brodsky et al, 1979

Platelets
Platelets from healthy donors of known blood group were isolated by differential centrifugation from EDTA-anticoagulated blood as previously described (Santoso et al., 1989). Platelets were used immediately for radioimmunoprecipitation and immunoblotting or stored in isotonic saline containing 0.1% NaN_3 at 4°C for MAIPA assay (see below).

Radioimmunoprecipitation
Platelets were surface-labelled with ^{125}I using the lactoperoxidase catalyzed method of Phillips and Poh Agin (1977). Immunoprecipitation was performed as described (Santoso et al., 1989). The immunoprecipitates were analyzed by 2D-gel electrophoresis according to the method of O'Farell (1975).

Immunoblotting
Immunoblotting was performed as described (Santoso et al., 1990 b). In brief, 4×10^9 washed platelets were solubilized in 10 mM tris buffer (TB) containing 150 mM NaCl, 3 mM EDTA, 30 mM ethylmaleinimide, 1 mM phenylmethylsulfonylfluoride, 40 µg leupeptin, 2% SDS for 1 h at 37°C. 1.5 mg protein of platelet lysates were separated on 7.5% SDS-PAGE and blotted to nitrocellulose membranes by the method of Towbin et al. (1979). After blocking in 20 mM TB containing 3% bovine serum albumine (BSA-TB) for 90 min at room temperature, strips were incubated 2 h with 30 µl antibody eluates in 2 ml 1% BSA-TB, washed with TB and expossed to ^{125}I-labelled sheep anti-human IgG (Amersham Buchler, Braunschweig, FRG). Strips were then washed and autoradiographed.

Monoclonal antibody-specific immobilization of platelet antigens (MAIPA assay)
The MAIPA assay was performed as published in detail (Kiefel et al., 1987). Mabs against platelet glycoproteins were used for antigen immobilization (Table 1).

Acid elution
Anti-A and anti-B were purified by absorption with platelets and acid elution as described by Hotchkiss et al (1986)

RESULTS

Identification of blood group A, B determinants on platelet glycoproteins

Fig. 1 shows the immunoprecipitation pattern of anti-A with iodine-labelled platelets of a blood group A1 donor on two-dimensional gel electrophoresis. Four platelet glycoproteincomplexes Ia/IIa, Ic'/IIa, Ib/IX and IIb/IIIa recognized by anti-A could be precipitated.
The same pattern was obtained from blood group B donor with anti-B (data not shown). To determine which glycoprotein(s) carried the blood group antigenic determinants recognized by anti-A, immunoblotting analysis was performed with purified anti-A obtained through absorption and elution with platelets. By this technique, the epitopes defined by anti-A could be assigned to GP IIa, GP IIIa and GP Ib (Fig. 2).

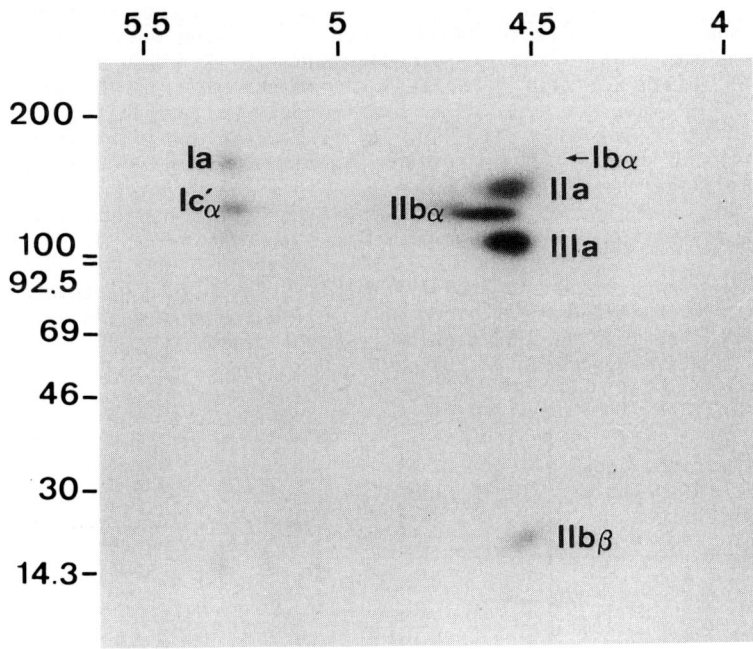

Fig. 1: Autoradiogram of reduced ^{125}I-labelled glycoproteins from a blood group A1 donor immunoprecipitated by anti-A serum. Immunoprecipitates were analyzed by two-dimensional gel electrophoresis. First dimension: isoelectric focussing pH 4-5.6; second dimension: 7.5% SDS-PAGE.

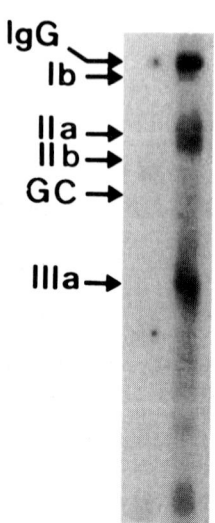

Fig. 2:

Immunoblot of platelet membranes from a blood group A1 donor. Platelets were solubilized on 7.5% SDS-PAGE under non-reduced conditions. After transfer to nitrocellulose membranes and incubation with control eluate (lane 1) and anti-A eluate (lane 2) bound antibody were detected with ^{125}I sheep anti-human IgG.

Reactivity and glycoprotein specificity of anti-A and anti-B in MAIPA assay

Table 2 show the results of MAIPA experiments using anti-A and anti-B sera with platelets from donors of blood groups A1, B and O and mabs directed against GP Ib/IX, IIb/IIIa, IIa, Ia, Ic' and HLA class I for antigen immobilization. The blood group A1 determinants could be immobilized by mabs specific for GP Ib/IX, IIb/IIIa, IIa, Ia, Ic' from platelets of blood group A1, but not of B and O donors. All these mabs also immobilized blood group B determinants from platelets of B donor only.

In contrast, blood group A and B determinants could not be immobilized with the mab specific for HLA class I molecules.

Table 2: The reactivities of anti-A and anti-B serum with platelets from individual donors of blood group A1, B and O in MAIPA assay using mabs against various platelet glycoproteins. Negative reactions are below 0.150.

human serum containing	blood group of platelet donors	glycoproteins immobilized with mab specific for					
		Ib/IX	IIb/IIIa	IIa (VLAβ)	Ia (VLAα2)	Ic' (VLAα6)	HLA class I
anti-A	A1	0.58	0.52	1.54	1.19	0.29	0.13
	B	0.07	0.08	0.06	0.10	0.04	0.13
	O	0.14	0.07	0.09	0.02	0.01	0.12
anti-B	A1	0.06	0.03	0.02	0.03	0.03	0.04
	B	0.37	0.25	1.35	0.61	0.19	0.05
	O	0.00	0.07	0.05	0.02	0.01	0.01

DISCUSSION

The precise structural assigment of blood group A and B determinants to platelet glycoproteins is still under debate. Mollicone et al. (1988) recently demonstrated that the anti-A monoclonal antibody (3-3A) recognizes major bands around 130-140 kd. Minor bands ranging from 160 to 60 kd were also detected. The authors therefore considered it likely that glycocalicin represented the major band, but the true glycoproteins were not identified.

We now show that blood group A, B determinants reside on intrinsic platelet glycoproteins IIa, IIIa and Ib.
Using human immune anti-A, B IgG antibodies and a battery of murine glycoprotein-specific monoclonal antibodies, the MAIPA results indicate that A, B determinants are present on at least four different glycoprotein complexes. i.e. GP Ia/IIa, Ic'/IIa, IIb/IIIa and Ib/IX (Table 2).
The strongest reactions of anti-A, B were observed using mabs against GP Ia (VLA α 2) and GP IIa (VLAß), intermediate reactivity with those directed against the glycoprotein complexes IIb/IIIa and Ib/IX, while the lowest values were obtained with anti GP Ic' (VLA α 6).
Since GP IIa represents the common ß subunit of VLA antigens in the platelet membrane, known to be associated in heterodimeric complexes with GP Ia (VLA α 2), GP Ic (VLA α 5) and GP Ic' (VLA α 6) (Hemler et al., 1988), our results suggest that GP IIa is the major carrier of AB determinants on these complexes.
These findings were corroborated in radioimmunoprecipitation experiments. At least four different platelet glycoprotein complexes Ia/IIa, Ic'/IIa, IIb/IIIa and Ib/IX were precipitated by anti-A (Fig. 1).
A more precise localization on platelet glycoproteins was accomplished by immunoblotting. By this technique, the blood group A determinants could be clearly assigned to GPs IIa, IIIa and Ib (Fig. 2).
Our data provide a rational biochemical basis for the clinical experience that immune anti-A/anti-B may occasionally cause platelet transfusion refractoriness in ABO-incompatible donor recipient pairs (Duquesnoy et al., 1979; Brand et al., 1986) and neonatal alloimmune thrombocytopenia (Mueller-Eckhardt et al., 1981; 1989).
Further studies are warranted to determine if the condition of refractoriness to A, B incompatible, HLA compatible platelet transfusions and neonatal alloimmune thrombocytopenia is realibly indicated by immune anti-A, B reactive with immobilized platelet glycoproteins.

ACKNOWLEDGEMENTS

This work was supported by the Deutsche Forschungsgemeinschaft (Mu 277/9-7). The technical assistance of Ms. Micaela Zickert and the secretarial expertise of Ms. Tanja Ille is appreciated.

REFERENCES

Berndt, M.C., Chong, B.H., Bull,H.A., Zola, H., Castaldi, P.A. (1985): Molecular characterization of quinine/quinidine drug-dependent antibody platelet interaction using monoclonal antibodies. Blood 66, 1292.

Brand, A., Sintnicolaas, K., Claas, F.H.J., Eernisse, J.G. (1986): ABH antibodies causing platelet transfsuion refractoriness. Transfusion 26, 463.

Brodsky, F.M., Parham, P. Barnstable, C.J., Crumpton, M.J., Bodmer, W.F. (1979): Monoclonal antibodies for analysis of the HLA-system. Immunol. Rev. 47, 3.

Dunstan, R.A., Simpson, M.B., Knowles, R.W., Rosse, W.F. (1985): The origin of ABH antigens on human platelets. Blood 65, 615.

Dunstan, R.A. & Mansbach, C.M. (1985): Biochemical characterisation of a blood group activity on human platelets. Vox Sang. 49, 149.

Duquesnoy, R.J., Anderson, A.J., Tomasulo, P.A., Aster, R.H. (1979): ABO-compatibility and platelet transfusions of alloimmunized thrombocytopenic patients. Blood 54, 595.

Hemler, E.M., Ware, C.F., Strominger, J.L. (1983): Characterization of a novel differentiation antigen complex recognized by a monoclonal antibody (A-1A5): Unique activation-specific molecular forms on stimulated T cells. J. Immunol. 131, 334.

Hemler, M.E, Crouse, C., Takada, Y., Sonnenberg, A. (1988): Multiple very late antigen (VLA) heterodimers on platelets. Evidence for distinct VLA-2, VLA-5 (fibronectin receptor), and VLA-6 structures. J. Biol. Chem. 263, 7660.

Hotchkiss, A.J., Leissinger, C.A., Smith, M.E., Jordan, J.V., Kautz, C.A., Shulman, N.R. (1986): Evaluation by quantitative acid elution and radioimmunoassay of multiple classes of immunoglobulins and serum albumin associated with platelets in idiopathic thrombocytopenic purpura. Blood 67, 1126.

Kiefel, V., Santoso, S., Weisheit, M., Mueller-Eckhardt, C. (1987): Monoclonal antibody-specific immobilization of platelet antigens (MAIPA): A new tool for the identification of platelet-reactive antibodies. Blood 70, 1722.

Mollicone, R., Caillard, T., Le Pendu, J., Franois, A., Sansonetti, N., Villarroya, J., Oriol, R. (1988): Expression of ABH and X (Le^x) antigens on platelets and lymphocytes. Blood 71, 1113.

Moreaux, P. & Andre, A. (1954): Blood groups of human blood platelets. Nature 174, 88.

Mueller-Eckhardt, C., Kayser, W., Förster, C., Mueller-Eckhardt, G. (1981): Improved assay for detection of platelet-specific Pl(A1) antibodies in neonatal alloimmune thrombocytopenia. Vox Sang. 43, 76.

Mueller-Eckhardt, C., Kiefel, V., Grubert, A., Kroll, H., Weisheit, M., Schmidt, S., Mueller-Eckhardt, G., Santoso, S. (1989): 348 cases of suspected neonatal alloimmune thrombocytopenia. Lancet 1, 363.

O'Farell, P.H. (1975): High resolution two-dimensional electrophoresis of proteins. J. Biol. Chem. 250, 4007.

Phillips, D.R., Poh Agin, P. (1977): Platelet plasma membrane glycoproteins. Evidence for the presence of nonequivalent disulfide bonds using non-reduced reduced two-dimensional gel electrophoresis. J. Biol. Chem. 252, 2121.

Santoso, S., Kiefel, V., Mueller-Eckhardt, C. (1989): Immunochemical characterization of the new platelet alloantigen system Br(a)/Br(b). Br. J. Haematol. 72, 191.

Santoso, Su., Kiefel, V., Santoso, S., Mueller-Eckhardt, G., Mueller-Eckhardt, C. (1990a; submitted for publication): Crossmatching and serological studies in patients on platelet-substitution therapy.

Santoso, S., Kiefel, V., Mueller-Eckhardt, C. (1990b; submitted for publication): Blood group A and B determinants are expressed on platelet glycoproteins IIa, IIIa and Ib.

Sonnenberg, A., Janssen, H., Hogervorst, F., Calafat, J., Hilgers, J. (1987): A complex of platelet glycoproteins Ic and IIa identified by a rat monoclonal antibody. J. Biol. Chem. 262, 10376.

Towbin, H., Stachelin, T., Gordon, J. (1979): Electrophoretic transfer of proteins from polyacrylamide gels to nitrocellulose shetts: Procedure and some applications. Proc. Natl. Acad. Sci. USA 76, 4350.

Résumé

Nous démontrons la localisation des déterminants des groupes sanguins A et B sur les glycoprotéines plaquettaires (GP) en utilisant des anticorps anti A et B de nature IgG. Par radioimmunoprécipitation et analyse en gel 2 dimensions (isoelectrofocalisation SDS-PAGE) l'anti A précipite 3 spots avec des mobilités identiques aux complexes glycoprotéique Ia/IIa, Ic'/IIa, Ib/IX et IIb/IIIa. Les résultats sont confirmés par les données, obtenues dans une technique utilisant l'immobilisation spécifique des antigènes plaquettaires par des anticorps monoclonaux (MAIPA). Grâce à cette technique, les déterminants des groupes sanguins A et B ont été immobilisés par des anticorps monoclonaux (Mabs) spécifiques de GPIa, Ic', IX, IIb/IIIa et très fortement par des Mabs spécifiques pour GPIIa mais non pas des Mabs spécifiques pour les molécules HLA de classe I. La localisation plus précise sur les glycoprotéines plaquettaires a été effectuée par immoblotting montrant la localisation du déterminant du groupe sanguin A sur le GP IIa, IIIa et Ib.

Posttransfusion purpura

C. Mueller-Eckhardt, H. Kroll, V. Kiefel and the members of the European PTP Study Group*

Institute of clinical Immunology and Transfusion Medicine, Justus-Liebig-University, Langhansstrasse 7, D-6300 Giessen, Germany

ABSTRACT

Posttransfusion purpura (PTP) is a rare, but serious complication of blood transfusion. In a joint European study, data from a total of 104 PTP cases from 14 centers in 9 European countries were collected and analyzed. Ninety-nine patients were women. The mean age of patients was 58.4 years. The interval between administration of blood products containing platelet material and onset of PTP was 6 to 8 days (range 1 to 14 days). Bleeding symptoms were severe in most cases with an initial platelet count below 10,000/µl at diagnosis in 81%. No immediate deaths were reported. The most effective therapy appeared to be high-dose IgG. Platelet-specific antibodies incriminated for elicitation of PTP were anti-Zw(a)(n=88), anti-Zw(b)(n=5), anti-Bak(a)(n=6), anti-Bak(b)(n=1), uncertain antibodies (n=5). Possible pathogenetic mechanisms are discussed.

INTRODUCTION

Posttransfusion purpura (PTP) was recognized as a clinical and pathophysiological entity by Shulman et al in 1961 (1). The syndrome is characterized by a sudden onset of thrombocytopenic purpura approximately one week after blood transfusion containing platelet material. PTP is rarely encountered. Until 1986, a total of about 150 cases had been published (2), but the incidence is unknown. Although the clinical features of PTP have now been well established, it has remained an enigmatic disease with regard to

---

*Members of the European PTP Study Group are: A.E.G.Kr. von dem Borne (Amsterdam); P. Bierling (Créteil); J.V. Clough (Chester); C. Entwistle (Oxford); C. Kaplan (Paris, CNTS); A. Majsky (Prague); C. Mueller-Eckhardt (Giessen); E. Muniz-Diaz (Barcelona); R. Nordhagen (Oslo); P. Perrier (Nancy); E. Taaning (Copenhagen); A. Waters (London); J.L. Wautier (Paris, Lariboisière); B.Zupanska (Warsaw)

immunological as well as pathophysiological problems. It was for this reason that we recently initiated a Joint European PTP Study attempting to retrospectively collect all available information of PTP patients observed in European countries. Preliminary data of this study will be presented.

PATIENTS AND CONTRIBUTING CENTERS

A detailed questionnaire was sent out in December 1989 to all European centers known to be involved in platelet immunology. Data from a total of 104 PTP patients investigated at 14 different centers in nine European countries were obtained and are summarized in Table 1.

CLINICAL DATA

Out of 104 patients, 99 (95.2%) were women and 5 were men. The mean age of patients at diagnosis (n=90) was 58.4 years with a range of 16 to 83 years. Indications for blood transfusions were documented in 85 patients and were perioperative blood loss (n=62), anemia (n=16), acute hemorrhages, mostly from the gastrointestinal tract (n=6), and delivery (n=1). Transfusion reactions (chills, fever) were noted in 28 out of 51 patients. The interval between administration of blood products and onset of PTP was 1 to 14 days, with a peak incidence of purpura at days 6 to 8. Platelet counts at commencement of PTP were provided in 84 cases. The mean platelet count was 8,800/µl, and in 68 out of 84 patients (81%) the initial count was less than 10,000/µl. The duration and severity of purpura is influenced by treatment. Information as to the clinical course of PTP was available in 30 cases. Hemorrhagic signs lasted for a mean duration of 10.2 days, with a range of 3 to 37 days. The mean time until platelet counts reached a level of 50,000/µl (n=63) was 14.6 days with a range of 3 to 90 days, and platelet counts of 100,000/µl were observed at day 19.5 (n=58; range 3 to 130 days).

Treatment of PTP is mandatory because purpura at onset is usually severe and fatalities have been described in the acute hemorrhagic period (2). In the present material corticosteroids were given to 50 patients, 30 received high-dose IgG (in 16 cases together with corticosteroids). Plasmapheresis was performed in 10 patients. Thirty-one patients were treated with random platelet concentrates, 12 of whom reacted with untoward side effects.

Although the effectiveness of the different treatment modalities could not be clearly delineated in many of the presented cases, there is now convincing evidence that the treatment of choice for PTP is probably high-dose IgG. In our recent survey of 17 PTP patients treated with adequate doses of IgG (3), 16 had a good or excellent response. Plasmapheresis often is also effective, but with a lower success rate and at the cost of a higher risk for the patients. Administration of corticosteroids or platelet transfusions usually show little or no effect. Since recurrence of PTP has been described in several instances, only antigen-poor blood products, i.e. washed packed red cells or platelet antigen-negative components, should be utilized further.

The prognosis of PTP is undeterminable. Approximately 5-10% of published cases deceased from intracerebral hemorrhages within the first 10 days (2). However, this may be an overestimation, since among the 104 cases of this study no immediate deaths due to PTP were documented.

SEROLOGICAL DATA

The specificities of platelet-reactive antibodies presumed to be involved in the elicitation of PTP are listed in Table 2. About 85% of cases had Zw(a) antibodies, either alone or, more frequently, together with HLA antibodies. One serum also had platelet autoantibodies of undetermined specificity. Bak(a) antibodies were recognized in 6, respectively in 7 cases, and therefore this specificity is the second most frequent antibody involved in PTP. Zw(b) antibodies were diagnosed in 5 cases (4.8%). The Bak(b) antibody was described in detail by Kiefel et al (4). HLA antibodies alone (once in conjunction with an undefined "platelet-specific antibody") were detected in 4 cases. Their pathogenetic role is still uncertain. If one disregards the latter, all PTP cases of our study were caused by platelet antibodies directed against epitopes on the glycoprotein complex IIb/IIIa.

PATHOPHYSIOLOGY

The pathophysiology is still unclear. One precondition for precipitation of PTP appears to be an anamnestic immune response, either by pregnancy and/or by blood transfusions. In all cases of the present study in which relevant information was provided there was evidence for pre-immunization, mainly by pregnancies. This explains why the great majority of PTP patients are elderly women with a history of childbearing. Another typical feature of PTP is that the platelet-specific antibodies (at least so far as Zw(a) antibodies are concerned) always appear to be complement-fixing at initiation of PTP (5), quite different from Zw(a) antibodies in neonatal alloimmune thrombocytopenia which are always of the noncomplement-fixing ("blocking") type. Also a switch of IgG subclasses from IgG1 to IgG3 has been proposed as a pathogenetic factor (6).

The pathogenetic mechanism by which destruction of autologous platelets is brought about by an alloantibody directed against antigens of the transfused platelets is as yet obscure. Four mechanisms are considered: 1. The production of an autoantibody, arising with specific alloantibody that crossreacts with autologous platelets; 2. the generation of immune complexes which are being formed from transfused platelet fragments or soluble plasma antigen with subsequently formed alloantibodies that bind with high affinity to autologous platelets; 3. the "coating" of autologous platelets with acquired alloantigens, either transfused soluble in plasma or released from platelets, allowing them to be sensitized by subsequently formed alloantibody; 4. the production of alloantibodies with "pseudospecificity" and subsequent complement activation. The evidence for such a mechanism stems from observations in a very similar condition in the red cell system, i.e. delayed hemolytic transfusion reactions. We postulate that in PTP inital alloantibodies may be produced in the early anamnestic phase that combine with autologous platelets ("pseudospecific" alloantibodies) and elicit transitory complement activation. This notion is supported by data of von dem Borne & van der Plas-van Dalen (7) who found Zw(a) antibodies in all three eluates prepared from platelets of PTP patients between days 9 and 21. We have had similar experiences (V. Kiefel, unpublished data).

COMMENTS

The Joint European PTP Study 1990 comprising 104 PTP cases is the largest body of PTP patients so far reported. Although it is a retrospective study, the preliminary analysis of data has corroborated many of the typical clinical and immunological features of PTP. It is hoped that the questionnaire designed for complete clinical and immunogenetic documentation of PTP will assist in the future analysis of such cases in a more prospective manner. From a clinical point of view it is likely that most cases of PTP still remain undiagnosed as reflected in the great variation of numbers within the various countries und regions. In our experience, the correct diagnosis is most commonly missed. A broadened awareness for this syndrome by the attending clinicians is a prerequisite for a clearer delineation of therapeutic guidelines. Collaboration among laboratories and exchange of antibody-containing sera can help to improve serological technology obligatory for rapid clinical diagnosis. It will furthermore promote our unterstanding of the role of these antibodies in the pathogenesis of PTP. It is in this sense that we express our expectation that the European PTP Study 1990 is not an end, but the beginning of a joint European venture aiming at the resolution of some of the yet challenging problems of PTP.

ACKNOWLEDGEMENTS

This work was supported by the Deutsche Forschungsgemeinschaft (Mu 277/9-7). We greatly appreciate the generous cooperation of all members of the European PTP Study Group and their associates. A full account of data is now being prepared and will be published after completion of the study elswhere.

REFERENCES

1) Shulman, N.R., Aster, R.H., Leitner, A., Hiller, M.C. (1961): Immunoreactions involving platelets. V. Post-transfusion purpura due to a complement-fixing antibody against a genetically controlled platelet antigen. A proposed mechanism for thrombocytopenia and its relevance in "autoimmunity". J. Clin. Invest. 40, 1597-1620.

2) Mueller-Eckhardt, C. (1986): Posttransfusion Purpura. Br. J. Haematol. 64, 419-424.

3) Mueller-Eckhardt, C., Kiefel, V. (1988): High-dose IgG for post-transfusion purpura-revisited. Blut 570, 163-167.

4) Kiefel, V., Santoso, S., Glöckner, W.M., Katzmann, B., Mayr, W., Mueller-Eckhardt, C. (1989): Post-transfusion purpura associated with anti-Bak(b). Vox Sang 56, 93-97.

5) Aster, R.H. (1989): The immunologic thrombocytopenias. In Platelet Immunobiology, ed. T.J. Kunicki, J.N. George, 387-435. Philadelphia: J.B. Lippincott Company.

6) Taaning, E., Killmann, S.-A., Morling, N., Ovesen, H., Svejgaard, A. (1986): Post-transfusion purpura (PTP) due to anti-Zw(b) (-PlA2): the significance of IgG3 antibodies in PTP. Br. J. Haematol. 64, 217-225.

7) Borne, A.E.G.Kr. von dem, Plas-van Dalen, C.M. van der (1985): Further observations on post-transfusion purpura (PTP). Br. J. Haematol. 61, 374-375.

Table 1: Countries, centers, number of PTP patients and senior authors of the European PTP Study 1990

country	center	no.of patients	senior authors
Czechoslovakia	Prague	1	A. Majsky
Denmark	Copenhagen	10	E. Taaning et al
France	Paris (CNTS)	14	C. Kaplan et al
	Paris (Lariboisière)	2	J.-L. Wautier et al
	Créteil	4	P. Bierling et al
	Nancy	2	P. Perrier et al
Germany	Giessen	31	C. Mueller-Eckhardt et al
Great Britain	London	18	A. Waters et al
	Oxford	3	C. Entwistle et al
	Chester	1	J.V. Clough
Netherlands	Amsterdam	10	A. von dem Borne et al
Norway	Oslo	4	R. Nordhagen
Poland	Warsaw	2	B. Zupanska et al
Spain	Barcelona	2	E. Muniz-Dias et al

Table 2: Specificities of platelet-reactive antibodies presumably involved in elicitation of 104 cases of PTP

Antibody specificities	n	%
Zw(a)	29	
Zw(a) + HLA	58	84.6
Zw(a) + autoantibodies	1	
Zw(b) + HLA	3	
Zw(b) + Bak(a) + HLA	1	4.8
Zw(b) + Br(a) + HLA	1	
Bak(a)	1	
Bak(a) + HLA	5	5.8
Bak(b) + HLA	1	
HLA only	3	
HLA + "platelet-specific antibody"	1	

RESUME

Le purpura post transfusionnel est un accident rare mais grave. Les résultats d'une étude européenne, regroupant 14 centres dans 9 pays différents ont été collectés et analysés. 99 malades étaient des femmes. L'âge moyen était de 58.4 ans. L'intervalle entre l'administration de produits sanguins contenant des plaquettes et la date d'apparition du purpura était de 6 à 8 jours (1-14 jours). Les symptomes hémorragiques étaient sévères dans la plupart des cas avec une numération plaquettaire initiale inférieure à 10 000/l (81 % des cas). Des décès précoces n'ont pas été rapportés, le traitement le plus efficace semble être les injections intraveineuses d'immunoglobulines à haute dose. Les antigènes plaquettaires incriminés étaient anti-Zw^a (N = 88), anti Zw^b (N = 5), anti Bak^a (N = 6), anti Bak^b (N = 1). Dans certains cas les anticorps n'ont pu être clairement identifiés. Les mécanismes physiopathologiques sont discutés.

Fetal primary hemostasis

F. Forestier*, F. Daffos*, Y. Solé*, N. Catherine*, P. Champeix** and C. Kaplan**

*Service de Médecine et de Biologie Fœtales, Institut de Puériculture de Paris, 26, bd Brune, 75014 Paris, France
**INTS, Laboratoire d'Imumunologie Plaquettaire, 6, rue Alexandre Cabanel, 75015 Paris, France

Our knowledge of fetal biology is limited due to the fact that the most earlier studies were performed on aborted fetuses or under sampling conditions which may have altered biological values. Having developed an easy and safe technique for fetal blood sampling, we retrospectively selected normal fetuses to establish reference values and to study fetal primary hemostasis. Fetal platelets normally respond to presence of ADP, thrombin, collagen and arachidonic acid. No aggregation is observed in the presence of epinephine. Glycoprotein IIb-IIIa is immunologically detectable as early as the 18th week of gestation. Platelet glycoproteins (quantified by monoclonal or polyclonal antibodies) where in the same range in fetuses as in adults. Main platelet antigens are expressed very early in the gestation allowing prenatal diagnosis of alloimmunisation.

FETAL PLATELETS

I - PLATELET COUNT AND AGGREGATION

Platelet counts did not change during the second and the third trimester of pregnancy and did not correlate with gestational age (Table I) (Forestier et al 1986)

Table I - Evolution of platelet count in 1.233 normal fetuses during gestation (mean ± SD)

Gestational age weeks	Platelet 10^9/liter
18 - 23 (n = 771)	241 ± 45
24 - 29 (n = 407)	267 ± 49
30 - 35 (n = 55)	265 ± 59

Fetal platelets normally respond to presence of ADP, thrombin, collagen and arachidonic acid. No aggregation is observed in the presence of epinephrine (Forestier 1987).

II - BIOCHEMICAL PROPERTIES OF PLATELET MEMBRANES AND GLYCOPROTEINS

Materials and Methods

Platelet preparation

Fetal, maternal or control (adult) platelets were isolated from 1 ml EDTA-anticoagulated blood by standard procedures (KIEFFER et al 1984) and resuspended in a solution containing 10mM Tris HCl, 150 mM Nacl, 3 mM EDTA, 30 mM N-ethylmaleimide and 1 mM phenyl methylsufonyl fluoride (Buffer I) at pH 7,0.

Neuraminidase treatment was performed by incubating 30 ul of platelet suspension (10^9/ml) for 60 minutes at 37^0 C, in a solution containing 50 mM Na acetate, 150 mM NaCl, 9 mM CaCl2 PH 5,5 to which 0,1 or 0,5 unit/ml of neuraminidase from Vibrio cholerae (Boehringwerke AG, Marburg-Lahn, Germany) was added. The supernatant obtained after centrifugation (15 minutes, 1400 g) was submitted to sialic acid analysis.

Solubilisation of the platelets

Platelets (2.10^9/ml) were solubilized in SDS Buffer (2 % wt/vol SDS in Buffer I). The samples were then heated at 100^0 C for 5 minutes, aliquoted and stored at -20^0 C. The protein content of the samples was estimated by the Lowry-Folin technique as reported by GEIGER and BESSMAN (1972) using cristalline bovine serum albumin as a standard.

Electrophoresis and related techniques

60 ug of proteins from native or neuraminidase treated platelets were separated by homogeneous 7 % SDS polyacrylamide slab gel electrophoresis according to the method of Laemmli (1970), using a commercial mini-slab apparatus (Proteau, Bio-rad, USA, 6 mm x 8 mm x 0,75 mm gel, 15 mA per slab gel for 1 hour 1/2). After electrophoresis, sialoglycoproteins were revealed by periodic/acid/schiff (PAS) staining described by FAIRBANKS et al (1971). Separated proteins were then electrophoretically transferred to nitrocellulose membranes (Schleicher and Schull, 0,1 um Ceralabo France) using the LKB transblot apparatus (LKB, Bromo, Sweden) according to TOWBIN et al (1979). The transfer was performed at 35 volts for 4 hours in 20 mM Tris HCl, 150 mM glycine at pH 8,3. The remaining non-specific protein binding sites on the nitrocellulose paper were blocked by overnight incubation, at room temperature, with 100 ml of 10 mM Tris HCl containing 0.9 % wt/vol NaCl and 0.6 % wt/vol gelatin at pH 7,4 (Buffer A). Lectin staining procedures were performed according to MOROI et al (1984), modified as follows : for native transferred proteins, saturated nitrocellulose sheets were submitted to neuraminidase treatment by incubation for 60 minutes at room temperature with 1 ml of neuraminidase solution (see above) in a plastic bag with rotatory agitation (10 rpm). After three washes (15 minutes each) in Buffer A containing 0.1 % wt/vol Tween 20 (Serva-FRG) (Buffer B), nitrocellulose strips were then incubated for 4 hours with peroxidase conjugated lectin (10 ug/ml, Miles scientific-USA) in 10 mM Tris HCl at pH 7.4 containing 0.9 % wt/vol. The glycoproteins (GP) were visualised by incubating nitrocellulose membranes with 0.05 % wt/vol 3-3' diaminobenzidine (Serva-FRG) dissolved with 10 mM Tris HCl at pH 7.6 containing 0.5 % vol/vol hydrogen peroxide.

Results

Analysis on SDS PAGE

Fetal, maternal or control solubilized platelets were submitted to electrophoresis in a 7 % polyacrylamide minislab gel in non reducing conditions. After PAS staining of control platelets (fig. 1A, 3), three bands could be detected and identified as GP Ib (160 kDa), GP IIa/b (134 KDa) and GP IIIa/b (90 KDa) according to JENNINGS (1982). Molecular weights (MW) were assigned by reference to molecular markers from Bio-rad. Maternal and control platelets showed similar results (fig. IA, lanes 1 and 3) whereas platelets migrated differently (fig.1A, lane 2). The electrophoretic profile for fetal sialoglycoproteins showed a higher molecular weight compared to the maternal profile, especially for GP Ib which was estimated 165 kda. However, the proportions of sialoglycoproteins were the same on fetal and maternal platelets.

Western blot analysis of platelet GP Ib

Using peroxydase coupled peanut agglutinin (Miles), platelet GP Ib can be specifically revealed on nitrocellulose sheets. After electrophoresis and transfer on a nitrocellulose membrane, followed by neuraminidase treatment (0.1 U/ml), GP Ib was revealed as shown fig. 2A, lane 3, by incubation with peroxidase coupled peanut agglutinin and staining with 3-3' diaminobenzidine. Maternal and control platelets GP Ib (fig. 2A, lanes 1 and 3) were revealed at the same level on the nitrocellulose sheets. For the fetal sample (fig.2A, lane 2) the GP Ib specifically revealed, migrated differently from the control, with a higher MW as described above. This experiment was performed on nine different fetal samples and identical results were obtained. Prior, Neuraminidase treatment (0,50/ml) before platelet lysis, abolished the difference of mobility between fetal and maternal GP Ib (Fig. 2 B).

Sialic acid content

Sialic acid content in the supernatant after neuraminidase treatment (0.5 U neuraminidase/ml), was estimated by the technique described by Warren using neuraminic acid as standard. For maternal platelets, the removed sialic acid.content was estimated to 24 ug/10^9 platelets, whereas it was 44 ug/10^9 platelets for fetal platelets.

Discussion

The SDS-PAGE profile showed a major difference in mobility between maternal and fetal samples, mainly for GP Ib. The identification of each band was confirmed by analyzing

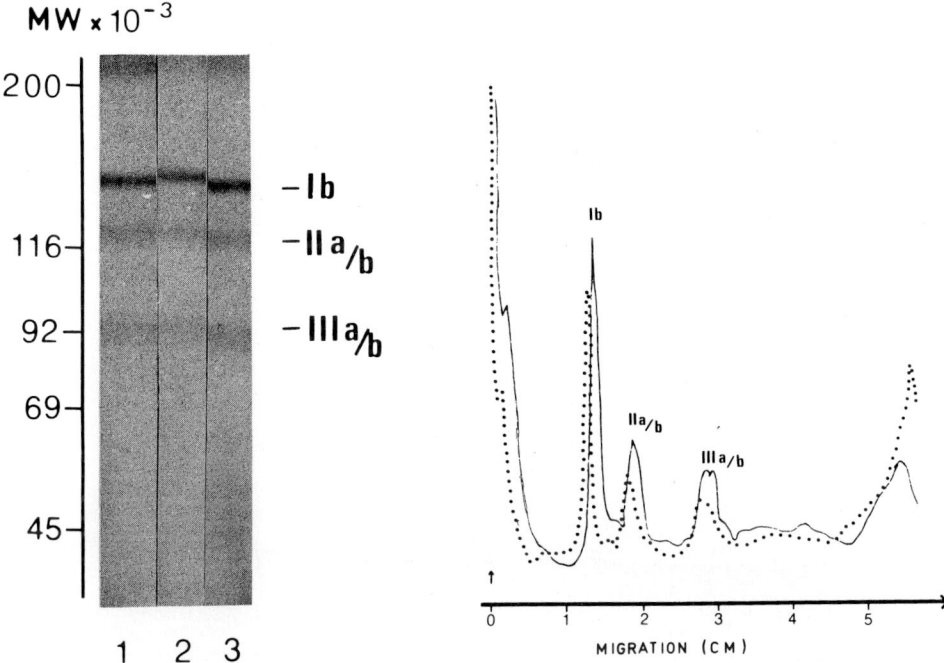

Figue 1

Electrophoresis analysis of normal platelet proteins on SDS polyacrylamide gel (7%) in non reducing conditions. Results after PAS ataining.

A. Lane 1 : Maternal platelets
   Lane 2 : Fetal platelets
   Lane 3 : Control platelts (adult)
Molecular weights were assigned by references to molecular markers from Bio-rad

B. Gels scans analysis :
   .... Fetal platelts
   ___ Maternal platelets

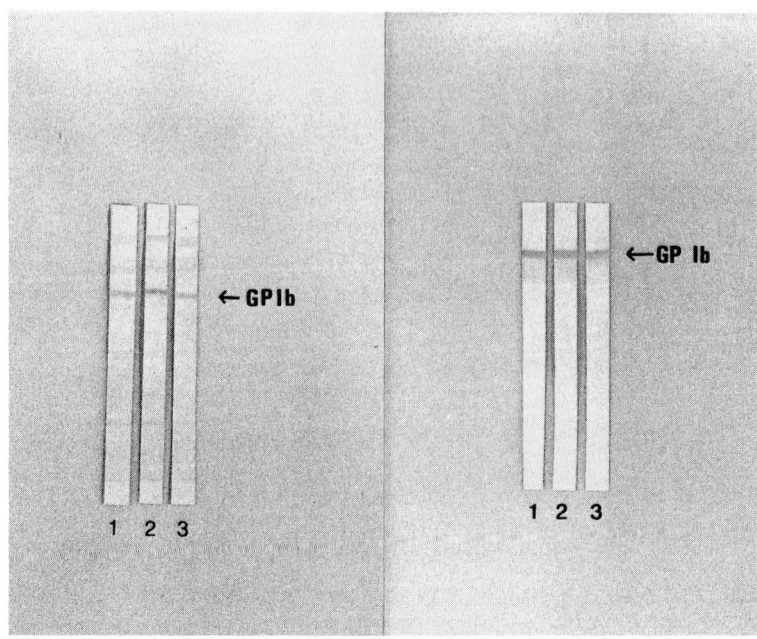

Figure 2

Western-blot analysis of platelet GP Ib using peroxydase coupled peanut agglutinin :

Platelet proteins were electrophoresed on SDS polyacrylamide gel (7%) onto nitrocellulose sheets
  Lanes 1 : maternal platelets
  Lanes 2 : Fetal platelets
  Lanes 3 : Control (adult) platelets

A : Neuraminidase treatment (0.1 u/ml) after transfer on nitrocellulose membrane

B : Neuraminadase treatment (0.5 u/ml) on whole platelets before lyain and electrophoresis the autoradiography. Fetal platelets contained more sialic acid than adult ones ; However no significant difference was found between the volume of maternal and fetal platelets. The results were the same at all gestational ages. Our data using immunoblotting and biochemical assays indicated that a greater sialic acid content is responsible for the higher MW of fetal GPIb

In erythrocyte membranes, a change in sialic acid has been observed at birth (CALATRONI et al 1984) and appears to be involved in the control of both the production of red cells and survival time. Its specific role has not yet been elucidated. Similarly sialic acid could play a role in the regulation of platelet function, maturation and regulation throughout fetal life.

III - DETERMINATION OF PLATELET ANTIGENS AND GLYCOPROTEINS

Materials and Methods

Three polyclonal antibodies of human origin were used : Anti-PLA^I, anti-Lek^a, and IgGL. The anti-PLA^I serum was obtained from the mother of a child with neonatal allimmune thrombocytopenia. Its specificity was assessed by the study of platelets from PLA^I positive and PLA^I negative subjects and by a immunoblot procedure (KIEFFER 1984) The anti-Lek^a serum, which was obtained from a patient with posttransfusion purpura defined a new platelet-specific alloantigen, Lek^a (BOIZARD 1984), which is carried by membrane GPIIb, as demonstrated by immunoblotting. IgGL reacted predominantly with GPIIb/IIIa complex, as demonstrated by immunoprecipitation (ROSA 1984). Platelets GPs were characterized using four monoclonal antibodies : AP-2 (supplied by T.Kunicki) is a murine monoclonal antibody which reacts specifically with the complex formed by human platelet membrane GPIIb and GPIIIa but not with the individual GPs (PIDARD 1983). AP-3 (supplied by P.Newman) as recently demonstrated by indirect immunoprecipitation, reacts solely with GPIIIa (NEWMAN 1985). AN51 (supplied by G.Tobelem) is a monoclonal antibody directed against the glycocalicin region of GPIb (Mc MICHAEL 1981, RUAN 1981). 6DI (supplied by B.Coller) is also directed against the glycocalicin part of GPIb, but its specificity is probably different since it inhibits totally the binding of the von Willebrand factor to platelets by 100 % whereas inhibition obtained with AN51 is only 40 % to 50 % (COLLER 1983).

These monoclonal antibodies were studied using platelet suspension immuno-fluorescence tests. The binding of each antibody was quantified using a cytofluorograph (Ortho 50H).

Results

PL^{A1} and Lek^a antigens were expressed in normal amounts on fetal platelets as early as 16 weeks of intrauterine life. The GPIIb IIIa complex quantified by polyclonal or monoclonal antibodies was in the same range in fetuses (IgGL = 427 ± 23 AUF, AP-2 = 459.5 ± 8.5 ; AP-3 = 536 ± 14) and in adults (IgGL = 420 ± 30 ; AP-2 = 498 ± 11 ; AP-3 = 515 ± 13). The platelet binding of antibodies that recognized GPIb was higher in fetuses (AN51 = 491,5 ± 14 ; 6D1 = 479 ± 15) than in adults (AN51 = 426.5 ± 9 ; 6D1 = 449 ± 8.7).

These results summarized in Table II suggest that immunological techniques can be applied as early as 18 weeks of gestation for the antenatal diagnosis of Glanzmann Thrombasthenia and Bernard Soulier Syndrome (GRUEL 1986).

Table II - Mean Fluorescence Values (± SEM)

Platelets	Immunofluorescence Intensity (AUF)	
	Fetuses (Mean ± SD)	Adults (Mean ± SD)
Antigens		
PL^1_A	433.0 ± 30.0	427 ± 13.5
LeK^a	441.5 ± 25.0	459 ± 15.0
Glycoproteins		
GPIIb IIIa, IgG	427.0 ± 23.0	420.0 ± 30.0
GPIIb IIIa, AP-2	459.5 ± 8.5	498.0 ± 11.0
GPIIIa, AP-3	536.0 ± 14.0	515.0 ± 13.0
GPIb, AN51	491.5 ± 14.0	426.5 ± 9.0
GPIb, 6D1	479.0 ± 15.0	443.0 ± 8.7

Values measured with the specific antibodies directed against platelet antigens PL^1_A, Lek^a and platelet glycoproteins (Gp) IIb, IIIa, Ib, in 10 to 13 fetuses and 23 adults. Only three fetuses were tested with 6D1.

REFERENCES

Boizard B., Wautier JL. Lek[a], a new platelet antigen absent in Glanzmann's thrombasthenia. Vox Sang. 1984, 46, 47

Coller BS., Peerschke EL., Scudder LE., Sullivan CA. Studies with a murine monoclonal antibody that abolishes ristocetin-induced binding of von Willebrand factor to platelets : Additional evidence in support of GPIb as a platelet receptor for von Willebrand factor. Blood, 1983, 51, 99

Daffos F., Forestier F. Médecine et Biologie du Foetus Humain. Maloine Edit. Paris, 1988

Fairbanks G. et al. Electrophoretic analysis of the major polypeptides of the human erythrocyte membrane. Biochemistry. 1971, 10, 2606-2617

Forestier F., Daffos F., Galactéros F., Bardakjian J., Rainaut M., Beuzard Y. Hematological values of 163 normal fetuses between 18 and 30 weeks of gestation. Pediat Res. 1986, 20, 342-346

Forestier F. Some aspects of fetal biology. Fetal Therapy. 1987, 2, 181-187

Geiger PJ., Bessman SP. Protein determination by Lowry's method in the presence of sulfhydryl reagents. Analyt Biochem. 1972, 49, 467-473

Kieffer N., Didry D., Nurden A. Application de l'immunoblotting à l'étude des protéines plasmatiques ; in Lévy Toledano. Nouvelles techniques d'études d'hémostase et de thrombose, pp. 13-29 (INSERM, Paris 1984)

Moroi M., Jung SM., Yoshida N. Genetic polymorphism of platelet glycoprotein Ib. Blood. 1984, 64, 622-629

Pidard D., Montgomery RR., Bennett JS., Kunicki TJ. Interaction of AP-2, a monoclonal antibody specific for the human platelet glycoprotein IIbIIIa complex, with intact platelets. J Biol Chem. 1983, 258, 12582

Rosa JP., Kieffer N., Didry D., Pidard D., Kunicki TJ., Nurden AT. The human platelet membrane glycoprotein complex GPIIb-IIIa expresses antigenic sites not exposed on the dissociated glycoproteins. Blood. 1984, 64, 1246

Towbin H., Staehelin T., Gordon J. Electrophoretic transfer of proteins from polyacrylamide gels to nitrocellulose sheets : procedure and some applications. Proc Nath Acad Sci. 1979, USA 76, 4350-4354

Résumé

Nos connaissances en biologie foetale étaient limitées en raison des difficultés techniques de prélèvement, et des conditions susceptibles d'altérer la biologie. Grâce à une technique simple et fiable permettant de prélever du sang in utero dès le 2ème trimestre de la grossesse, nous avons pu établir des valeurs de référence en hémostase et étudier l'hémostase primaire. Quantitativement et qualitativement les plaquettes foetales sont très proches de celles de l'adulte et la reconnaissance de certaines glycoprotéines ou de motifs antigéniques par des anticorps monoclonaux permet le diagnostic prénatal des pathologies héréditaires de l'hémostase primaire ainsi que le diagnostic et la thérapeutique des allo et/ou auto-immunisations antiplaquettaires.

Current trends in neonatal alloimmune thrombocytopenia : Diagnosis and therapy

C. Kaplan*, F. Daffos**, F. Forestier**, M.C. Morel*, N. Chesnel* and G. Tchernia***

*INTS, 6, rue Alexandre Cabanel, 75015 Paris, France
**Institut de puériculture, 26, bd Brune, 75014 Paris, France
***Hôpital Antoine Béclère, 157, rue de la Porte-de-Trivaux, 92141 Clamart, France

SUMMARY

Maternal alloimmunization against fetal platelets can cause severe fetal and neonatal thrombocytopenia (NAIT). These infants are at risk of hemorrhage particularly in the central nervous system leading to death (10% of the cases) or neurological sequellae (20%). We report here our data concerning anti-PL^{A1} allo-immunization and preliminary results concerning NAIT due to anti-Br^a antibodies. The definition of immune factors associated with maternal immunization allows detection and management of pregnancy at risk of NAIT. Antenatal diagnosis is now feasible as early as 21 weeks of gestation.This facilitates appropriate management and in utero therapy.

Neonatal alloimmune thrombocytopenia (NAIT), due to maternal immunization against fetal platelets affects approximately one in 3000 live birth and accounts for 20 % of neonatal thrombocytopenias (Blanchette et al., 1986). This affection can cause severe bleeding in the central nervous system and death or severe neurologic sequelae. The risk of life-threatening hemorrhage must lead to a prompt diagnosis and effective therapy.

---

* This work was supported in part by a grant from Fondation de France , from the "Société d 'Etudes et de Soins pour les Enfants Paralysés et Polymalformés" (S.E.S.E.P).and by the Collaborative project PROCOPE 1988-1989.

I - PATHOGENESIS

NAIT is considered to be the platelet counterpart of the red cell hemolytic disease. The maternal IgG antibodies directed against paternal antigens present on fetal platelets can cross the placenta as soon as 14th week of gestation. The resulting fetal thrombocytopenia is variable, the sensitized fetal platelets are removed from the circulation by the fetal reticulo endothelial system.

As the HPA-1a (PL^{A1}) antigen is expressed as soon as 19 weeks of gestation (Kaplan et al., 1985 ; Gruel et al., 1986), thrombocytopenia can occur very early during pregnancy. Sonographies, have shown in utero intracranial hemorrhage and fetal blood samplings revealed severe thrombocytopenia as early as the 20th week of pregnancy (Kaplan et al., 1988).

II - PLATELET ANTIGENS IMPLICATED

NAIT results from the destruction of fetal platelets by maternal alloantibodies directed against platelet specific antigens (Harrington et al., 1953 ; Shulman et al., 1964). ABO incompatibility or HLA alloimmunizations have not been causally related to NAIT. One possible explanation is that HLA antigens are widely distributed, especially on placental tissues and that the antibodies are adsorbed on them. Currently eight platelet alloantigens are described. Among those implicated in NAIT (table 1), sensitization against HPA-1a (PL^{A1}) and HPA-5b (Br^a) occurs most frequently. The antigen "Duzo" was the first to be described (Moulinier 1958) but until now, as no more serum is available neither serological nor biochemical characterization is possible.

Recently due to the progress of serology and immunobiochemistry reliable methods for the detection of antibodies and characterization of the antigens are available.

- *HPA-1 (PL^A, Zw) system :*

The epitopes (Van Loghem 1959) are located on glycoprotein IIIa-(GP IIIa) (Kunicki and Aster, 1979).
There are 40,000 HPA-1a (PL^{A1}) epitopes per platelet for an homozygous subject corresponding to the estimated number of GP IIb-IIIa complexes at the platelet surface, half for an heterozygous one. These data are in favour of only one HPA-1a (PL^{A1}) epitope per GP IIIa molecule (Kunicki and Beardsley, 1989).
The platelet phenotypings are usually done with an anti-HPA-1a alloantiserum. Homozygous HPA-1a (PL^{A1})/HPA-1a (PL^{A1}) and heterozygous HPA-1a (PL^{A1})/HPA-1b (PL^{A2}) subjects are then considered HPA-1a (PL^{A1}) positive, the HPA-1b/ HPA-1b (PL^{A2}/PL^{A2}), HPA-1a (PL^{A1}) negative. In most cases immunizations are observed in HPA-1b/HPA-1b mothers

incompatible with their HPA-1a (PL^{A1}) positive fetuses. Only NAIT rarely is due to anti HPA-1b (PL^{A2} antibody). HPA-1a (PL^{A1}) is by far the most frequent in NAIT.

- *HPA-2 (Ko, Sib) system :*

This system has been essentially implicated in transfusion alloimmunization. But recently a case of NAIT has been reported (Bizzaro and Dianese, 1988).

- *HPA-3 (Bak, Lek) system :*

The platelet alloantigen HPA-3a (Bak^a=Lek^a) is on glycoprotein IIb. (Von Dem Borne et al., 1980 ; Von Dem Borne and Van Der Plas, 1986) Only few NAIT are due to this system (Von Dem Borne et al., 1980 ; Mc Grath et al., 1989).

- *HPA-4 (Yuk, Pen) system:*

This di-allelic system is frequently implicated in NAIT among Japanese (Shibata et al., 1986). One case due to "Pen^a" has been reported in a latin-american woman (Friedman and Aster, 1985). This antigen was further identified as Yuk^b and localized on GP IIIa in a site distinct from HPA-1a(PL^{A1}) (Santoso et al., 1987). It is the second platelet specific alloantigen described on this glycoprotein. We have in our series one case of alloimmunization in a caucasoid french family due to anti Yuk^a antibody.

- *HPA-5 (Br, Hc, Zav) system:*

The application of a recent technique, monoclonal antibody platelet antigen immobilization (MAIPA) (Kiefel et al., 1989), leads to the identification of this new system located on GPIa-IIa. It could be the second most important system implicated in NAIT.

TABLE 1:

PLATELET SPECIFIC ALLOANTIGENS			
SYSTEM		ANTIGENS	GLYCOPROTEINS
HPA-1 Zw,PL^A	HPA-1a HPA-1b	Zw^a,PL^{A1} Zw^b,PL^{A2}	IIIa
HPA-2 Ko,Sib	HPA-2a HPA-2b	Ko^b Ko^a,Sib^a	Ib
HPA-3 Bak,Lek	HPA-3a HPA-3b	Bak^a,Lek^a Bak^b	IIb
HPA-4 Pen,Yuk	HPA-4a HPA-4b	Pen^a Yuk^b Pen^b,Yuk^a	IIIa
HPA-5 Br,Hc Zav	HPA-5a HPA-5b	Br^b,Zav^b Br^a,Zav^a, Hc^a	Ia-IIa

The platelet membrane glycoproteins play a fundamental role in platelet function: adhesion (GPIb) and aggregation (the GP IIb-IIIa complex). It has been shown that anti-HPA-1a (PL^{A1}) (Kunicki and Beardsley, 1989) and anti-Pen^a alloantibodies interfere with platelet aggregation. So, the potential impact of these alloantibodies upon primary haemostasis must be taken into consideration when judging the severity of the affection. This majors the risk of thrombocytopenia itself.

III - IMMUNE RISK FACTORS

The frequency of PL^{A2}/PL^{A2} women is estimated at 2,5 % and calculations suggest that there is an 84 % chance that the fetus will be HPA-1a (PL^{A1}) positive, but the incidence of NAIT is much lower. Prospective and retrospective studies reported that the HLA type was of importance. The HLA B8-DR3 phenotype has been implicated as an important risk factor for the development of maternal immunization (Reznikoff et al., 1988) and recently involvement of the DR52a allele has been reported. (Valentin et al., 1990)

The definition of this high risk group allows the detection and follow up of such pregnancies in which NAIT can affect the first child and the incidence of recurrence is estimated at 90 %. It is very important to screen the sisters considered to be at risk. For Br^a immunization, DRw6 has been implicated (Mueller-Eckhardt et al., 1989). So far, little is known about the role of immune factors in NAIT due to other platelet antigens.

IV - CLINICAL ASPECTS OF NAIT

Diagnosis must be suspected in healthy full-term neonates who unexpectedly present petechia and are found severely thrombocytopenic, in spite of uneventful pregnancy. The clinical features are present at birth or shortly after. In some cases the thrombocytopenia is asymptomatic (13 % for anti-PL^{A1} immunization), discovered by a systematic platelet count. Visceral or central nervous system hemorrhages are not a rare event (20%). In utero intracerebral hemorrhages (ICH) have been estimated to have an incidence of 10 %, brain damages such as hydrocephalus, porencephaly can be assessed by sonographies (Mueller-Eckhardt et al., 1989 ; Herman et al., 1986).

The physical examination excludes other causes of neonatal thrombocytopenia in particular there is no evidence of hepatosplenomegaly, absent radii, cutaneous hemangionas.

V - DIFFERENTIAL DIAGNOSIS

The diagnosis is usually one of exclusion. The thrombocytopenia is isolated, there are no signs of disseminated intravascular coagulation nor viral infection. The mother is well with a normal platelet count. Maternal drug induced thrombocytopenia, autoimmunity and systematic lupus erythematosus, must also be considered and excluded.

NAIT due to alloimmuzation is then suspected.

VI- GENERAL CHARACTERISTICS OF NAIT

- Anti-HPA-1a (PL^{A1}) immunization.

We report here the clinical evaluation of our series concerning 137 cases. The clinical symptoms were purpura or haematoma in 65,4 % of the cases and visceral hemorrhage and/or intracerebral hemorrhage in 21 % of the infants. 13 % of the affected children were asymptomatic (Table 2). The sex ratio (74 boys/56 girls) was similar to that of the control group.

TABLE 2:

CLINICAL SYMPTOMS IN 127 CHILDREN WITH NAIT		
None	17	(13.4%)
Purpura, Haematomas	83	(65.4%)
Visceral or intracerebral hemorrhages	27	(21.2%)

The first offspring was affected in 50 % of the cases. Previous abortion was positive in 36 % of the cases. Recurrence has an incidence of 90 %. NAIT has a significant risk of morbidity, 21 % neurological sequellae , and mortality, 7 % deaths. The mortality rate was comparable for the first affected cases compared to their subsequent affected siblings. We noticed that the incidence of neurological sequellae was higher in the subsequent cases. Actually therapy may have a significant impact on the course of the disease and this evaluation could be modified in the future. The prognosis relies upon the severity of the initial symptomatology and the precocity of the therapy. We observed that the course was uneventful in 76 % of the cases when purpura or petechia was present, and in only 18,5 % when there were visceral or cerebral hemorrhages (table 3).

TABLE 3:

EVOLUTION OF 137 CHILDREN WITH NAIT ACCORDING TO THE INITIAL CLINICAL STATUS			
EVOLUTION	HEMORRAGIC SYMPTOMS		
	NONE	PURPURA HAEMATOMA	VISCERAL OR INTRACEREBRAL HEMORRHAGE
UNEVENTFUL	16	68	5
NEUROLOGICAL SEQUELLAE	0	14	12
DEATH	0	1	8
UNKNOWN	1	10	2

Hematologic recovery is usual, the thrombocytopenia is temporary and resolves within the first two weeks of life because the progressive disparition of the mother alloantibodies in the infant's circulation.

- Anti-HPA-5b (Br^a) immunization

In our series, the first offspring was affected only in 5 of 15 cases. The thrombocytopenia is often moderate (70 % of cases) and the nadir is usually reached a few days after birth. But in 5 cases, the infants were severely affected, with platelet counts less than 30.10^9/L. We observed two cases of visceral bleeding and one death due to intracerebral hemorrhage.

In all cases of NAIT, as severe hemorrhage is a serious concern, prompt diagnosis and therapy are imperative.

VII- LABORATORY DIAGNOSIS OF NAIT

The diagnosis depends upon the demonstration of maternal antibodies reacting with the paternal platelets, directed against an antigen, inherited by the fetus, absent from the mother. Currently different methods are available (Von Dem Borne *et al.*, 1978 ; Soulier *et al.*, 1975).

Due to difficulties such as:
- severe infant thrombocytopenia
- coexistence of anti HLA or ABO antibodies
- Absence of circulating maternal antibodies (30 % of the cases in our series)
the following tests must be included:
- screening of the maternal serum sample against paternal platelets and platelets phenotyped in the most frequent antigenic systems
- distinction between platelet specific and anti HLA antibodies
- platelet phenotyping of both parents

Later, it can be necessary to phenotype the infant. Additional testings may be of value, and include mother HLA phenotyping (HLA DR3/DR6), biochemical characterization of platelet-specific antibodies by western-blot (Champeix and Kaplan, 1988), immunoprecipitation and MAIPA technique (Kiefel *et al.*, 1987).

However in some cases such as the absence of circulating maternal antibodies, or involvement of rare or new antigens, the laboratory diagnosis may be equivocal. In these situations, retesting is important as improved methods become available. In any case, the biological difficulties should not interfere with a therapy particularly when thrombocytopenia is very severe.

VIII -CURRENT TRENDS IN THERAPY

Two situations will be considered as the management is different: unexpected NAIT when diagnosis and effective therapy must be established promptly, and management of future pregnancies in which NAIT can be anticipated.

1) Unexpected NAIT

When thrombocytopenia is severe, ICH is a major risk, therefore maternal platelet transfusion is the treatment of choice, it is always compatible with the circulating antibody. The platelets are washed to eliminate the antibody and resuspended in normal AB plasma. They should be irradiated to prevent graft versus host disease in the newborn (Martin et al., 1983).

In cases of immunization due to anti HPA-1a (PL^{A1}) antibodies platelets compatible donors can be available. At the present time there are no blood banking stores for platelets of other phenotypes. In these cases, the mother's siblings can be typed to find potential donors.

In emergency situation, exchange transfusion is valuable, as it removes in part the circulating antibody and secures improved hemostasis.

As an alternative treatment, infusion of intravenous gammaglobulins had been advocated but the effect is not perceptible until 12 to 24 hours later and doesn't prevent hemorrhage during this period.

2) Management of future pregnancies

The risk of subsequent pregnancies being affected is very high (88 % to 97 %) and management must be aimed at preventing severe complications especially ICH during gestation and birth trauma. Detection of thrombocytopenia early in pregnancy is important if a woman has a previous history of NAIT, or if she is at high risk, because her first child may be affected. The level of maternal antibody is not of predictive value since 20 % of the mothers lacked circulating antibodies in our series. We had shown in a previous study that there was no correlation between the antibody level and the severity of the fetal thrombocytopenia (Kaplan et al., 1988). In consequence, there is no adequate means for detecting and assessing the severity of fetal thrombocytopenia without performing fetal blood sampling. Percutaneous umbilical blood sampling (PUBS) is a much less invasive procedure than fetoscopy and provides precise information on the fetal platelet status.

Usually the first PUBS is performed at 20 weeks of gestation allowing detection of fetal thrombocytopenia and fetal platelet phenotyping in case of a father's heterozygoty for the considered antigen.

In utero therapy of fetal thrombocytopenia is actually discussed and is reviewed in this book (Bussel J.). Studies have reported the benefit of high doses intravenous gammaglobulin, corticosteroids (Daffos et al., 1988) a combination of both (Bussel et al., 1988), or weekly in utero transfusions (Murphy et al. 1990). In our series therapy did not appear to be uniformly effective, whatever we treated the mother with corticosteroïds or IVGG (Fig 1).

The second FBS is performed at 32 weeks of gestation to assess the effect of maternal therapy on the fetal thrombocytopenia. According to the results obtained, the treatment can be modified. The 3rd FBS is usually done in the preterm period allowing in utero maternal platelet transfusion in case of therapy failure (KAPLAN et al. 1988). The maternal platelets must be washed and irradiated. Such transfusions promptly increase the in utero platelet count, therefore protecting the infant during delivery and immediately afterwards, which is the period of greatest risk for ICH.

FIGURE 1:

ANTENATAL TREATMENT OF NEONATAL ALLOIMMUNE THROMBOCYTOPENIA

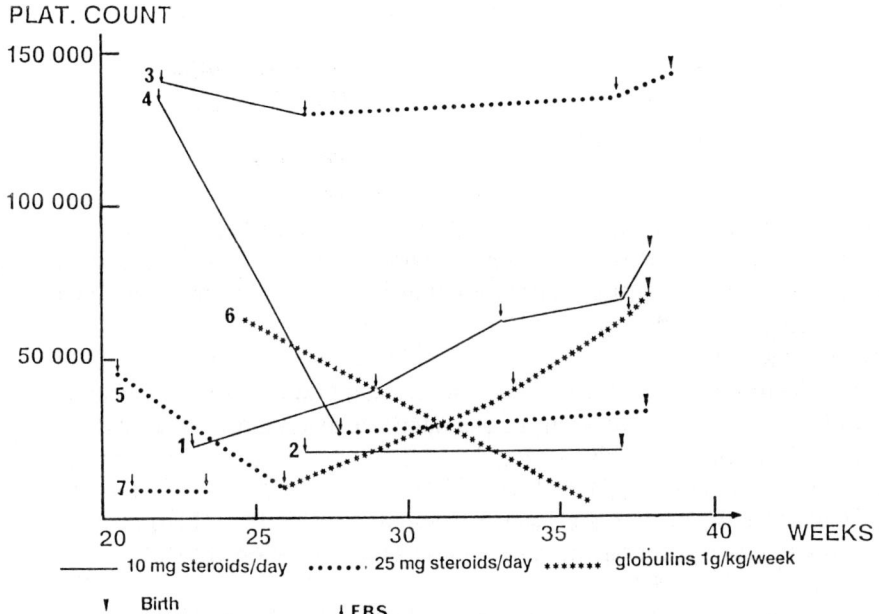

Considering high risk groups without prior NAIT many questions remain without response:
- What are the mechanisms of immunization?
- Should FBS be performed and at what time?

The risk of antiplatelet immunization due to the procedure itself should be considered, although the dose of platelets necessary for sensitization is unknown. As in 50 % of cases, NAIT occurs in the first pregnancy, it is suggested that the mechanism of immunization may be very complex and be different from the Rh- hemolytic disease of the newborn.

It must be emphasized in the future that the improvement of new serological methods and characterization of genetic markers would help in diagnosis, definition of high risk groups and thus lead to a better prevention of this severe disease. Further clinical research is necessary to rule on the best in utero therapy, thereby reducing the morbidity and mortality of this affection.

REFERENCES

. Bizzaro N., Dianese G.(1988) : Neonatal alloimmune amegakaryocytosis. *Vox Sang.*, *54* : 112 - 114

. Blanchette V.S., Peters M.A., Pegg-Feige K.(1986) : Alloimmune thrombocytopenia in *Current Studies in Hematology and Blood Transfusion* , *52* : 87 - 96. Decary F. Rock GA (eds).

. Bussel J.F., Berkowitz R.L., Mc Farland J.G., Lynch L., Chitbara N. (1988) : Antenatal treatment of neonatal alloimmune thrombocytopenia. *New Engl. J. Med.,319* : 1374 - 1378

. Champeix P., Kaplan C.(1988) : Biochemical characterization of Zw^a antigen using the immunoblotting technique. In *Curr. Stud. Hematol. Blood. Transf.*, *55* : 104 - 111. C. Kaplan-Gouet - Ch. Salmon (Eds), Karger Basel.

. Daffos F., Forestier F., Kaplan C, (1988) · Prenatal treatment of fetal alloimmune thrombocytopenia. *Lancet, II* : 910

. Friedman J.M., Aster R.H.(1985) : Neonatal alloimmune thrombocytopenic purpura and congenital porencephaly in two siblings associated with a new maternal antiplatelet antibody. *Blood*, *65* : 1412 - 1415.

. Gruel Y.,Boizard B.,Daffos F.,Forestier F.,Caen J.,Wautier J-L. (1986) : Determination of platelet antigens and glycoproteins in the human fetus. *Blood,68*:488-492

. HarringtoN W.J., Sprague C.C., Minnich V., Moore C.V., Aulvin R.C., Dubach R.(1953) : Immunologic mechanisms in idiopathic and neonatal thrombocytopenic purpura. *Ann. Inter. Med.* , *38* : 433-469

. Herman J.H., Jumbelic M.I., Ancona R.J., Kickler T.S. 1986 : In utero cerebral hemorrhage in alloimmune thrombocytopenia. *Am. J. Pediatr. Hematol. Oncol.*, *8* : 312 - 317

. Kaplan C., Patereau C, Reznikoff-etievant M.F., Muller J.Y., Dumez Y., Kesseler A.(1985) : Antenatal PL^{A1} typing and detection of GP IIb-IIa complex. *Br. J. Haematol.*, *60* : 586 - 588

. Kaplan C., daffos F., Forestier F., Cox W.L., Lyon-caen D., Dupuy-Montbrun M.C., salmon Ch.(1988) : Management of alloimmune thrombocytopenia: antenatal diagnosis and in utero transfusion of maternal platelets. *Blood* , *72* : 340 - 343

. Kiefel V., Santoso S., Weisheit M., Mueller-eckhardt C.(1987) : Monoclonal antibody-specific immobilization of platelet antigens (MAIPA) : a new tool for the identification of platelet reactive antibodies. *Blood, 70* : 1722 - 1726

. Kiefel V., Santoso S., Katzmann B., Mueller-eckhardT C.(1989) : The Br^a/Br^b alloantigen system on human platelets. *Blood., 73* : 2219 - 2223

. Kunicki T.J., Aster R.H.(1979) : Isolation and immunologic characterization of the human platelet alloantigen PL^{A1}. *Mol. Immunol., 16* : 353 - 360

. Kunicki T.J., Beardsley S.D. (1989) : The alloimmune thrombocytopenias : Neonatal alloimmune thrombocytopenia. Purpura and post transfusion purpura. p.203-232 In *Progress in Hemostasis and Thrombosis* B.S. Coller Ed., Saunders Philadelphia

. Martin B., Robins H., Williams R., Ornelias W. (1983) : Neonatal graft vs host disease following transfusion of maternal platelets. *Transfusion., 23* : 417

. Mc Grath K.,Minchinton R.,Cunningham I., Ayberk H.(1989) : Platelet anti-bak^b antibody associated with neonatal alloimmune thrombocytopenia. *Vox. Sang.,57* :182-184

. Moulinier J.(1958) : Iso-immunisation maternelle antiplaquettaire "Duzo". *Proc. 6th Congr. Eur. Soc. Haematol.* : 817 - 820

. Mueller-Eckhardt C., Grubert A., Weisheit M., Mueller-EckhardT G., Kiefel V., Kroll H., Schmidt S., Santoso S.(1989) : 348 cases of suspected neonatal allo-immune thrombocytopenia. *The Lancet,I*: 363 - 366

. Mueller-Eckhardt C., Kiefel V., Kroll H., Mueller-Eckhardt G. (1989) : HLA-DRw6, a new immune response marker for immunization against the platelet alloantigen Br^a. *Vox. Sang., 57* :90 - 91

. Muller J..Y., Patereau C., Reznikoff-Etievant M.F., Kaplan C., Simonney N.(1985) : Les thrombopénies néonatales alloimmunes. *Rev. Fr. Transf. Immunohématol., 28* : 625 - 641

. Murphy M.F., Pullon H.W.H., Metcalfe P.,Chapman J.F., Jenkins E., Waters A.H., Nicolaides K.H., Mibashan R.S. (1990) : Management of fetal alloimmune thrombocytopenia by weekly in utero platelet transfusions *Vox Sang., 58* : 45 - 49

. Reznikoff-Etievant M.F., Kaplan C., Muller J.Y., Daffos F., Forestier F.(1988) : Allo-immune thrombocytopenias, definition of a group at risk: a prospective study. In *Curr. Stud. Hematol. Blood Transf.* C.Kaplan-Gouet Ch. Salmon (Eds). Karger Basel., *55* : 119 - 124

. Santoso S., Shibata Y., Kiefel V., Mueller-Eckhardt C.(1987) : Identification of the Yuk^b alloantigen on the platelet glycoprotein IIIa. *Vox. Sang., 53* : 48 - 51

. Shibata Y., Miyaji T., Ichikaya Y, Matsuda I.(1986) : A new platelet antigen system Yuk^a/Yuk^b. *Vox. Sang., 51* : 334 - 336

. Shulman R.R., Marder V.J., Hiller M.C., Collier E.M.(1964) : Platelet and leukocyte isoantigens and their antibodies. Serologic, physiologic and clinical studies. Moore C.V., Brown E.B. (eds). *Progress in Hematology , 4 :* 222 - 304

. Soulier J.P., Patereau, C., Drouet J.(1975) : Platelet indirect radioactive Coombs test. Its utilization for PL^{A1} grouping. *Vox Sang., 29 :* 253 - 268

. Valentin N., Vergracht A., Bignon J.D., Cheneau M.L., Blanchard D., Kaplan C., Reznikoff-Etievant M.F., Muller J.Y. (1990) : HLA DRw52a is involved in alloimmunisation against PL-^{A1} antigen. *Human Immunology* : *27* : 73-79

. Van Loghem J.J., Dorfmeijer H., Van Der Hart M., Schreuder F.(1959) : Serological and genetical studies on a platelet antigen (Zw). *Vox Sang., 4* : 161 - 169

. Von Dem Borne A.E.G.K., Verheugt F.W.A., Oosterhof F., Von Riez E., Brutel De La Riviere A., Engelfriet C.P.(1978) : A single immunofluorescence test for the detection of platelet antibodies. *Br. J. Haematol., 39* : 195 - 207

. Von Dem Borne A.E.G.K., Von Leeuven E.F., Von Riesz L.E., Verheugt F.W., Tencate J.W., Koppe J.G., Engelfriet C.P., Nijenhuis L.E.(1980) : Bak^a, a new platelet-specific antigen involved in neonatal alloimmune thrombocytopenia. *Vox. Sang., 39* : 113 - 120

. Von Dem Borne A.E.G.K., Van Der Plas C.(1986) : Bak^a and lek^a are identical antigens (letter). *Br. J. Haematol, 62* : 404 - 405

Résumé

Les thrombopénies néonatales allo-immunes (NAIT) résultent de la destruction des plaquettes foetales par les anticorps maternels. Les enfants sont à risques hémorragiques particulièrement dans le système nerveux central, entrainant soit des décès (10%),soit des séquelles neurologiques graves (20%). Nous présentons ici nos données concernant l'alloimmunisation anti-PL^{A1} ainsi que les résultats préliminaires des thrombopénies néonatales dues à des anticorps anti-Br^a . La définition de facteurs génétiques associés à l'immunisation foeto-maternelle a permis de définir des groupes de femmes à risques de NAIT lors de grossesses. Des progrès décisifs thérapeutiques ont été accomplis très récemment grâce aux possibilités de diagnostic anténatal dès 21 semaines de gestation, et à la mise en place de traitements in utéro.

Management of fetal alloimmune thrombocytopenia : the place of intrauterine platelet transfusions

A.H. Waters, R.S. Mibashan*, K.H. Nicolaides*, M.F. Murphy, R. Ireland* and H.W.H. Pullon*

St. Bartholomew's Hospital and Medical College West Smithfield, London EC1A 7BE, UK
*King's College Hospital Denmark Hill, London SE5 8RX, UK

Feto-maternal incompatibility for platelet specific alloantigens (notably $Pl^{A1}=Zw^a=HPA-1a$) may immunise the mother and cause alloimmune thrombocytopenia in the baby.

Most cases are diagnosed after birth; hence the terminology neonatal alloimmune thrombocytopenia (NAIT). However, improvements in fetal blood sampling techniques have shown that severe thrombocytopenia may be present by 20 weeks gestation (Kaplan et al, 1988) and serious intracranial haemorrhage (ICH) may occur in utero before delivery in as many as 5 per cent of cases (Bussel, 1987). These observations draw attention to the importance of the antenatal period in the overall management of NAIT.

Antenatal management of the pregnancy at risk has concentrated on attempts to minimise thrombocytopenia and protect the fetus from its complications, in particular serious ICH. The optimal treatment is currently under study and the therapeutic options include intravenous immunoglobulin (IVIgG) to mother or fetus (Bussel et al, 1988), low dose prednisone to mother (Daffos et al, 1988), and intrauterine platelet transfusions. Two platelet transfusion strategies are being explored - either a single transfusion prior to delivery (Daffos et al, 1984; Kaplan et al, 1988) or repeated transfusions during the latter part of pregnancy (Waters et al, 1987; Kaplan et al, 1988; Nicolini et al, 1988; Pullon et al, 1989). All of these approaches are dependent on direct fetal blood sampling to administer treatment and/or to monitor its effects.

This report describes our experience with three pregnancies at risk for NAIT treated with intrauterine platelet transfusions and considers the place of platelet transfusions in the antenatal management of NAIT.

CASE REPORTS

Case 1 (see de Vries et al, 1988)

The index case of NAIT (due to anti-Pl^{A1}) in this family suffered severe neurological consequences of ICH$_{A1}$ which probably occurred late in utero. The father was homozygous for Pl^{A1} and plans were made to manage a further pregnancy with intrauterine platelet transfusions. Ultrasound scans of the fetal head at 10, 22, 28 and 32 weeks gestation were all normal. Maternal anti-Pl^{A1} titre increased from 16 before pregnancy to 64 at 22 weeks and remained at this level. At 35 weeks she was admitted for further ultrasound studies and fetal blood sampling (FBS). On this occasion the ultrasound scan suggested ICH which was not seen at 32 weeks. FBS showed severe thrombocytopenia (platelets 12 x 10^9/l). Platelets from a selected Pl^{A1} negative donor were transfused into the umbilical vein under ultrasound guidance (Nicolaides et al, 1986); the post-transfusion platelet count was 139 x 10^9/l. The baby was delivered by caesarean section; the cord blood platelet count was 120 x 10^9/l and there were no superficial signs of thrombocytopenic bleeding. Subsequent clinical assessment by CT scanning and NMR indicated both recent (1-2 weeks) and older (>4 weeks) cerebral haemorrhages, and the baby suffered severe neurological damage

This case emphasised the unpredictable occurrence of ICH in utero and the difficulty of timing the first platelet transfusion to prevent this.

Case 2 (see Pullon et al, 1989)

Past history

This patient first became pregnant at the age of 16. The pregnancy was terminated for psychosocial reasons. At the age of 23 she again became pregnant and subsequently delivered a 2.5 kg male infant by spontaneous vaginal delivery at 38 weeks gestation. The infant was found to be profoundly thrombocytopenic and had a left-sided hemiparesis and developmental delay due to ICH$_{A1}$ Further investigation revealed that the mother's platelets typed as Pl^{A1}-negative, the baby's as Pl^{A1}-positive and that the mother's serum contained platelet-specific antibodies of anti-Pl^{A1} specificity. The maternal HLA type was:- A1, A3, B7, <u>B8</u>, Bw6, <u>DR3</u>, DR4, <u>DRw52</u>, DRw53, DQw2, DQw3.

Third pregnancy

She became pregnant again at the age of 24. The father was found to be homozygous for Pl^{A1} using the platelet immunofluorescence test and immunoblotting. This pregnancy was followed carefully with regular ultrasound scans from 20 weeks' gestation. At 26 weeks, FBS revealed severe thrombocytopenia (platelet count 32 x 10^9/l).

Intrauterine transfusions of Pl^{A1}-negative platelets were started earlier than in Case 1. At 26 weeks the fetal platelet count was 32 x 10^9/l, rising to 160 x 10^9/l after platelet transfusion. This was repeated at 27 weeks (25 to 280 x 10^9/l) and 29 weeks (5 to 320 x 10^9/l). Before the third platelet transfusion, the mother also received IVIgG 0.4g/Kg/d for 5 days, which had no effect on the fetal platelet count. At 30 weeks, the mother fell and a few days later fetal death was diagnosed. She delivered a 1.2 kg stillborn infant and post-mortem examination did not reveal any evidence of haemorrhage.

Fourth pregnancy

Her next pregnancy was at the age of 25. The fetus was monitored with regular ultrasound scans from 16 weeks. At 29 weeks FBS revealed severe thrombocytopenia (platelet count $17 \times 10^9/l$).

Intrauterine transfusions of Pl^{A1}-negative platelets were started at 29 weeks' gestation and continued at weekly intervals for six weeks; a greater number of platelets were given with each transfusion than in her third pregnancy (Table 1). Good immediate platelet increments were obtained and, by using higher platelet doses than in the previous pregnancy, platelet counts after one week were successfully maintained above $30 \times 10^9/l$ in all but one case (Fig 1). After the 5th transfusion, fetal distress was noted with brief episodes of bradycardia and tachycardia. One week later after the 6th transfusion at 34 weeks and 5 days' gestation, the fetus again had bradycardia. A 2.1 kg female infant was delivered by caesarean section on the following day.
Cord blood sampling after delivery revealed a haemoglobin of 6.8 g/dl and a platelet count of $102 \times 10^9/l$. The baby's platelet count was $66 \times 10^9/l$ on the next day. The baby had mild respiratory distress and was given a red cell exchange transfusion and a further platelet transfusion; after this procedure the haemoglobin was 13.3 g/dl and the platelet count was $198 \times 10^9/l$. A satisfactory platelet count was maintained without further transfusions and the baby left hospital 7 days after birth with a platelet count of $235 \times 10^9/l$. Follow-up examinations have shown no evidence of neurological damage.

Platelet serology

The maternal anti-Pl^{A1} titre was 16 to 32 during the third pregnancy and 8 to 16 during the last pregnancy. Maternal HLA antibodies were detected for the first time at the end of the last pregnancy. HLA and platelet-specific antibodies were not detectable in fetal blood samples taken prior to each platelet transfusion in both the third and fourth pregnancies, apart from on one occasion at 32 weeks in the fourth pregnancy when weak anti-Pl^{A1} was found.

DISCUSSION

The advent of fetal blood sampling has made it possible to confirm the diagnosis of alloimmune thrombocytopenia and assess its severity in the fetus; in addition, it provides a means of transfusing platelet concentrates to the fetus to correct the thrombocytopenia prior to delivery (Daffos et al, 1984).

Platelet transfusion strategies

In most affected pregnancies, fetal thrombocytopenia is already present at 20 weeks gestation (Kaplan et al, 1988). The possibility that repeated platelet transfusions from 20 weeks until term might provide complete protection from intrauterine haemorrage has been discounted because of the putative need for transfusions every 4 or 5 days (Daffos et al, 1988). On the other hand, some cases of NAIT do not develop severe thrombocytopenia until after 20 weeks gestation (Kaplan et al, 1988; Lynch et al, 1988), and there are only two documented cases of intrauterine haemorrhage before 30 weeks' gestation (Hermann et al, 1986; Reznikoff-Etievant, 1988),

Table 1. Case 2. Details of intrauterine platelet transfusions and changes in cord blood haemoglobin.

Gestation weeks	PLATELET TRANSFUSION		CORD PLATELETS		RECOVERY FACTOR	CORD Hb	
	Platelets x 10^9	Volume ml	Pre x10^9/l	Post x10^9/l		Pre g/dl	Post g/dl
29	110	50	17	374	0.43	13.1	10.5
30	87	65	75	281	0.43	11.9	9.7
31	149	54	31	510	0.54	11.2	9.3
32	169	69	80	563	0.55	11.4	9.8
33	153	90	69	*	*	10.6	*
34	104	72	24	269	0.54	10.2	8.3

* Clotted sample

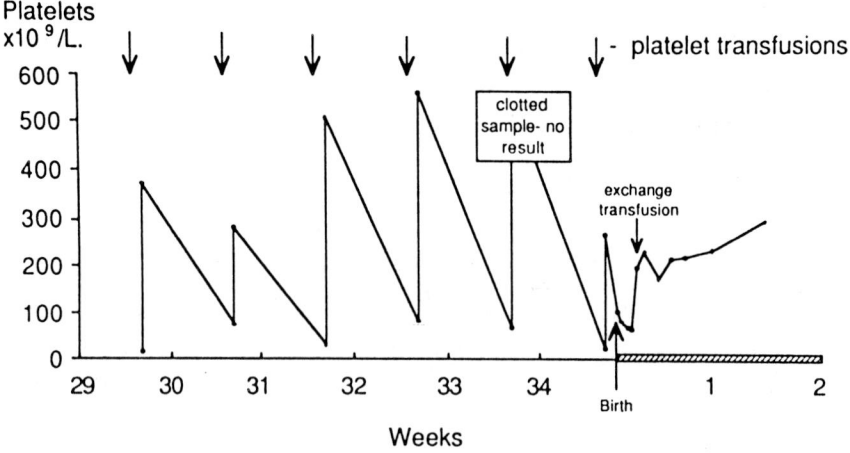

Fig. 1 Case 2. Fetal platelet counts before and after weekly intrauterine platelet transfusions. A further platelet transfusion was given the day after birth in association with a red cell exchange transfusion.

suggesting that the greatest risk of haemorrhage may be in the last trimester of pregnancy. This is the rationale for a compromise strategy using repeated platelet transfusions, beginning between the 26th and 30th weeks of pregnancy, and continuing until fetal maturity is reached, when an elective caesarean section is performed.

In the fourth pregnancy of Case 2 described in the present paper, it was possible to maintain the fetal platelet count above $30 \times 10^9/l$ for almost the whole of the last trimester of pregnancy by increasing the number of platelets transfused. Nicolini et al (1988) and Kaplan et al (1988) have also used this approach. However, further studies are needed to confirm the efficacy of this strategy in preventing antenatal haemorrhage.

An alternative platelet transfusion strategy and involves giving a single platelet transfusion just before delivery to protect the infant from trauma at birth and immediately afterwards, which is the time of greatest risk for ICH (Daffos et al, 1984; Kaplan et al, 1988). This option might be considered suitable for pregnancies thought to be at low risk of antenatal haemorrhage; such pregnancies are difficult to identify with certainty and this approach would not protect against the risk of thrombocytopenic bleeding in the last trimester (de Vries et al, 1988).

Intrauterine platelet transfusions - practical aspects

Platelet concentrates can be prepared by plateletpheresis of compatible donors. For single transfusions, the mother is a convenient donor, but this approach is not practical for repeated platelet transfusions and it is necessary to establish a panel of selected donors. The identification of sufficient numbers of such donors could present a logistical problem, especially if the platelet antibody specificity was not anti-Pl^{A1}. All platelet concentrates should be gamma irradiated to prevent transfusion-induced graft-versus-host disease in the fetus.

A routine platelet concentrate should be further centrifuged to achieve a platelet count of at least $2000 \times 10^9/l$, to enable an adequate platelet dose to be given to the fetus in an acceptable transfusion volume. An important consideration in the use of repeated platelet transfusions is calculation of the volume of platelet concentrate required to maintain the platelet count for one week at the required 'safe' level. The calculation is based on a simple mathematical formula:

$$\text{Volume of concentrate} = \frac{\text{Desired platelet increment} \times \text{Feto-placental blood volume}}{\text{Platelet count of concentrate}}$$

The feto-placental blood volume for gestational age was derived from previously constructed charts (Nicolaides et al, 1987). The immediate platelet increment (after 1-1.5 minutes) was only about 50 per cent of that expected i.e. 50 per cent recovery of transfused platelets (Table 1), which should be taken into consideration in calculating the volume of platelet concentrate. The lower recovery was probably due to pooling of transfused platelets in the fetal liver, spleen and placenta, and to the effect of dilution associated with the significant increase in fetal blood volume produced by the transfusion. An additional factor that needs to be considered is the half-life of the transfused platelets which was found to be approximately 3 days.

In experienced hands the procedure itself has minimal risk for the fetus (Daffos et al, 1985), but repeated transfusions increase the risk of complications. Transfusion-transmitted infection may be avoided by the use of maternal platelets, but this approach is not practical for repeated transfusions. This risk may be minimised by careful screening of platelet donors, including CMV testing in addition to standard microbiological testing.

In addition, in the fourth pregnancy of Case 2 described in this report, there was a progressive fall in the fetal haemoglobin level. This may have been the result of repeated fetal blood sampling and dilution. If intrauterine platelet transfusions are started earlier in pregnancy, then fetal anaemia may necessitate intrauterine transfusion of red cells. Another possible complication of repeated transfusions is the development of alloantibodies to platelet antigens resulting in poor responses to subsequent platelet transfusions, but there was no evidence that this occurred in the two pregnancies described in this report. Moreover, a recent study has demonstrated that neonates do not form red cell alloantibodies after multiple red cell transfusions (Ludvigsen et al, 1987).

Non-invasive strategies

Repeated intrauterine platelet transfusions may prove to be too invasive and a single pre-delivery transfusion, although protecting the fetus against bleeding from birth trauma, would leave it at risk of possible ICH during late pregnancy. For these reasons non-invasive methods for antenatal treatment of NAIT have been attempted. Daffos et al (1988) reported an apparent increase in the fetal platelet count after maternal treatment with prednisone 10 mg daily from the 23rd week of pregnancy until delivery. Bussel et al (1988) treated seven high-risk cases of NAIT with weekly maternal administration of high-dose intravenous IgG (1 g/kg infused over 4-7 hours once a week), with or without dexamethasone (3-5 mg/day), for a period of 6-17 weeks until delivery. In all cases fetal platelet counts (monitored by FBS) were increased and there were no bleeding complications; by contrast, platelet counts were lower at birth in all seven of their respective untreated siblings, three of whom had had ICH (antenatal in two). However, the effect of this treatment is not always predictable and in two other cases of NAIT (Kaplan et al, 1988; Mir et al, 1988), and in Case 2 reported here, the use of high-dose IVIgG alone had no effect on the fetal platelet count.

Optimal management of pregnancies at risk

The optimal management of NAIT to prevent ICH in utero is currently under study. To accelerate progress the Neonatal Immune Thrombocytopenia Working Party (Chairman: Dr. J. Bussel, New York) of the ICTH Neonatal Hemostasis and Thrombosis Sub-committee is collecting data from many centres as a basis for interim guidelines on the management of NAIT.

The cases described in this report, and similar cases reported by Nicolini et al (1988) and Kaplan et al (1988), illustrate the potential value of intrauterine transfusions for raising the fetal platelet count, but emphasise the short duration of this effect. Repeated platelet transfusions at approximately weekly intervals are necessary to maintain a "safe" platelet count to reduce the risk of ICH. As the procedure is so invasive and labour-intensive, further studies are needed to identify the high risk pregnancies that would benefit most from such an aggressive approach. FBS makes it possible to identify a severely thrombocytopenic fetus, but apart from the occurrence of ICH in a previously affected infant, there is no other indication of these high risk cases. The timing of the first platelet transfusion is crucial to prevent ICH, and further information about the frequency and time of occurrence of ICH in utero is required. Although a single pre-delivery platelet transfusion would protect against bleeding due to birth trauma, the fetus would still be at risk of ICH during late pregnancy.

Concern about the invasiveness of multiple prophylactic platelet transfusions and the limitations of a single pre-delivery transfusion has focussed attention on the potential advantages of non-invasive strategies. In particular, maternal treatment with intravenous IgG and/or steroids should be further evaluated as first line treatment to prevent ICH in utero in NAIT. However, if non-invasive methods fail to raise the platelet count, intrauterine platelet transfusions may be used to achieve this. Optimal management of the pregnancy at risk for NAIT is therefore more exacting than previously envisaged, and not yet resolved. A combination of non-invasive strategies and intrauterine platelet transfusions may prove to be most effective in preventing ICH in utero.

These potential improvements in antenatal management of NAIT draw attention to the plight of the first baby at risk, in whom the diagnosis is usually unexpected and made after birth. A severely affected baby may already have had an ICH in utero or during delivery. This raises the question of routine antenatal screening for the most common form of NAIT due to fetomaternal incompatibility for the Pl^{A1} antigen. A preliminary economic evaluation in Canada concluded that NAIT screening might be able to compete with other health screening programmes for funding (Gafni and Blanchette, 1988). Before such programmes are initiated, it will be important to determine the frequency and time of occurrence of ICH in utero and the efficacy of antenatal management in preventing this complication.

REFERENCES

Bussel, J.B. (1987): Neonatal alloimmune thrombocytopenia (NAIT): information derived from a prospective international registry. Blood 70 (Suppl.): 336a (Abstract 1199).
Bussel, J.B., Berkowitz, R.L., McFarland, J.G., Lynch, L. and Chitkara, U. (1988): Antenatal treatment of neonatal alloimmune thrombocytopenia. New Engl. J. Med. 319: 1374-1378.
Daffos, F., Forestier, F., Muller, J.Y., Reznikoff-Etievant, M.F., Habibi, B., Capell-Pavlovsky, M., Maigret, P. and Kaplan, C. (1984): Prenatal treatment of alloimmune thrombocytopenia. Lancet 2: 632.
Daffos, F., Capella-Pavlovsky, M. and Forestier, F. (1985): Fetal blood sampling during pregnancy with use of a needle guided by ultrasound: a study of 606 consecutive cases. Am. J. Obstet. Gynecol. 153: 655-660.
Daffos, F., Forestier, F. and Kaplan, C. (1988): Prenatal treatment of fetal alloimmune thrombocytopenia. Lancet 2: 910.
de Vries, L.S., Connell, J., Bydder, G.M., Dubowitz, L.M.S., Rodeck, C.H., Mibashan, R.S. and Waters, A.H. (1988): Recurrent intracranial haemorrhages in utero in an infant with alloimmune thrombocytopenia. Case report. Br. J. Obstet. Gynaecol. 95: 299-302.
Gafni, A. and Blanchette, V.S. (1988): Screening for neonatal thrombocytopenia: an economic perspective. Curr. Stud. Hematol. Blood Transfns. 54: 140-147. Basel: Karger.
Herman, J.H., Jumbelic M.I., Ancona, R.J. and Kickler, T.S. (1986): In utero cerebral haemorrhage in alloimmune thrombocytopenia. Amer. J. Ped. Hematol. Oncol. 8: 312-317.

Kaplan, C., Daffos, F., Forestier, F., Cox, W.L., Lyon-Caen, D., Dupuy-Montbrun, M.C. and Salmon Ch. (1988): Management of alloimmune thrombocytopenia: antenatal diagnosis and in utero transfusion of maternal platelets. Blood 72: 340-343.

Ludvigsen, C.W., Swanson, J.L., Thompson, T.R. and McCullough, J. (1987): The failure of neonates to form red blood cell alloantibodies in response to multiple transfusions. Amer. J. Clin. Path. 87: 250-251.

Lynch, L., Bussel, J., Goldberg, J.D., Chitkara, U., Wilkins, I., Macfarland, J. and Berkowitz, R.L. (1988): The in utero diagnosis and management of alloimmune thrombocytopenia. Prenat. Diagn. 8: 329-331.

Mir, N., Samson, D., House, M.J., and Kovar, I.Z. (1988): Failure of antenatal high-dose immunoglobulin to improve fetal platelet count in neonatal alloimmune thrombocytopenia. Vox Sang. 55: 188-189.

Nicolaides, K.H., Clewell, W.H. and Rodeck, C.H.. (1987). Measurement of human fetoplacental blood volume in erythroblastosis fetalis. Amer. J. Obstet. Gynecol. 157: 50-53.

Nicolaides, K.H., Rodeck, C.H., Soothhill, P.W. and Campbell, S. (1986): Ultrasound-guided sampling of umbilical cord and placental blood to assess fetal wellbeing. Lancet 1: 1065-1067.

Nicolini, U., Rodeck, C.H., Kochenour, N.K., Greco, P., Fisk, N.M., Letsky, E. and Lubenko, A. (1988): In utero platelet transfusion for alloimmune thrombocytopenia. Lancet 2: 506.

Pullon, H.W.H., Murphy, M.F., Mibashan, R.S., Waters, A.H., Jenkins, E. and Nicolaides, K.H. (1989): Successful management of fetal alloimmune thrombocytopenia (AIT) by weekly in utero platelet transfusions. Br. J. Haemat. 71 (Suppl. 1): 11 (Abstract 40).

Reznikoff-Etievant, M.F. (1988): Management of alloimmune neonatal and antenatal thrombocytopenia. Vox Sang. 55: 193-201.

Waters, A.H., Ireland, R., Mibashan, R.S., Murphy, M.F., Millar, D.S., Chapman, J.F., Metcalfe, P., de Vries, L.E., Rodeck C.H. and Nicolaides, K.H. (1987): Fetal platelet transfusions in the management of alloimmune thrombocytopenia. Thromb. Haemostas. 58: 323 (Abstract 1178).

Résumé

L'incompatibilité plaquettaire foeto-maternelle est à l'origine de thrombopénie néonatale (TNA). La plupart des cas sont diagnostiqués après la naissance. Cependant, l'amélioration des techniques de prélèvements de sang foetal a permis de mettre en évidence des thrombopénies sévères dès 20 semaines de gestation (Kaplan et Coll. 1988) et des hémorragies intracérébrales sévères peuvent survenir in utero avec une fréquence de 5 % (Bussel, 1987). Ces observations soulignent l'importance de la surveillance anténatale dans les TNA et les problèmes posés quant au choix d'un traitement optimal.

Antenatal treatment of neonatal alloimmune thrombocytopenia with intravenous gammaglobulin

J.B. Bussel

Division of Pediatrics N-740, The New York Hospital – Cornell Medical Center, 525 East 68th Street, New York, NY 10021, USA

Introduction: Neonatal alloimmune thrombocytopenia was first described in the late 1950's and early 1960's (1,2,3). By 1964 several publications had characterized the serologic findings of the disease and reported a total of more than 20 cases. These reports recognized the preeminent clinical importance of intracranial hemorrhage and a mortality rate of 14% was estimated and has since been widely quoted (2). In 1979 the first cases with antenatal intracranial hemorrhage were described and subsequently other cases were also reported, often in sibling pairs. In 1986 a review of antenatal hemorrhage was able to summarize 10 previously published cases and add 2 new cases (4).

At approximately the same time a review of all published cases of alloimmune thrombocytopenia appeared which included a comparison of outcomes in first versus subsequent cases in families (5). The overly high figures in first affected cases for intracranial hemorrhage (47%) and for mortality (24%) clearly reflects the known bias of case reports to represent unduly dramatic cases. However the figures for the second affected siblings were striking in that they revealed a 15% rate of intracranial hemorrhage and a 5% mortality. While in part this might be due to the failure of the treating physician to manage the second case differently ie delivery by cesarean section, these numbers also reflect the failure of cesarean section at term to affect the outcome of antenatal intracranial hemorrhage.

Results of Pilot Studies: Our experience with antenatal treatment began with the presentation of a pregnant woman whose first child had been born at 38 weeks of gestation with an intracranial hemorrhage that dated to approximately 32 weeks gestation (6 weeks prior to birth). The baby had died at 24 hours of age after having been born with a platelet count of 3,000/ul. Management of the second gestation consisted of dexamethasone at a dose of 5 mg/day and intravenous gammaglobulin (IVIG) at a dose of 1 gm/kg/week (6). Elective early delivery was accomplished at 31 weeks of gestation after a mature L/S ratio was demonstrated using fluid obtained by amniocentesis. The cord blood platelet count was 30,000/ul and no intracranial hemorrhage had occurred. The baby received a double volume exchange transfusion followed by matched platelet transfusion, all accomplished within 2 hours of birth, and never again had a platelet count < 100,000/ul. The baby weighed 1400 gms, had an uneventful neonatal course, and went home at approximately 3 weeks of age.

After successful treatment of this initial case, a protocol was instituted for treatment of subsequent cases. Requirements were that the patient have proven alloimmune thrombocytopenia and that the previous affected sibling have been severely affected ie platelet count < 30,000/ul after birth. Treatment was initiated for fetal platelet counts of less than 100,000/ul with IVIG at 1 gm/kg/week with or without concomitant steroids. The report of the first 7 cases demonstrated impressive increases in the fetal platelet counts as a result of antenatal treatment administered to the mother (6,7). These responses were measured in two ways. First the fetal platelet counts were directly measured by fetal blood sampling and the fetal count prior to beginning treatment was compared to the fetal count obtained 4 to 6 weeks later after treatment had been initiated. Second, the platelet count at birth in the treated fetuses could be compared to the platelet count at birth in the previous untreated siblings. In addition, and of the utmost importance, the previous untreated sibling could be compared to the treated sibling in regard to the occurrence of intracranial hemorrhage. In the initial series 3 previous siblings had had intracranial hemorrhages, at least two of which had occurred prior to delivery. No intracranial hemorrhages were seen in the treated cases now including a total of 6 in which the previous untreated sibling had suffered an intracranial hemorrhage.

At the present time approximately 15 cases have been treated on our protocol with 12 responses, defined as good platelet increases occurring as a result of antenatal treatment (8). Additional anecdotal cases exist where the exact treatments and other case details are uncertain. Some appear to have responded while others clearly have not. What are some of the factors that may determine response in these cases ?

One factor appears to be the dose of intravenous gammaglobulin. Doses other than repeated weekly infusions of IVIG 1 gm/kg/week appear not to be successful; I am unaware that are there any cases where there was an effect at a lower dose. One case of ours, 1 case report (9), and two cases reported only in abstract form (10,11) using /either 400-500 mg/kg/week or a single infusion of 2 gm/kg all failed to demonstrate any platelet increase with IVIG treatment.

Another factor may be the use of adjunctive glucocorticoids. The original 5 cases that we treated included dexamethasone first at a dose of 5 mg (3 cases) and then 3 mg (2 cases). This was discontinued because of development of oligohydramnios in 4 of the 5 cases (6,7). Subsequently 1 of 2 cases treated with combined IVIG and low dose prednisone (10 mg/day) also responded (8). Analysis of the data remains unclear regarding whether or not there was an adjunctive effect of the steroids. The overall platelet increases were comparable between the two groups suggesting that there may not have been an effect but the steroid treated cases may have been more severe implying that the combined effect was greater since equal responses were seen with more severe cases. In one anecdotal case no response was seen to IVIG alone but when dexamethasone was then added, a response was seen to the combined treatment. Oligohydramnios also developed. A trial has now been launched to compare IVIG alone and IVIG plus low dose dexamethasone. This will serve to answer the question of the additive effect of corticosteroids at the same time as providing significant adidtional prospective data concerning both the natural history of antenatal thrombocytopenia and the morbidities of fetal sampling in thrombocytopenic fetuses and of platelet transfusions administered to fetuses. For both rms of the trial we will continue the IVIG and add 60 mg of prednisone a day if there is a failure as defined by an insufficient platelet response between the first and second fetal counts.

Finally a critical question is whether or not the most severe cases are as responsive to treatment as the less severe cases. One way to restate this is to emphasize that the only unequivocal reason to provide antenatal treatment is to avoid antenatal hemorrhage. This then raises the question of which fetus is at greatest risk to suffer an antenatal hemorrhage. Clearly a family where the previous fetus suffered a hemorrhage is at very high risk and treatment has been effective in preventing hemorrhage in 5 of these cases in our series (8). This is based upon the concept that a subsequent affected case in a family will be at least as severely affected as the previous affected case (12,14). One anecdotal case suffered an intracranial hemorrhage at 23 weeks of gestation (presumably) after having started treatment at 21 weeks which may have been too soon to see an effect. In the first 11 cases there was a strong correlation of the platelet count at the time of the first sampling to the count at birth (8). Since all of the cases were treated, this says that the more severe cases (those with the lowest in utero platelet counts) responded the least to treatment. This is a clear reason to perform the controlled steroid trial to see if treatment could be augmented especially for the more severe cases. An added part of this treatment is maternal avoidance of aspirin and untoward physical activity; as suggested by Kaplan, this may reduce the risk of antenatal hemorrhage by itself.

Objective prediction of antenatal hemorrhage (other than by the history of the previous sibling) is still in its infancy but is improving. We surmise, without hard evidence, that the earlier in gestation the platelet count becomes very low the more likely is the chance of intracranial hemorrhage (6). It appears plausible at the current time that the platelet count per se acts as a permissive (necessary but not sufficient) factor in regard to intracranial hemorrhage. Trauma (including at delivery or before) or inhibition of platelet function ie by aspirin may supervene to result in hemorrhage but properties of the antibodies may play a role in addition to their effects on the platelet count. Serologic indicators, such as complement fixation, may provide evidence of an antibody likely to cause hemorrhage beyond merely the platelet count itself (15). Perhaps higher titer antibodies and/or those which mediate endothelial damage as well as thrombocytopenia may result in a greater likelihood of hemorrhage. This will clearly need to be more carefully studied in the future.

Returning to the previous sibling, a crucial piece of elusive information would be which mother is likely to have a worse affected fetus the second time compared to the first. While HLA type has been shown to be related to the development of thrombocytopenia in PlA1- women (16,17), no known factor predicts which woman will have a worse affected fetus. This is important in assessing the risk of early severe fetal thrombocytopenia and of antenatal hemorrhage in a subsequent pregnancy. Possibly a mother who has a high titer anti-platelet antibody early in gestation will be at greater risk but this remains to be confirmed. Furthermore it is unclear what are the chances that a woman whose first child did not have an intracranial hemorrhage the first time will have a second child with a hemorrhage if delivery is by cesarean section.

The last area to comment upon regards the neonatal outcome in pregnancies during which the mother was treated. Surprisingly, four of the neonates were between the 3rd and 10th percentiles for age even when corrected for gestational age at birth. This was completely unrelated to steroid use despite the occurrence of oligohydramnios in only the dexamethasone-treated cases. Growth after birth was normal and no growth retardation was seen in 6 fetuses treated on an identical protocol for Rh disease. Furthermore no postnatal vulnerability to infections or abnormal development was seen.

Other forms of antenatal treatment are also being investigated. Two fetuses have been successfully treated with weekly in utero platelet transfusions (18); this however appears too invasive for any but highly selected cases which have first failed medical management. Steroids alone do not appear to be sufficient although data is limited (19). Early delivery alone will not be effective in all cases since hemorrhage can occur prior to 34 weeks gestation (4).

In summary therefore the awareness of the possibility of antenatal hemorrhage and the implicit need for antenatal treatment are crucial to optimizing outcome of fetuses affected with neonatal alloimmune thrombocytopenia. The preliminary data presented with the use of IV Gammaglobulin are encouraging but much remains to be studied including controlled trials of management and the development of better serologic predictors of hemorrhage as distinct from thrombocytopenia alone.

1. Loghem J van, Dorfmeijer H, Hart M van der. Serological and genetical studies on a platelet antigen (Zw). Vox Sang 1959, 4:161

2. Pearson HA, Shulman RM, Mader VJ, Cone TE. Isoimmune neonatal thrombocytopenia purpura. Clinical and therapeutic considerations. Blood 1964;23:154-177

3. Shulman NR, Nader VJ, Hiller MC, Collier EM. Platelet and leucocyte isoantigens and their antibodies. Serologic and clinical studies. Progress in haematology 1964; 4:222

4. Herman JH, Jumbelic MI, Amcona RJ, Kicklet TS. In utero cerebral hemorrhage in alloimmune thrombocytopenia. Am J Ped Hematol Oncol 1986; 8: 312-317

5. Deaver JE, Leppert P, Zaroulis CG. Neonatal alloimmune thrombocytopenic purpura. Am J of Perinatol 1986;3:127-131

6. Bussel JB, Berkowitz R, McFarland J, Lynch L, Chitkara U: Antenatal Treatment of Neonatal Alloimmune Thrombocytopenia. New Engl J of Med 1988;319:1374-1378

7. Bussel JB, McFarland JG, Berkowitz RL. Antenatal management of fetal alloimmune cytopenias. In Press Blut 1989;58:1-3

8. Bussel JB, McFarland J, Berkowitz R. Antenatal management of fetal alloimmune and autoimmune thrombocytopenia. Transf Med Rev April;1990

9. Mir N, Samson D, House MJ, Kovar IZ. Failure of antenatal high-dose immunoglobulin to improve fetal platelet count in neonatal all-immune thrombocytopenia. Vox Sang 1988;55:188-189

10. Waters AH, Ireland R, Mibashan RS, et al. Fetal platelet transfusion in the management of alloimmune thrombocytopenia. Thromb Haemost 1987;58:323

11. Kaplan C, Daffos F, Forestier F. Fetal blood sampling in patients with autoimmune thrombocytopenia Abstract presented at International Committee of Thrombosis. Tokio, Japan 1989

12. Bussel JB. Neonatal Immune Thrombocytopenia Study Group. Neonatal Alloimmune Thrombocytopenia: A prospective case accumulation Study. Pediatr Res 12:337A (abs)

13. Muller JY, Reznikoff-Etievant MF, Paterau C, Dangu C. Thrombocytopenies neonatales alloimmunes. Etude clinique et biologique de 84 cas. Nouv. Presse med 1985;14:83-84

14. Schulman NR, Jordan JV. Platelet Immunology. In Coleman RW, Hirsh J, Marder VJ, Salzman EW eds. Hemostasis and thrombosis 1982;274-342

15. Bussel JB, McFarland JG. The Chromium release assay correlates with intracranial hemorrhage (ICH) in neonatal alloimmune thrombocytopenia (NAIT). Presented at the SPR meeting 1990

16. Reznikoff-Etievant M, Dangu C, Lobet R. HLA-B8 antigen and anti-P1A1 alloimmunization. Tissue Antigens 1981;18:66-68

17. Taaning E, Antosen H, Petersen S, Svejgaard A, Thompsen M. HLA antigens and maternal antibodies in alloimmune neonatal thrombocytopenia. Tissue Antigens 1983;21:351-359

18. Nicolini U, Rodeck CH, Kochenour NK, et al. In utero platelet transfusion for alloimmune thrombocytopenia. Lancet 1988;ii:506

19. Daffos F, Forestier F, Kaplan C, Prenatal treatment of fetal alloimmune thrombocytopenia. Lancet 1988;ii:910

Neonatal Alloimmune Thrombocytopenia occurs in approximately 1/1000-1/2000 births. In the United States with approximately 4-6,000,000 deliveries per year. If the rate of intracranial hemorrhage is approximately 10-20 % of all cases, then there would be 200 to 1200 cases with ICH per year. If 1/4 to 1/2 of all ICH occur prenatally, then there would be 50 to 600 cases of prenatal hemorrhage born per year in the United States. Some of the prenatal hemorrhages occur in the first affected child in the family and therefore cannot be prevented but these women may wish to have another child. Since the next affected child in a family is virtually always at least as seriously affected as the previously affected child, prenatal treatment may be required if there is a risk of prenatal hemorrhage. We have treated in pilot studies 27 women with intravenous gammaglobulin at a dose of 1 gm/kg/infusion administered weekly with or without concomitant steroids. 22 have had at least a clinically important increase in their platelet count. No recurrence of 6 antenatal intracranial hemorrhages that occurred in previous siblings has been seen. We are currently performing a controlled trial of IVGG with or without concomitant steroids to see if they have a synergistic effect.

Résumé

Les thrumbopénies néonatales alloimmunes ont une fréquence de 1/1000 à 1/2000 naissances. Aux Etats Unis cela représente 2000 à 6000 cas/an. Si le taux d'hémorragies intracérébrales est de 10 à 20 %, cela signifie que 200 à 1200 enfants seront atteints/an. Si 25 à 50 % de ces hémorragies surviennent in utéro 50 à 600 enfants naîtront déjà atteints. Lorsque l'hémorragie intracérébrale prénatale touche le 1er enfant elle ne peut être prévenue ; mais les mères peuvent désirer une autre grossesse. Etant donné que les autres enfants peuvent être aussi sinon plus atteints que le 1er, les traitements in utero doivent être mis en place s'il existe un tel risque. Dans une étude pilote nous avons traité 27 femmes avec des immunoglobulines à la dose de 1 mg/kg/injection/semaine avec ou sans adjonction de corticoïdes. Chez 22 foetus on a observé une correction de la thrombopénie. Aucun enfant n'a eu d'hémorragie intracérébrale contrairement à leurs aînés dans les 6 cas où cela avait été diagnostiqué. Nous proposons actuellement deux protocoles avec ou sans adjonction de corticoïdes afin de tester un éventuel effet synergique.

Antibody detection in autoimmune thrombocytopenic purpura

V. Kiefel, S. Santoso and C. Mueller-Eckhardt

Institute of Clinical Immunology and Transfusion Medicine, Justus Liebig University, Langhansstrasse 7, D-6300 Giessen, Germany

ABSTRACT

Platelet autoantibodies (aabs) causing autoimmune thrombocytopenic purpura (AITP) have so far been studied with assays detecting immunoglobulin binding to intact platelets. Results of indirect binding tests employed for demonstration of free aabs may be affected by platelet reactive alloantibodies. Elevated amounts of platelet associated IgG (PAIgG) on autologous platelets are a frequent finding also in patients with non-immune thrombocytopenia. Target antigens of aabs have been localized on platelet glycoproteins (GPs). Assays which allow determination of GP specificity of both free and platelet bound aabs are more reliable diagnostic tools for thrombocytopenic patients.

INTRODUCTION

In clinical practice the diagnosis of AITP is usually made be excluding conditions of impaired thrombocytopoiesis, enhanced platelet pooling in the enlarged spleen and accelerated platelet destruction due to non-immunological mechanisms. However, these clinical criteria for "idiopathic" immune thrombocytopenia cannot be applied to patients with AITP accompanying other diseases. Conditions found to be associated with "secondary" AITP include lymphomas, systemic lupus erythematosus, carcinoma without impairment of thrombocytopoiesis due to bone marrow in filtration. Therefore, the immunohematologist has to provide reliable assays for assessment of platelet specific aabs as a diagnostic aid in thrombocytopenic patients.

Specificity of antibodies involved in AITP

Observations made by Harrington et al. (1953) and Shulman et al. (1965) suggested that idiopatic thrombocytopenic purpura (ITP) is most probably caused by antibodies found in the 7S gamma globulin fraction of plasma. Other authors supposed that ITP might be caused by circulating immune complexes (CICs). Aggregated IgG or ICs become attached in vitro to platelets (Helmerhorst et al. 1983, Winiarski et al., 1985) and can induce platelet activation (Mueller-Eckhardt & Lüscher, 1968). CICs have been found by some authors in sera of patients with ITP (Lurhuma et al. 1977, Clancy et al.,

1980, Wautier et al., 1980), but these findings were not confirmed by others (Ercilla et al., 1982, Kiefel et al., 1986). Van Leeuwen et al. 1982 first localized the antigenic determinant recognized by many platelet specific aabs on the GPIIb/IIIa complex. These findings were later confirmed by others (Woods et al., 1984a, McMillan et al., 1987). Using the immunoblotting technique, Beardsley et al., (1984) could identify aabs reacting with GPIIIa and Tomiyama et al. (1987) found aabs specific for GPIIb. Woods et al. (1984b), McMillan et al. (1987) observed aabs against the GPIb/IX complex in rare patients with AITP. GPV was identified as target antigen in acute varicella associated immune thrombocytopenia (Beardsley, 1989). An antibody causing both AITP and impairment of collagen induced platelet functions (Sugiyama et al. 1987) was shown to react with platelet GPVI (Moroi et al., 1989). It is not known if this is identical to the 56 kDa protein identified using direct radioimmunoprecipitation by Tomiyama et al (1990).

Less is known about aabs reacting with other constituents of the platelet membrane. Harris et al. (1985) found anticardiolipin antibodies in ITP patients and van Vliet et al. detected antibodies against glycosphingolipids. However, it remains to be shown, if phospholipid or glycolipid antigens play an important role in the pathogenesis of AITP.

Methods for platelet aab detecton

First attempts to characterize platelet aabs were made with the platelet agglutination test (Harrington et al., 1953) and the complement fixation test (Shulman et al., 1964). Both assays are not adequate for the reliable detection of platelet aabs: many sera from individuals without thrombocytopenia contain agglutinating antibodies and nearly all platelet specific aabs do not fix complement, although rare exceptions have been described.

In the last years it became general practice to study both free platelet aabs in the patient's plasma and aabs on the autologous platelets.

Binding of antibodies to platelets can be determined with anti-human immunoglobulins labelled with fluorescent dyes, enzymes and radioisotopes. A vast number of assays have been described of which the platelet suspension immunofluorescence assay (PSIFT, von dem Borne et al., 1978) became the most widely applied procedure. But antibodies against HLA-class I antigens also react with platelets and therefore interfere with platelet aab detection. This problem was in part overcome by chloroquine treatment of test platelets which reduces the amount of HLA determinants on the platelet surface (Blumberg et al., 1984, Nordhagen & Flaathen, 1985).

More recently some laboratories including our own have begun to determine the GP specificity of platelet reactive antibodies in thrombocytopenic patients to obtain more reliable results. This is possible by incubating platelet GPs immobilized on nitrocellulose with the diluted patient sera following separation by SDS polyacrylamide gelelectrophoresis (SDS PAGE) (immunoblotting: Beardsley et al., 1984, Huisman, 1986). By this technique some, but not all platelet specific auto- and alloantibodies may be visualized. Antibodies, which react with conformational antigens may be destroyed by SDS-treatment at 100°C and will therefore be missed in IB. In indirect radioimmunoprecipitation (RIP), the sequence of protein separation and antibody binding to antigen is inverted (Mulder et al., 1984): Platelet reactive antibodies are allowed to react with radioactively labelled platelets. Antibody-GP complexes can be precipitated from the platelet lysate with immobilized protein A and after elution in SDS, the molecular weight of the purified GPs is determined by SDS-PAGE, followed by autoradiography of the gel. An advantage of RIP is that antibody binding occurs before SDS treatment. Therefore also those antibodies recognizing conformational epitopes are detected by RIP.

Both techniques, RIP and IB, use SDS-PAGE, which is rather time-consuming and requires some skill and experience. Therefore, other authors used monoclonal antibodies (mabs) with defined GP specificity for isolation of the target antigens. Woods et al. (1984a) described the first of this type of assays: platelet GPs from a platelet lysate are fixed to the well of a microtiter plate with a mab. After washing, the wells are exposed to the patient serum and then to radiolabelled anti-human IgG. However, in our hands this procedure proved to be rather insensitive due to high background signals. Moreover, conformation of antigens may be changed by platelet lysis which occurs prior to antibody binding. All these problems are overcome by assay configurations which allow antibody binding to intact platelets prior to sulubilization. Such assays have been developed by McMillan et al. (1987) and by our group (Kiefel et al., 1987). The principle of our monoclonal antibody specific immobilization of platelet antigens (MAIPA) assay: test platelets are incubated with the serum containing an antibody reacting with a platelet GP and a mab binding to another epitope on the same GP. Platelets are then washed, lysed in buffer, containing the nonionic detergent Triton X-100 and insoluble material is removed by centrifugation. The supernatants are then diluted and pipetted into wells of microtiter plates which had been coated with anti-mouse immunoglobulin. After washing, human antibody bound to the immobilized GP can be detected withe enzyme-labelled anti-human IgG. This assay and the immunobead assay (McMillan et al., 1987) are not only suited for characterization of free platelet specific autoantibodies, but also for detection autoantibodies bound to the patient's autologous platelets. Using the MAIPA assay, the autologous platelets of the patient already sensitized with autoantibody are then incubated with monoclonal anti-GPIb/IX or anti-GPIIb/IIIa. Whereas elevated amounts of platelet associated immunoglobulins measured on intact platelets are often also found in patients with non-immune thrombocytopenia (Mueller-Eckhardt et al., 1980, Kelton et al., 1982, Kiefel et al., 1986, Vos et al., 1987), platelet bound GPIIb/IIIa- or GPIb/IX-specific aabs are a specific finding in AITP (McMillan et al., 1987, own unpublished observations). Therefore, this type of assays should be preferred in the future to methods measuring the overall amount of PAIgG. A similar approach was recently published by Tomiyama et al. (1990), using the method of direct radioimmunoprecipitation. In addition, sera containing platelet reactive aabs (detected by platelet immunofluorescence) should be further analyzed by glycoprotein specific immunoassays.

ACKNOWLEDGEMENT

The authors wish to thank Ms. P. Völker for her secretarial expertise.

REFERENCES

Beardsley, D. S., Spiegel, J. E., Jacobs, M. M., Handin, R. J., Lux, S. E. (1984): Platelet membrane glycoprotein IIIa contains target antigens that bind anti-platelet antibodies in immune thrombocytopenia.
J. Clin. Invest 74, 1701-1707

Beardsley, D. S. (1989): Platelet autoantigens. In Platelet Immunobiology, ed. T. J. Kunicki, J. N. George, pp. 121-131. Philadelphia: J. B. Lippincott company.

Blumberg, N., Masel, D., Mayer, T., Horan, P., Heal, J. (1984): Removal of HLA-A, B, antigens from platelets.
Blood 63, 448-450

von dem Borne, A. E. G. Kr., Verheugt, F. W. A., Oosterhof, F., von Riesz, E., Brutel de la Rivière, A., Engelfriet, C. P. (1978): A simple immunofluorescence test for the detection of platelet antibodies.
Brit. J. Haematol. 39, 195-207

Clancy, R., Trent, R., Danis, V., Davidson, R. (1980): Autosensitization and immune complexes in idiopathic thrombocytopenic purpura.
Clin. exp. Immunol 39, 170-175

Ercilla, M. G., Borche, L., Vives, J., Castillo, R., Gelabert, A., Rozman, C. (1982): Circulating immune complexes in immune thrombocytopenic purpura.
Brit. J. Haematol. 52, 679-682

Harrington, W., Sprague, C. C., Minnich, V., Moore, C. V., Aulvin, R. C., Dubach, R. (1953): Immunologic mechanisms in idiopathic and neonatal thrombocytopenic purpura.
Ann. Intern. Med. 38, 433-400

Harris, E. N., Gharavi, A. E., Hegde, U., Derue, G., Morgan, S. H., Englert, H., Chan, J. K. H., Asherson, R. A., Hughes, G. R. V. (1985): Anticardiolipin antibodies in autoimmune thrombocytopenic purpura.
Brit. J. Haematol. 59, 231-234

Helmerhorst, F. M., Smeenk, R. J. T., Hack, C. E., Engelfriet, C. P., von dem Borne, A. E. G. Kr. (1983): Interference of IgG, IgG aggregates and immune complexes in tests for platelet autoantibodies.
Brit. J. Haematol. 55, 533-545

Huisman, J. G. (1986): Immunoblotting: an emerging technique in immunohaematology.
Vox Sang. 50, 129-136

Kelton, J. G., Powers, P. J., Carter, C. J. (1982): A prospective study of the usefulness of the measurement of platelet-associated IgG for the diagnosis of idiopathic thrombocytopenic purpura.
Blood 60, 1050-1053

Kiefel, V., Spaeth, P., Mueller-Eckhardt, C. (1986): Immune thrombocytopenic purpura: autoimmune or immune complex disease?
Brit. J. Haematol. 64, 57-68

Kiefel, V., Santoso, S., Weisheit, M., Mueller-Eckhardt, C. (1987): Monoclonal antibody-specific immobilization of patelet antigens (MAIPA): A new tool for the identification of platelet reactive antibodies.
Blood 70, 1722-1726

van Leeuwen, E. F., van der Ven, J. T. M., Engelfriet, C. P., von dem Borne, A. E. G. Kr. (1982): Specificity of autoantibodies in autoimmune thrombocytopenia.
Blood 59, 23-26

Lurhuma, A. Z., Riccomi, H., Masson, P. L. (1977): The occurrence of circulating immune complexes and viral antigens in idiopathic thrombocytopenic purpura.
Clin. exp. Immunol. 28, 49-55

Moroi, M., Jung, S. M., Okuma, M., Shinmyozu, K. (1989): A patient with platelets deficient in glycoprotein VI that lack both collagen-induced aggregation and adhesion.
J. Clin. Invest. 84, 1440-1445

McMillan, R., Tani, P., Millard, F., Berchtold, P., Renshaw, L., Woods, V. L. (1987): Platelet-associated and plasma anti-glycoprotein autoantibodies in chronic ITP.
Blood 70, 1040-1045

Mueller-Eckhardt, C., Lüscher, E. F. (1968): Immune reactions of human blood platelets. I. A comparative study on the effects on platelets of heterologous antiplatelet antiserum, antigen-antibody complexes, aggregated gammaglobulin and thrombin.
Thrombosis et Diathesis Haemorrhagica 20, 155-167

Mueller-Eckhardt, C., Kayser, W., Mersch-Baumert, K., Mueller-Eckhardt, G., Breidenbach, M., Kugel, H. G., Graubner, M. (1980): The clinical significance of platelet associated IgG: A study on 298 patients with various disorders.
Brit. J. Haematol. 46, 123-131

Mulder, A., van Leeuwen, E. F., Veenboer, G. J. M., Tetteroo, P. A. T., von dem Borne, A. E. G. Kr. (1984): Immunochemical characterization of platelet-specific alloantigenes.
Scand. J. Haematol. 33, 267-274

Nordhagen, R., Flaathen, S. T. (1985): Chloroquine removal of HLA antigens from platelets for the platelet immunofluorescence test.
Vox Sang. 48, 156-159

Shulman, N. R., Marder, V. J., Hiller, M. C., Collier, E. M. (1964): Platelet and leukocyte isoantigens and their antibodies: serologic, physiologic and clinical studies.
Progress in Hematology 4, 222-304

Shulman, N. R., Marder, V. J., Weinrach, R. S. (1965): Similarities between known antiplatelet antibodies and the factor responsible for thrombocytopenia in idiopathic purpura. Physiologic, serologic and isotopic studies.
Ann. N. Y. Acad. Sci. 124, 499-542

Sugiyama, T., Okuma, M., Ushikubi, F., Sensaki, S., Kanaji, K., Uchino, H. (1987): A novel platelet aggregating factor found in a patient with defective collagen-induced platelet aggregation and autoimmune thrombocytopenia.
Blood 69, 1712-1720

Tomiyama, Y., Kurata, Y., Kanakura, Y., Mizutani, H., Tsubakio, T., Yonezawa, T., Tarui, S. (1987): Platelet glycoprotein IIb as a target antigen in two patients with chronic idiopathic thrombocytopenic purpura.
Brit. J. Haematol. 66, 535-538

Tomijama, Y., Take, H., Honda, S., Furubayaski, T., Mizutani, H., Tsubakio, T., Kurata, Y. (1990): Demonstration of platelet antigens that bind platelet-associated autoantibodies in chronic ITP by direct immunoprecipitation procedure.
Brit. J. Haematol. 75, 92-98

van Vliet, H. H. D. M., Kappers-Klunne, M. C., van der Hel, J. W. B., Abels, J. (1987): Antibodies against glycosphingolipids in sera of patients with idiopathic thrombocytopenic purpura.
Brit. J. Haematol. 67, 103-108

Vos, J. J. E., Huisman, J. G., van der Lelie, J., von dem Borne, A. E. G. Kr. (1987): Platelet-associated IgG in thrombocytopenia: a comparison of two techniques.
Vox Sang. 53, 162-168

Wautier, J. L., Boizard, B., Wautier, M. P., Kadeva, H., Caen, J. P. (1980): Platelet-associated IgG and circulating immune complexes in thrombocytopenic purpura.
Nouv. Rev. Fr. Hématol. 22, 29-36

Winiarski, J. (1985): Immunoglobulin binding to platelets. The effect of aggregated IgG.
Blut 51, 259-266

Woods, V. L., Oh, E. H., Mason, D., McMillan, R. (1984a): Autoantibodies against the platelet glycoprotein IIb/IIIa complex in patients with chronic ITP.
Blood 63, 368-375

Woods, V. L., Kurata, Y., Montgomery, R. R., Tani, P., Mason, D., Oh, E. H., McMillan, R. (1984b): Autoantibodies against platelet glycprotein Ib in patients with chronic immune thrombocytopenic purpura.
Blood 64, 156-160

Résumé

Les auto-anticorps anti-plaquettaires à l'origine du purpura thrombopénique autoimmum on été jusqu'à présent étudiés avec des techniques mettant en évidence la fixation des anticorps sur les plaquettes entières. Les résultats des tests indirects, employés pour mettre en évidence les anticorps libres circulants, peuvent être perturbés par l'existence d'alloanticorps. L'élévation du taux des anticorps fixés sur les plaquettes autologues est souvent rencontrée chez des patients avec une thrombopénie non immune. Les cibles antigéniques de ces anticorps ont été localisées sur les glycoprotéines plaquettaires (GPS). Les métodes permettant de préciser la spécificité glycoprotéique à la fois des anticorps libres et liés sont d'un grand intérêt diagnostic pour ces malades.

Autoimmune platelet destruction in pregnancy and its relationship to neonatal thrombocytopenia

D.S. Beardsley and B.Y. Thompson

Pediatric Hematology Division, Yale University School of Medicine, 333 Cedar Street, New Haven, Connecticut, USA

SUMMARY

Destruction of fetal platelets by maternal antiplatelet antibodies can cause severe thrombocytopenia during fetal and neonatal life. Although the platelet counts of affected newborns return to normal within the first few weeks of life, these infants are at risk for central nervous system hemorrhage leading to death or severe neurological sequelae. Current perinatal management when the mother has immune thrombocytopenic purpura (ITP) may include fetal scalp platelet counts during labor, elective Cesarean section, or percutaneous umbilical cord blood sampling. In many cases, these interventions may be overly invasive, but there is currently no way to predict which infants will be thrombocytopenic by simpler methods. We summarize here background material relevant to the clinical problem and discuss preliminary results of our ongoing study of the antibodies and antigens involved in platelet destruction in these newborn infants. We are comparing a number of parameters involved in immune platelet destruction in pregnancies resulting in affected versus unaffected infants. The overall hypothesis being tested in these studies is that biochemical characteristics of the target autoantigen and the antiplatelet antibody determine whether a particular autoantibody will lead to destruction of fetal platelets. Our goal is to determine factors important for the destruction of fetal platelets and thus to improve the perinatal management of these pregnancies.

CLINICAL BACKGROUND

In 1953, Harrington et al. recognized that maternal autoantibodies can cross the placenta and cause fetal thrombocytopenia; he also proposed that fetal platelet destruction might result from alloantibodies directed against fetal platelets. The clinical syndrome now known as neonatal alloimmune thrombocytopenic purpura ("NATP") was reported shortly thereafter (Moulinier, 1958; Shulman et al., 1962; Pearson et al., 1964). That condition, characterized by transient, severe thrombocytopenia and hemorrhage in an otherwise healthy infant, is associated with maternal antibodies against a fetal platelet antigen absent from the maternal platelets. Deaths or significant morbidity due to intracranial hemorrhage have occurred in 10-15% of the cases studied (Kunicki & Beardsley, 1988; Muller et al., 1985). Intracranial hemorrhage can occur in utero (reviewed by Herman et al. 1986), but the greatest risk is during delivery. Generally prenatal therapy (Kaplan et al., 1988; Bussel et al., 1988) or surgical delivery is recommended if a pregnancy is complicated by alloimmune thrombocytopenia, and the factors associated with a high risk for NATP have been reported (Reznikoff-Etievant et al. 1983).

Increased understanding of the basic immunology of NATP has allowed for improved perinatal diagnosis and management. There is less known about another cause of neonatal immune thrombocytopenia, mothers who have idiopathic (autoimmune) thrombocytopenia purpura (ITP). Maternal ITP can also cause fetal and neonatal thrombocytopenia, although the precise incidence is unclear. In this situation, maternal autoantibodies cross the placenta and destroy fetal platelets. Several authors have reported that about one third of pregnancies complicated by maternal ITP result in thrombocytopenic infants (Scott et al., 1983; Kelton et al., 1982). However, Scioscia et al.(1988) recently reported a prospective series of 19 pregnancies complicated by maternal ITP; only two infants had platelet counts <100,000/mm3· Unfortunately, neither maternal platelet count nor assays of antiplatelet antibody by standard methods can accurately predict which individual mothers with ITP will give birth to thrombocytopenic newborns and which will be unaffected.

Not all pregnant women who have platelet counts below the normal range have autoimmune thrombocytopenia. In 1986, Freedman and colleagues reported an entity termed "periparturient thrombocytopenia" which had a benign outcome for both mother and infant; the etiology and mechanism for the observed mild thrombocytopenia during pregnancy was unclear. Two other series have been reported (Hart et al., 1986; Burrows & Kelton, 1988). Burrows and Kelton (1988) followed 1357 pregnancies prospectively, and found no adverse outcomes in the 112 (8.3%) affected by mild thrombocytopenia (platelet counts of 97-150,000/mm3). Thus, when studying the effects of maternal ITP upon fetal or neonatal platelet counts, it is important to define the diagnosis precisely. For our study, we chose to include only those women in whom the diagnosis of chronic ITP of greater than six months' duration had been made prior to pregnancy. The differential diagnosis of thrombocytopenia during pregnancy is included in Table 1.

Table 1
Thrombocytopenia During Pregnancy
Differential Diagnosis

ITP
Toxemia
Sepsis
Splenomegaly
Disseminated intravascular coagulation
Periparturient thrombocytopenia
Systemic lupus erythematosus
Vasculitis
Thrombotic thrombocytopenic purpura
Drug-induced thrombocytopenia
Obstetric complications
Congenital thrombopathy
Type IIb von Willebrand's disease
Vascular anomalies
Bone marrow failure

Not all of the types of maternal thrombocytopenia can affect fetal platelets; in this discussion we will be limited to maternal ITP.

The thrombocytopenic infant is at risk for intracranial hemorrhage, although the frequency of this complication in maternal ITP is not clear. Reports vary from 0-25%, but intracranial bleeding is probably less common in this condition than in NATP. Routine Cesarean section is not appropriate for all cases of maternal ITP, particularly since these mothers are at risk for hemorrhage themselves. Fetal scalp platelet counts have been used to determine if operative delivery is indicated (Scott et al., 1980). However, the sample cannot be obtained until active labor has progressed, and it is possible that labor could initiate serious CNS bleeding. Scioscia et al. (1988) have used percutaneous umbilical blood sampling (PUBS) to determine the fetal platelet count. This has an advantage over scalp sampling in that can be done prior to the onset of labor, although this is a more invasive technique. There is an obvious need for simple, noninvasive methods to predict which pregnancies are at highest risk for neonatal thrombocytopenia so that perinatal management can be optimized.

Maternal platelet counts cannot be used to predict the fetal platelet count, since a mother may have a compensated thrombolytic state, while the infant may be severely thrombopenic. The best correlation with neonatal platelet counts reported has been that with levels of circulating plasma antiplatelet antibodies as determined by radiolabelled antiglobulin test (Cines et al. 1982). However, this assay can be confused by the presence of anti-HLA antibodies unless a panel of test platelets is examined, and the indirect correlation may not hold for other assays of circulating antiplatelet antibodies. Although these results suggest that free plasma antibody is a requirement for destruction of fetal platelets, we sought to identify antigen and antibody characteristics correlated with the greatest risk to the fetus.

PLATELET AUTOANTIGENS

Much has been learned about the antigenic targets of platelet autoantibodies in ITP (for a review, see Beardsley, 1989). Using an immunofluorescence test, van Leeuwen et al. (1982) concluded that some ITP antibodies are directed against GPIIb/IIIa since they reacted with platelets from 8 normal donors, but not with Glanzmann's thrombasthenic platelets which were totally deficient in GPIIb/IIIa. Woods and McMillan (1984, 1984a) isolated platelet glycoproteins with monoclonal antibodies and found autoantibodies against GPIIb/IIIa and GPIb in a radioimmunoassay. We have determined by immunoblotting that GPIIIa specifically contains the most frequent antigenic target for ITP antibodies (Beardsley et al., 1884). Since autologous platelets obtained during a period of remission also contain the specific antibody-binding protein, these antibodies are truly autoantibodies, rather than alloantibodies. When Pl^{A1} negative platelets have been used, the anti-GPIIIa antibodies reacted with the same intensity as with Pl^{A1} positive platelets; thus, the target epitope for these antibodies is not identical to Pl^{A1}. Toniyama et al. (1987) found that some other anti-GPIIb/IIIa autoantibodies are specifically directed against GPIIb. Using ITP patients' lymphocytes, Nugent and colleagues (1987,1988) have created human hybridomas which produce monoclonal antibodies directed against GPIb and a senescence antigen on GPIIIa (28). Our laboratory (Beardsley et al. 1985) and Stricker et al. (1986) have found antibodies against GPV in cases of acute ITP of childhood. The platelet autoantigens are considered to be "public" antigens, present on all normal platelets, however, there have been no reported studies of these antigens on fetal platelets.

Different proteins and even different epitopes on the GPIIIa molecule can be target antigens for ITP autoantibodies. In a study of 48 patients with ITP, we found that 36 of them had circulating antibodies against platelet proteins. However, there were a variety of bands by immunoblotting. The most frequently observed target protein was a 100 kD band, although bands at 85, 110, and 140kD were also observed (Beardsley et al. 1984a) as indicated in Table 2.

Table 2

Immunoblotting Results - 48 Cases of ITP:

Specific Antigenic Bands	Frequency
100kD only	12/48
100kD + 85, 110, or 140kD	21/48
85kD only	3/48
no specific band	12/48

The ITP autoantibodies which we have identified as directed against GPIIIa do not all react with the same antigenic epitope. In fact, two of these antibodies, isolated from patients with unusually severe bleeding symptoms in spite of only mild thrombocytopenia, interfered with ADP-stimulated fibrinogen binding to GPIIIa (Beardsley et al., 1984b).

Table 3 summarizes some of the platelet proteins which have been identified as targets of antiplatelet autoantibodies occurring in ITP.

Table 3
Platelet Proteins Containing Autoantigens

Antigenic Protein	Reference
GPIIb/IIIa	van Leeuwen et al. 1982 Woods et al. 1984
GPIIIa	Beardsley et al. 1984 Nugent et al. 1987
GPIIb	Tomiyama et al., 1987
GPIb	Woods et al., 1984a Nugent, 1987 Szatkowski et al., 1986
GPV	Beardsley et al., 1985 Stricker et al., 1986
25 kD	Stricker et al., 1985
66 & 108 kD	Kaplan et al., 1987

PERINATAL IMMUNE MEDIATED BLOOD CELL DESTRUCTION

Erythroblastosis fetalis, first recognized by Hippocrates, serves as a model cytopenia caused by transplacental antibodies. IgM antibodies no not cross the placental barrier, so they are not involved in destruction of fetal erythrocytes. This occurs via IgG binding and non-complement-dependent phagocytosis by macrophages of the reticuloendothelial system, primarily in the spleen. The same mechanism is involved in platelet destruction in ITP. Macrophage uptake depends upon specific Fc receptors for IgG subclasses 1 and 3. Subclasses 2 and 4 also interact with the Fc receptors, but their binding affinity is too low to be clinically significant (Hay et al., 1972). In general, increased antibody titer is associated with an increased risk of hemolysis due to Rh antibodies. However, for individual pregnancies, titer alone is not predictive of occurence or severity of hemolytic disease (Schneider et al., 1967). All subclasses of IgG can cross the placenta (Sidiropoulos et al., 1986). However, anti-Rh antibodies of the IgG_1 subclass, particularly those of the Glm(4) GM allotype are associated with the most severe fetal hemolysis (Taslimi et al., 1986; Parinaud et al., 1985). The antiplatelet autoantibodies implicated in ITP can be either IgG or IgM. All subclasses of IgG circulating antiplatelet antibodies have been detected, although the IgG_3 subclass predominates in the antibody bound to platelets. There have been no reported studies of which subclasses or GM allotypes of ITP antibodies can destroy fetal platelets.

THE CURRENT STUDY

Pregnant women who have been diagnosed as having immune thrombocytopenic purpura (ITP) by platelet counts and bone marrow examination prior to pregnancy and their infants are the subjects of this study. The Yale High Risk Obstetrics Service is a major referral center, seeing approximately 25 pregnant women with ITP each year. We characterize the antibodies and antigens of mothers whose infants are thrombocytopenic and contrast them with those of mothers whose infants are unaffected.

A monoclonal antibody inhibition of platelet antigen ("MAIPA") technique has been developed by Keiffel et al. (1987) for the identification of platelet alloantibodies. The technique involves simultaneous incubation of intact platelets with a monoclonal antibody against one of the platelet glycoproteins (e.g. GPIIb/IIIa, GPIIIa, GPIb) and the patient plasma, followed by solubilization in nonionic detergent. Anti-mouse IgG coating microtiter wells is then used to isolate the glycoprotein of interest. Human antibodies attached to the same protein that the monoclonal antibody immobilizes are detected with an enzyme linked antiglobulin (anti-IgG or IgM). If the human antibody is directed against the same epitope as the mouse monoclonal, there can be competition for antibody binding. We therefore use two murine monoclonal antibodies (directed against different target epitopes) to screen patient samples.

HYPOTHESIS I: That there are biochemical differences in the target antigens of maternal platelet autoantibodies which cross the placenta and destroy fetal platelets and those antibodies that do not affect fetal platelets. Characteristics of the antigens involved include 1) which platelet glycoprotein contains the target antigen, 2) are these antigens present on fetal as well as maternal platelets, and 3) for the antigens on GPIIb/IIIa, which epitopes of the protein complex are involved? The antigenic target protein of the maternal antiplatelet antibodies are being assessed by the monoclonal antibody immobilization of platelet antigens (MAIPA) assay. Both IgG and IgM antibodies are identified using the MAIPA assay.

HYPOTHESIS II: That antibody titer as well as Ig class and IgG subclass and/or GM allotype are determinants of whether a maternal anti-platelet autoantibody will destroy fetal platelets. Although IgG antibodies can cross the placenta, IgM cannot. Maternal plasma samples are characterized as to class of antiplatelet antibody. It is hypothesized that those women with only IgM antiplatelet antibodies will have infants with normal platelet counts. However, among adults with ITP, IgG antibodies are more common than IgM. The simple presence of IgG antibodies may not correlate with whether or not an infant will be thrombocytopenic. Therefore, we also assay IgG subclass and GM allotype by the same techniques by using subclass specific reagents.

To date, we have performed MAIPA assays for anti-GPIIb/IIIa antibodies of both the IgG and IgM classes on serum from 30 mothers with documented ITP. Since all of these patients had a diagnosis of chronic ITP, it was not surprising to find that IgM antibodies were uncommon. In the two rare cases in which IgM could be identified, the infants were unaffected. These results support hypothesis II, but more cases will meed to be studied for confirmation. Further work is in progress to assess subclass specificity of the anti-GPIIb/IIIa antibodies identified and to identify the percise antigenic targets of these autoantibodies.

The biochemical characterization of autoimmune platelet destruction and further definition of the usual clinical course of pregnancies affected by maternal ITP as well as incidental thrombocytopenia should lead to more appropriate management of all these pregnancies and a better outcome for both infant and mother.

REFERENCES:

Beardsley, D.J.S, Spiegel, J.E., Jacobs, M.M., Handin, R.I. & Lux, S.E. (1984): Platelet membrane glycoprotein IIIa contains target antigens that bind anti-platelet antibodies in immune thrombocytopenias. J Clin Invest, 74, 1701-1707.

Beardsley, D.J.S., Taatjes, H. & Lux, S.E (1984a): Target antigens in immune thrombocytopenic purpura. Clin Res, 32: 494a.

Beardsley, D.J.S., Timmons, S., Bobeck, H. & Hawiger J (1984b): Human antiplatelet antibodies which interfere with fibrinogen binding. Blood, 64: 845a.

Beardsley, D.S., Ho, J. & Beyer, E.C. (1985): Varicella associated thrombocytopenia: Antibodies aganist an 85kD thrombin sensitive protein (GPV). Blood, 66: 1030a.

Beardsley, D.J.S. (1989): "Platelet autoantigens" in Platelet Immunobiology. T.J. Kunicki and J. George eds. J.B. Lippincott Company, Philadelphia, 121-131.

Burrows, R.F. & Kelton, J.G. (1988): Incidentally detected thrombocytopenia in healthy mothers and their infants. N. Engl. J. Med. 319: 142-145.

Bussel, J., Berkowitz, R., McFarland, J., Lynch, L., & Chitkara, U. (1988): Antenatal treatment of neonatal alloimmune thrombocytopenia. N. Engl. J. Med., 319: 1374-1378.

Cines, D.B., Dusak, B., Tomaski, A., Mennuti, M. & Schreiber, A.D (1982): Immune thrombocytopenic purpura and pregnancy. N Engl J Med, 306: 826-830.

Freedman, J., Musclow, E., Garvey, B. & Abbott, D. (1986): Unexplained periparturient thrombocytopenia. Am J Hematol. 21: 398-407.

Harrington, W.J., Sprague, C.C., Minnich. V., et al. (1953): Immunologic mechanisms in neonatal and thrombocytopenic purpura. Ann Intern Med, 38, 433-469.

Hart, D., Dunetz, C., Nardi, M., Porges, R.F., Weiss, A. & Karpatkin, M. (1986): An epidemic of maternal thrombocytopenia associated with elevated antiplatelet antibody. Am J Obstet Gynecol. 154: 879-883.

Hay, F.C., Torrigiani, G. & Roitt, J.M. (1972): The binding of human IgG subclass to human monocytes. Eur J Immunol, 2: 257-62. Herman JH, Humbelic MI, Ancona RJ, & Kickler TS, In utero cerebral hemorrhage in alloimmune thrombocytopenia. Am J Pediatr Hematol Oncol, 1986, 8, 312-317.

Kaplan, C., Champeix, Blanchard. D., Muller, J.Y. & Cartron, J.P. (1987): Platelet antibodies in systemic lupus erythematosis Br. J. Haematol. 67: 89-93.

Kaplan, C., Daffos, F., Forestier, et al. (1988): Management of alloimmune thrombocytopenia: antenatal diagnosis and in utero transfusion of maternal platelets. Blood, 70; 340-343.

Kiefel, V., Santoso, S., Weisheit, M. & Meuller Eckhardt, C. (1987): Monoclonal antibody-specific immobilization of platelet antigens (MAIPA): A new tool for the identification of platelet-reactive antibodies. Blood, 70: 1722-1726.

Kelton, J.G., Inwood, M.J., Barr, R.M., Effer, S.B., Hunter, D., Wilson, W.E., Ginsberg, D.A. & Power, P. (1982): The prenatal prediction of thrombocytopenia in infants of mothers with clinically diagnosed immune thrombocytopenia. Am J Obstet Gynecol, 144: 449-454.

Kunicki, T.J. & Beardsley, D.S. (1989): The alloimmune thrombocytopenias: Neonatal alloimmune thrombocytopenia and post-transfusion purpura. Prog. Hemost. Thromb., 9: 203-232.

Moulinier, P.J. (1958): Iso-immunization maternelle antiplaquettaire et purpura neonatal. Proceedings of the Sixth Congress of the European Society of Hematology. S Karger, New York, 817.

Muller, J.Y., Patereau, C., Reznikoff-Etievant, M.F., Kaplan, C. & Simonney, N. (1985a): Neonatal alloimmune thrombopenia. Rev Fr Transfus Immunohematol, 28, 625-641.

Nugent, D.J. (1987): Identification of antiplatelet antibody idiotypes associated with glycoprotein Ib specificity, present in ITP plasma and produced by human hybridomas from ITP spleen cell fusions. Thromb Haemost, 58a: 531.

Nugent, D.J., Kunicki, T.J., Berglund, C. & Bernstein, I.D. (1987): A human monoclonal antibody recognizes a neoantigen on glycoprotein IIIa expressed on stored and activated platelets.

Parinaud, J., Blanc, M., Grandjean, H., Fournie, A., Bierme, S. & Pontonnier, G. (1985): IgG subclasses and Gm allotypes of anti-D antibodies during pregnancies: Correlation with the gravity of the fetal disease. Am J Obstet Gynecol, 154: 1111-1115.

Pearson, H.A., Shulman, N.R., Marder, V.J. & Cone, T.E. (1964): Isoimmune neonatal thrombocytopenic purpura: Clinical and therapeutic considerations. Blood, 23, 154-177.

Reznikoff-Etievant, M.F., Muller, J.Y., Julien, F. & Patereau, C. (1983): An immune response gene linked to MHC in man. Tissue Antigens, 22, 312-314.

Schneider, M.J., Profsky, B., Hoskin, B.Y., et al. (1967): Prediction of intrauterine fetal involvement in erythroblastosis fetalis. Obstet Gynecol, 30: 432-437.

Scioscia, A.L., Grannum, P., Copel, J.A. & Hobbins, J.C. (1988): The use of percutaneous umbilical blood sampling in immune thrombocytopenia purpura. Am J Obstet Gynecol, 59: 1066-1068.

Scott, J.R., Rote, N.S. & Cruishank, D.P. (1983): Antiplatelet antibodies and platelet counts in pregnancies complicated by autoimmune thrombocytopenic purpura. Am J Obstet Gynecol, 145: 932-939.

Scott, J.R., Cruikshank, D.P., Kochenour, N.K., Pitkin, R.M. & Warenski, J.C. (1980): Fetal platelet counts in the obstetric management of immunologic thrombocytopenic purpura. Am J Obstet Gynecol, 136: 495-499.

Shulman, N.R., Aster, R.H., Pearson, H.A., & Hiller, M.C. (1962): Immunoreactions involving platelets. VI. Reactions of maternal isoantibodies responsible for neonatal purpura. Differentiation of a second platelet antigen system. J Clin Invest, 41, 1059-69.

Sidiropoulos, D., Herrmann, U., Morell, A., von Muralt, G. & Barandun, S. (1986): Transplacental passage of intravenous immunoglobulin in the last trimester of pregnancy. J Pediatr, 109: 505-508.

Stricker, R.B., Koerper, M.A., Bussel, J. & Shuman, M.A. (1986): Target platelet antigens childhood immune thrombocytopenic purpura. Blood 68: 118a.

Stricker, R.B., Abrams, D.I., Corash, L. & Shuman, M.A. (1985): Target antigens in homosexual men with immune thrombocytopenia. N. Engl. J. Med. 313: 1375-1378.

Szatkowski, N.S. & Aster (1986): Identification of glycoprotein Ib as a target for autoantibody in idiopathic (autoimmune) thrombocytopenic purpura. Blood 67: 310-315.

Taslimi, M.M., Sibail, B.M., Mason, J.M. & Dacus, J.V. (1986): Immunoglobulin G subclasses and isoimmunized pregnancy outcome. Am J Obstet Gynecol, 154: 1327-1330.

Tomiyama, Y., Kurata, Y., Mizutani, H., et al. (1987): Platelet glycoprotein IIb as a target antigen in two patients with chronic idiopathic thrombocytopenic purpura. Br J Haematol, 66: 535-540.

vanLeeuwen, E.F., vanderVen, J.Th.M., Engelfriet, C.P. & vondemBorne, A.E.G.Kr (1982): Specificity of autoantibodies in autoimmune thrombocytopenia. Blood, 59: 23-27.

Woods, V.L.Jr., Oh, E.H., Mason, D., et al. (1984): Autoantibodies against the platelet glycoprotein IIb/IIIa complex in patients with chrinic idiopathic thrombocytopenic purpura. Blood, 63: 368-71.

Woods, V.L., Kurata, Y., Montgomery, R.R., Tani, P., Mason, D., Oh, E.H. & McMillan, R. (1984a): Autoantibodies against platelet glycoprotein Ib in patients with chronic immune thrombocytopenia purpura. Blood, 64: 156-61.

Résumé

La destruction des plaquettes foetales par des anticorps maternels peut être à l'origine d'une thrombopénie sévère pendant la vie foetale et la période néonatale. Bien que la normalisation de la numération plaquettaire de ces enfants se situe dans les premières semaines de vie, ces enfants sont à risques hémorragiques notamment dans le système nerveux central conduisant à des décès ou à des des séquelles neurologiques graves. La surveillance des foetus des femmes atteintes de purpura autoimmun peut s'effectuer dans la période périnatale par numération au scalp en début de travail ou par ponction de sang foetal au cordon ombilical sous contrôle échographique. Des naissances par césarienne peuvent être proposées. Dans la plupart des cas ces examens peuvent être trop invasifs mais il n'existe pas actuellement de méthodes simples permettant la prédiction de la thrombopénie foetale. Nous faisons le point ici des données cliniques et discutons nos résultats préliminaires concernant l'étude des anticorps et des antigènes impliqués dans la destruction plaquettaire de ces nouveaux-nés. Nous comparons les différents paramètres en fonction de l'atteinte ou non de l'enfant.L'hypothèse testée dans ces études est que la caractérisation biochimique de l'autoantigène cible et de l'anticorps antiplaquettaire permettront de prédire qu'un auto-anticorps particulier peut entrainer la destruction des plaquettes foetales. Notre but est de déterminer les facteurs jouant un rôle important dans cette destruction plaquettaire foetale permettant ainsi d'améliorer la pris en charge de ces grossesses.

Autoimmune thrombocytopenic purpura and pregnancy : from threat to routine, a new danger ?

G. Tchernia*, C. Kaplan**, F. Daffos***, G. Tertian*, F. Forestier***, M. Dreyfus* and N. Catherine***

*Laboratoire d'Hématologie, Hôpital Antoine Béclère, 157, rue de la Porte-de-Trivaux, 92140 Clamart, France
**INTS, 6, rue Alexandre Cabanel, 75015 Paris, France
***Institut de Puériculture, 26, bd Brune, 75014 Paris, France

Auto immune thrombocytopenic purpura is frequent in women and thus often associated with pregnancy. Most of the maternal problems have been solved and concern is now focused on the small percentage of fetuses who, being severely thrombocytopenic at birth, are at risk for intra cerebral bleeding.
The antenatal prediction of fetal thrombocytopenia based on maternal biological or clinical criteria has been a complete failure. The risk of birth injury when delivery is vaginal has favoured attempts to recognize severe fetal thrombocytopenia in order to decide cesarean section when present. Fetal scalp sampling has been shown to be unreliable. The risk of percutaneous umbilical sampling must be weighed according to the risk of the disease itself. Antenatal treatments have not yet been shown to be effective. The borderlines between auto immune thrombocytopenic purpura and asymptomatic maternal thrombocytopenia are often ill defined and need a better definition.

Auto immune thrombocytopenic purpura (AITP) is related to an inappropriate synthesis of antibodies directed against platelet antigens. Antibodies coated platelets are destroyed by phagocytosing macrophages, mostly in the spleen (Mc Millan, 1981). AITP is frequent in women and thus often associated with pregnancy ; Platelet antibodies being usually of the IgG class can cross the placenta, recognize fetal platelets as targets and induce thrombocytopenia which can be responsible for bleeding. During the last 3 decades, the association of AITP and pregnancy has led to many controversial discussions, most of them being still unsettled.

1°) THE FIRST MAJOR CONCERN HAS BEEN WITH THE THROMBOCYTOPENIC MOTHERS. In the fifties their mortality rate was high and the questions were whether these patients should be advised to conceive and whether abortion or splenectomy should be discussed during pregnancy (Tancer, 1960). However, owing to the improvement of obstetrical and medical management and to the successive avaibilities of steroid therapy (O'Reilly and Taber, 1978) and of high dose IV immunoglobulin therapy (IV IgG) (Tchernia et al, 1984 ; Lavery, 1985), most of the maternal problems have been solved and no maternal death related to thrombocytopenia has been reported after 1960. Provided that the follow-up of such pregnancies can be achieved by obstetricians who are aware of the management of bleeding disorders, and that causes of chronic thrombocytopenia such as SLE or HIV infection have been ruled out it is of general agreement that pregnancy should not be discouraged in such patients. If maternal thrombocytopenia is severe before delivery or if bleeding occurs during pregnancy, steroid therapy or IV IgG or the association of both can be prescribed.

It must be stressed that fetal thrombocytopenia can be observed whatever is the maternal status : A woman who has AITP can be in a state of compensated thrombocytolysis (Karpatkin et a!., 1971) where the association of an increased medullary megakaryocytopoiesis with an ongoing synthesis antibodies can lead to a normal platelet count in spite pf a decreased life span. For that reason past history of platelet disorders or bleeding episodes should be sought for by all obstetricians, eventhough the routine biological status appears to be normal. Girls and women who have experienced AITP should be advised that subsequent pregnancies even after years of normalisation of platelet count, will require an adapted follow-up.

2°) DURING THE SIXTIES, MAJOR CONCERN WAS FOCUSED ON THE HIGH MORTALITY RATE AMONG THE INFANTS born of mothers with AITP which was estimated to range between 10 and 20% (O'Reilly and Taber, 1978 ; Murray and Harris, 1976). Morbidity was also important. Both deaths and neurologic sequelae were or to intracerebral bleeding initiated during delivery by the traumatism of labor.

In contrast, antenatal bleeding is seldom reported and although stillbirth is not uncommon in the previous obstetrical history of women with AITP (Daffos, 1990), the antenatal risk for fetuses appears to be far less important than it is in neonatal allo immune thrombocytopenia and the management of the two diseases must be appreciated in a totally different way.

Thrombocytopenia is often moderate at birth and worsens during the first week of life with a nadir on day 4-6 preceeding a spontaneous resolution which will occur within 10-60 days. This postnatal accentuation of thrombocytopenia could be related to a transient fetal hyposplenism illustrated by the presence of pocked erythrocytes and Howell-Jolly bodies or to a functional immaturity of the macrophages (Speer et al, 1986). However, unless initiated during delivery, postnatal bleeding is absent or moderate and most of the time easy to manage. Therefore the infants at risk for severe bleeding and especially intracranial hemorrhage are only those who exhibit an antenatal severe thrombocytopenia ($<50 \times 10^9$ platelets/l).

The vast majority of infants born of mothers with AITP will not exhibit severe thrombocytopenia at birth and will not need any other help than regular platelet counts until normalisation and possibly low dose steroid therapy or IV IgG if requested by any clinical event or by a surgical procedure (Chirico et al, 1983). Parents must be aware of the necessity of an adapted follow-up for the next pregnancy. It must be stressed that many studies report an overall percentage of severely thrombocytopenic infants, regardless of the age of onset of severe thrombocytopenia, which leads to an overestimation of the risk. In our experience the percentage of severe thrombocytopenia at birth averages 10-15% and we did not find any variation with years (Table 1). However the ratio of thrombocytopenic neonates, when compared to the first studies in this field appears to have markedly decreased in recent reports. This is probably due to the fact that mothers with low platelet counts deliver thrombocytopenic infants more often than mother with stabilized AITP and that only the former appeared in the first publications. Ultimately, concern must be focused on the *severely thrombocytopenic fetuses, at risk for intracerebral bleeding* related to *a passive and transient disease* in an otherwise normal infant.

Table I : Incidence of thrombocytopenia at birth

Platelet counts		$<50 \times 10^9$/l	50-150
1973-1986	(29)	5 (17%)	7 (24%)
1987-1990	(27)	4 (11%)	4 (11%)
Total	(56)	9 (16%)	11 (19%)

3°) FOR MANY YEARS, ALL THE GROUPS INVOLVED IN THE FIELD HAVE BEEN DESPERATLY SEARCHING FOR A CLINICAL OR A BIOLOGICAL MATERNAL PARAMETER PREDICTIVE OF THE OCCURRENCE OR OF THE ABSENCE OF FETAL THROMBOCYTOPENIA (FT). However all the clinical or biological indicators which have been claimed as possibly reliable have been subsequently proved to be irrelevant. Women with or without previous splenectomy have an equivalent risk of delivering thrombocytopenic offsprings (Scott et al, 1983). Thrombocytopenic women have a slightly higher risk of having affected infants but the overlap between the groups (Kelton, 1983) is more important than previously assumed (Territo, 1973). Maternal platelet-associated antibody levels and or antiplatelet antibody titers in maternal serum transiently considered as predictible in some studies, (Kelton et al, 1982, Logaridis et al, 1982, Cines et al, 1982 ; Kelton, 1983) have been shown to be disappointing when used on a larger scale (Scott et al, 1982 ; Laurian et al, 1987).

4°) WHEN IT BECAME OBVIOUS THAT FT COULD NOT BE PREDICTED, THE NEXT LOGICAL STEP WAS TO TRY TO PROTECT THE INFANTS FROM BIRTH INJURY. At that time <u>systematic cesarean section</u> (CS) in any parturient who had experienced ITP was advocated (Murray and Harris, 1976). However this attitude led to many useless cesarean sections for infants with cord blood samples exhibiting normal or moderately decreased platelet counts (Laros and Kagan, 1984). Recognition of fetal severe thrombocytopenia at the onset of labor has then been considered : *Fetal scalp sampling* proned in 1978 (Ayromlooi, 1978) and widely used during the following years provides platelet count by direct sampling performed at the initiation of labor and gives the opportunity to decide CS if thrombocytopenia is severe (Scott et al, 1980).
However scalp blood samples are often contaminated by amniotic fluid which leads to micro coagulation in vitro and to spurious low platelet counts (Tchernia, 1988). In all groups, including ours, once this practice had evolved from a clinical investigation to a routine procedure, the incidence of such artifactual thrombocytopenias increased and led to CS for normal infants : There is an agreement through most of the recent evaluations to reject the procedure (Christiaens and Helmerhorst, 1987).
Finally *percutaneous umbilical blood sampling* (PUBS) showed up (Daffos et al, 1983 ; Hobbins et al, 1985) in the years 1983-89 to work out the problem. It is a reliable procedure which, if performed during the last week of gestation, provides a good correlation between antenatal and cord blood or postnatal counts (Daffos et al, 1988 ; Moïse et al, 1988 ; Scioscia, 1988). But it is an invasive procedure with risks depending on the dexterity of the obstetricians. It should only be performed in referral centers in which the overall estimated lethal risks of PUBS varies from 0 to 0.2% according to the groups (Daffos et al, 1988 ; Pielet et al, 1988). Nevertheless, the low incidence of severe fetal thrombocytopenia (10-15%) and the fact that not all severely affected infants will develop an intracerebral bleeding must be taken into account. For these reasons recent warnings favour a disengagement from any active procedure (Sacks, 1986 ; Burrows and Kelton, 1989).

5°) ANTENATAL TREATMENTS, IF SHOWN TO BE EFFECTIVE IN ALL CASES AND WITH NO SECONDARY ADVERSE EFFECTS FOR MOTHERS AND FETUSES WOULD BE A LOGICAL ANSWER TO THE DIFFERENT DILEMMAS.
Low dose steroid therapy prescribed to the mother has been first considered as ineffective (Heys, 1966) and then claimed as effective in a small group of patients (Karpatkin et al, 1981). Subsequently all groups experienced negative results with this treatment (Yin et Scott, 1985) ; moreover it has been shown that if such treatment could decrease the amount of IgG bound to maternal platelets, and raise their platelet count, it increased consequently the free serum antibodies, making them available for a transplacental passage (Cines et al, 1982). High dose IV IgG have been prescribed to some thrombocytopenic mothers in order to raise their platelet count before delivery (Tchernia et al, 1984). These mothers gave birth to normal as well as to thrombocytopenic infants (Lavery et al, 1985). However it was suggested that such

passage of IgG is slow and IV IgG had been administered shortly before delivery. (Mc Nabb et al, 1976 ; Pitcher-Wilmott et al, 1980, Smith and Hammarstrom, 1985)

Actually the low incidence of severe thrombocytopenia at birth impedes any definitive appreciation of such antenatal treatments, unless early fetal samples obtained before the initiation of therapy can be compared to post treatment platelet counts after late or cord blood sampling.

We have performed such controls in some patients and failed to illustrate any effect either of low-dose steroid therapy or of IV IgG (Table 2). However this group of patients was small and treatments, some of them having been prescribed for maternal indications, were heterogeneous. We think that therapeutic trials should be conducted in some patients in referral centers, after informed consent. Should they confirm the failure of antenatal treatments, there would be no further justification for early PUBS in AITP.

Table 2 : Fetal and neonatal platelet counts after maternal treatments
(Numbers indicate fetal and neonatal platelet counts x 10⁹/l)

Patient N°	A	B	C	Treatment	
1	180	11	12	A-C	st 1mg/kg/day
2	166	32	40	A-B	st 1mg/kg/day
				B-C	st 1mg/kg/day + γ 0,4g/kg/day x 5
3	ND	8	5	B-C	γ 1g/kg/week x 2 weeks
4	60	11	28	A-C	st : 15 mg/day

A : first PUBS (21-24 weeks) - B : second PUBS (34-38 weeks) - C : Cord blood or post natal sampling - ST : Steroid therapy - γ : IV IgG treatment

6°) THE LAST CONTROVERSIAL ISSUE CAME WITH ASYMPTOMATIC MATERNAL THROMBOCYTOPENIA. It has been shown that some pregnant women, especially during the last trimester of gestation could exhibit moderate thrombocytopenia which resolved after delivery (Burrows and Kelton, 1988). The precise mechanisms and the fetal risk of AST are yet poorly known. Moreover some chronic ITP can be first discovered during pregnancy and considered as AST (Burns, 1988 ; Copplestone, 1988). In most of the recent studies the two entities are analyzed together which probably leads to an underevaluation of the fetal risk in ITP and can be responsible for the present tendency to avoid invasive procedures and admit vaignal delivery (VD) despite the risk of severe thrombocytopenia. AST is probably an heterogeneous disorder which can reflect the extreme variation of a physiological process (Fay et al, 1983), a pathologic event (Giles and Inglis, 1981), or the combination of the two, disrupting a long lasting equilibrium such as compensated thrombocytolysis. Its incidence could average 6% (Rasmus et al, 1989). The low incidence of obstetrical or fetal morbidity leads to erroneously consider AST as a trite event and to leave women without post partum assessment. We believe that such patients should be further explored, especially if another pregnancy is planned or if thrombocytopenia, even moderate, does not resolve, and be proposed for a platelet life span study(Yvart et al, 1988).

CONCLUSION
During the last 3 decades the association of thrombocytopenia and pregnancy has evolved from fear to routine. The attempt to further explore the natural history and the therapeutic approaches of fetal thrombocytopenia which has been made possible by PUBS, is fairly impeded by ethical questions concerning the relative risks of the disease and of the procedure. It is probably time to recall that some thrombocytopenic infants may die or have severe neurological impairment due to

thrombocytopenic infants may die or have severe neurological impairment due to intracranial hemorrhage and that on the other hand a procedure such as PUBS should be conducted only by those who are referee in the field. This attitude is probably the only way to increase our knowledge on in utero thrombocytopenia and to improve our management.

We consider that when a diagnosis of AITP has been previously established, on classical criteria in a pregnant woman, antenatal PUBS is still mandatory and can avoid neonatal intra cerebral hemorrhage during labor. Even if this event has a low incidence, all the groups who have experienced it do not wish such a preventable accident to occur again.

In contrast, moderate thrombocytopenia of unknown origin, when occurring during the last trimester of pregnancy, should probably not require a special management. However this entity is ill defined and claims for a better definition.

Figure 3 :

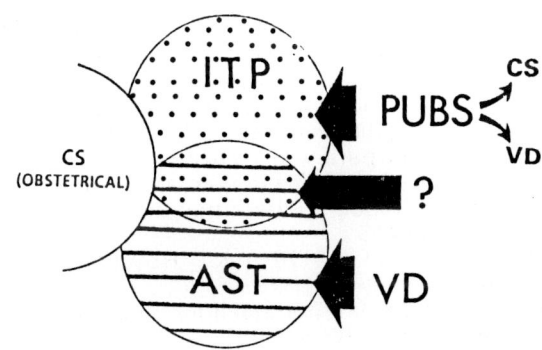

No clear cut attitude can be given for the borderline cases such as moderate thrombocytopenia early in pregnancy and individual decisions have to be achieved according to biological and obstetrical criteria and the availability of PUBS in experienced hands.

The decade will hopefully provide a better knowledge of the assessment of the fetal risk and thus a more adapted management.

REFERENCES

Ayromlooi J. (1978) : A new approach to management of immunologic thrombocytopenic purpura in pregnancy. *Am. J. Obstet. Gynecol.* 130, 235-236.

Burrows R.F., Kelton J.G. (1988) : Incidentally detected thrombocytopenia in healthy mothers and their infants. *N. Engl. J. Med.* 319, 142-145.

Burrows R.F., Kelton J.G. (1989) : Idiopathic thrombocytopenia purpura during pregnancy : Intervention for the fetus is not required. *Blood* 74, 187a.

Burns E.R. (1988) : Thrombocytopenia during pregnancy. *N. Engl. J. Med.*, 319, 1482.

Chirico G., Duse M., Ugazio A., Rondini G. (1983) : High dose intravenous gammaglobulin therapy for passive immune thrombocytopenia in the neonate. *J. Pediatr.* 103, 654-656

Christiaens G.C.M.L., Helmerhorst F.M. (1987) : Validity of intrapartum diagnosis of fetal thrombocytopenia. *Am. J. Obstet. Gynecol.* 157, 864-865

Cines D.B., Dusak B., Tomaski A., Mennuti M., Schreiber A.D. (1982): Immune thrombocytopenic purpura and pregnancy. *N. Engl. J. Med.* 306, 826-831

Copplestone J.A. (1988) : Thrombocytopenia during pregnancy. *N. Engl. J. Med.* 319, 1482

Daffos F., Capella-Pavlosky M., Forestier F. (1983) : A new procedure for fetal blood sampling in utero : preliminary results. *Am. J. Obstet. Gynecol.* 146, 985

Daffos F., Forestier F., Kaplan C., Cox W. (1988) : Prenatal diagnosis and management of bleeding disorders with fetal blood sampling. *Am. J. Obstet. Gynecol.* 158 : 939-946

Daffos F. (1990) : In the present book

Fay R.A., Hughes A.O., Farron N.T. (1983) : Platelets in pregnancy : hyperdestruction in pregnancy. *Obstet. Gynecol.* 61, 238-240

Giles C., Inglis T.C.M. (1981) : Thrombocytopenia and macrothrombocytosis in gestational hypertension. *Br. J. Obstet. Gynaecol.* 88, 1115-1119

Heys R.F. (1966) : Steroid therapy for idiopathic thrombocytopenic purpura during pregnancy. *Obstet. Gynecol. 28, 532-542*

Hobbins J.C., Grannum P.A., Romero R., Reece E.A., Mahoney M.J. (1985) : Percutaneous umbilical blood sampling. *Am. J. Obstet. Gynecol.* 152, 1-6

Karpatkin M., Porges R.F., Karpatkin S. (1981) : Platelet counts in infants of women with autoimmune thrombocytopenia : effect of steroid administration to the mother. *N. Engl. J. Med.* 305, 936-939

Kelton J.G., Inwood M.J. Barr R.M. et al (1982) : The prenatal prediction of thrombocytopenia in infants of mothers with clinically diagnosed immune thrombocytopenia . *Am. J. Obstet. Gynecol.* 144, 449-454

Kelton J.G. (1983) : Management of the pregnant patient with idiopathic thrombocytopenic purpura. *Ann. Intern. Med.* 99, 796-800

Laros Jr. R.K., Kagan R. (1984) : Route of delivery for patients with immune thrombocytopenic purpura. *Am. J. Obstet. Gynecol.* 148, 901-908

Laurian Y., Dreyfus M., Fernandez H., Kaplan C., Papiernik E., Tchernia G. (1987) : Purpura thrombopénique idiopathique auto-immun et grossesse. *Nouv. Rev. Fr. Hematol.* 29, 401-405

Lavery J.P., Koontz W.L., Liu Y.K., Howell R. (1985) : Immunologic thrombocytope-

nia in pregnancy ; use of antenatal immunoglobulin therapy : case report and review. *Obstet. Gynecol.* 66, 41S-43S

Logaridis T.E., Doran T.A., Scott J.G., Gare D.G., Comtesse C. (1983) : The effect of maternal steroid administration of fetal platelet count in immunologic thrombocytopenic purpura. *Am. J. Obstet. Gynecol.* 145, 147-151.

Mc Millan R. (1981) : Chronic idiopathic thrombocytopenic purpura. *N. Engl. J. Med.* 304, 1135-1147

Mc Nabb T., Koh T.Y., Dorrington K.J., Painter R.H. (1976) : Structure and function of immunoglobulin domains. V. Binding of immunoglobulin G and fragments to placental membrane preparations. *J. Immunol.* 117, 882-888.

Moise Jr KJ.., Carpenter Jr R.J., Cotton D.B., Wasserstrum N., Kirshon B., Cano L. (1988) : Percutaneous umbilical cord blood sampling in the evaluation of fetal platelet counts in pregnant patients with autoimmune thrombocytopenia purpura. *Obstet. Gynecol.* 72, 346-350

Murray J.M., Harris R.E. (1976) : The management of the pregnant patient with idiopathic thrombocytopenic purpura. *Am. J. Obstet. Gynecol.* 126, 449-451

O'Reilly R.A., Taber B.Z. (1978) : Immunologic thrombocytopenic purpura and pregnancy. Six new cases. *Obstet. Gynecol.* 51, 590-597

Pielet B.W., Socol M.L., Mc Gregor S.N., Ney J.A., Dooley S.L. (1988) : Cordocentesis : An appraisal of risks. *Am. J. Obstet. Gynecol.* 159, 1497-1500

Pitcher-Wilmott R.W., Hindocha P., Wood C.B.S. (1980) : The placental transfer of IgG subclasses in human pregnancy. *Clin. Exp. Immunol.* 41, 303-308

Rasmus K.T., Rottman R.L., Kotelko D.M., Wright W.C., Stone J.J., Rosenblatt R.M. (1989) : Unrecognized thrombocytopenia and regional anesthesia in parturients : a retrospective review. *Obstet. Gynecol.* 73, 943-946

Sacks D.A. (1986) : Percutaneous umbilical sampling in immune thrombocytopenic purpura. *Am. J. Obstet. Gynecol.* 154, 24-215

Scioscia A.L., Grannum P.A., Copel J.A., Hobbins J.C. (1988) : The use of percutaneous umbilical blood sampling in immune thrombocytopenic purpura. *Am. J. Obstet. Gynecol.* 159, 1066-1068

Scott J.R., Cruikshank D.P., Kochenour N.K., Pitkin R.M., Warenski J.C. (1980) : Fetal platelet counts in the obstetric management of immunologic thrombocytopenic purpura. *Am. J. Obstet. Gynecol.* 136, 495-499

Scott J.R., Rote N.S., Cruikshank D.P. (1983) : Antiplatelet antibodies and platelet counts in pregnancies complicated by autoimmune thrombocytopenic purpura. *Am. J. Obstet. Gynecol.* 145, 932-939

Smith C.I.E., Hammarstrom L. (1985) : Intravenous immunoglobulin in pregnancy. *Obstet. Gynecol.* 66, 395-405

Speer C.P., Wieland M., Ulbrich R., Gahr M. (1986) : Phagocytic activities in neonatal. monocytes. *Eur. J. Pediatr.* 145, 418-421

Tancer M.L. (1960) : Idiopathic thrombocytopenic purpura and pregnancy. *Am. J. Obstet. Gynecol.* 79, 148-153

Tchernia G., Dreyfus M., Laurian Y., Derycke M., Mirica C., Kerbrat G. (1984) : Management of immune thrombocytopenia in pregnancy. Response to infusions of immunglobulines. *Am. J. Obstet. Gynecol.* 148, 225-226

Tchernia G. (1988) : Immune thrombocytopenic purpura and pregnancy. *Curr Stud Hematol Blood Transf.* 55, 81-89

Territo M., Finklestein J., Oh W., Hobel C., Kattlove H. (1973) : Management of autoimmune thrombocytopenia in pregnancy and in the neonate. *Obstet. Gynecol.* 41, 579-584

Yin C.S., Scott J.R. (1985) : Unsuccessful treatment of fetal immunologic thrombocytopenia with dexamethasone. *Am. J. Obstet. Gynecol.* 152, 316-317

Yvart J., Archambeaud F., Laurian Y., Tchernia G. (1988) : Thrombopénie auto-immune et grossesse. Intérêt des études isotopiques. In : *Hémorragies et thromboses en Pédiatrie*, ed. N. Schlegel and F. Beaufils, pp. 113-115, Paris, Arnette.

Résumé

Le purpura thrombopénique autoimmum est fréquent chez les femmes et donc peut être souvent associé à la grossesse. La plupart des problèmes maternels ont été résolus et actuellement l'attention est portée sur le petit pourcentage de foetus qui étant très sévèrement thrombopéniques à la naissance risquent des hémorragies intracérébrales. La prédiction anténatale de la thrombopénie foetale fondée sur des paramètres maternels cliniques ou biologique a été un échec. Le risque de traumatisme obstétrical lors de l'accouchement par voie basse conduit à effectuer des prélèvements de sang foetal afin de reconnaître les thrombopénies foetales sévères et de décider des indications de la césarienne. La ponction de sang foetal au scalp s'est avérée difficile à appliquer. Les risques de ponction de sang foetal au cordon ombilical ne doivent pas être sous-estimés en regard du risque de la maladie elle-même. Les traitements anténataux ne sont pas tous efficaces. La frontière entre le purpura thrombopénique autoimmum et la thrombopénie asymptomatique est souvent mal définie et nécessite donc une meilleure définition.

Colloques **INSERM**
ISSN 0768-3154

Other *Colloques* published as co-editions by John Libbey Eurotext and INSERM

153 Hormones and Cell Regulation (11th European Symposium). *Hormones et Régulation Cellulaire (11e Symposium Européen).*
Edited by J. Nunez and J.E. Dumont.
ISBN : John Libbey Eurotext 0 86196 104 8
INSERM 2 85598 324 X

158 Biochemistry and Physiopathology of Platelet Membrane. *Biochimie et Physiopathologie de la Membrane Plaquettaire.*
Edited by G. Marguerie and R.F.A. Zwaal.
ISBN : John Libbey Eurotext 0 86196 114 5
INSERM 2 85598 345 2

162 The Inhibitors of Hematopoiesis. *Les Inhibiteurs de l'Hématopoïèse.*
Edited by A. Najman, M. Guignon, N.C. Gorin and J.Y. Mary.
ISBN : John Libbey Eurotext 0 86196 125 0
INSERM 2 85598 340 1

164 Liver Cells and Drugs. *Cellules Hépatiques et Médicaments.*
Edited by A. Guillouzo.
ISBN : John Libbey Eurotext 0 86196 128 5
INSERM 2 85598 341 X

165 Hormones and Cell Regulation (12th European Symposium). *Hormones et Régulation Cellulaire (12e Symposium Européen).*
Edited by J. Nunez, J.E. Dumont and E. Carafoli.
ISBN : John Libbey Eurotext 0 86196 133 1
INSERM 2 85598 347 9

167 Sleep Disorders and Respiration. *Les Evénements Respiratoires du Sommeil.*
Edited by P. Lévi-Valensi and D. Duron.
ISBN : John Libbey Eurotext 0 86196 127 7
INSERM 2 85598 344 4

169 Neo-Adjuvant Chemotherapy. *Chimiothérapie Néo-Adjuvante.*
Edited by C. Jacquillat, M. Weil, D. Khayat.
ISBN : John Libbey Eurotext 0 86196 150 1
INSERM 2 85598 349 5

171 Structure and Functions of the Cytoskeleton. *La Structure et les Fonctions du Cytosquelette.*
Edited by B.A.F. Rousset.
ISBN : John Libbey Eurotext 0 86196 149 8
INSERM 2 85598 351 7

Colloques INSERM
ISSN 0768-3154

172 The Langerhans Cell. *La Cellule de Langerhans.*
Edited by J. Thivolet, D. Schmitt.
ISBN : John Libbey Eurotext 0 86196 181 1
INSERM 2 85598 352 5

173 Cellular and Molecular Aspects of Glucuronidation. *Aspects Cellulaires et Moléculaires de la Glucuronoconjugaison.*
Edited by G. Siest, J. Magdalou, B. Burchell
ISBN : John Libbey Eurotext 0 86196 182 X
INSERM 2 85598 353 3

174 Second Forum on Peptides. *Deuxième Forum Peptides.*
Edited by A. Aubry, M. Marraud, B. Vitoux
ISBN : John Libbey Eurotext 0 86196 151 X
INSERM 2 85598 354 1

176 Hormones and Cell Regulation (13th European Symposium). *Hormones et Régulation Cellulaire (13e Symposium Européen).*
Edited by J. Nunez, J.E. Dumont, R. Denton
ISBN : John Libbey Eurotext 0 86196 183 8
INSERM 2 85598 356 8

179 Lymphokine Receptors Interactions. *Interactions Lymphokines-récepteurs.*
Edited by D. Fradelizi, J. Bertoglio
ISBN : John Libbey Eurotext 0 86196 148 X
INSERM 2 85598 359 2

191 Anticancer Drugs (1st International Interface of Clinical and Laboratory responses to anticancer drugs). *Médicaments anticancéreux (1re Confrontation internationale des réponses cliniques et expérimentales aux médicaments anticancéreux).*
Edited by H. Tapiero, J. Robert, T.J. Lampidis
ISBN : John Libbey Eurotext 0 86196 223 0
INSERM 2 85598 393 2

193 Living in the Cold (2nd International Symposium). *La Vie au Froid (2e Symposium International).*
Edited by A. Malan, B. Canguilhem
ISBN : John Libbey Eurotext 0 86196 234 9
INSERM 2 85598 395 9

Colloques INSERM
ISSN 0768-3154

194 Progress in Hepatitis B Immunization. *La Vaccination contre l'épatite B.*
Edited by P. Coursaget, M.J. Tong
ISBN : John Libbey Eurotext 0 86196 249 4
INSERM 2 85598 396 7

196 Treatment Strategy in Hodgkin's Disease. *Stratégie dans la maladie de Hodgkin.*
Edited by P. Sommers, M. Henry-Amar, J.H. Meezwaldt, P. Carde
ISBN : John Libbey Eurotext 0 86196 226 5
INSERM 2 85598 398 3

198 Hormones and Cell Regulation (14th European Symposium). *Hormones et Régulation Cellulaire (14e Symposium Européen).*
Edited by J. Nunez, J.E. Dumont
ISBN : John Libbey Eurotext 0 86196 229 X
INSERM 2 85598 400 9

199 Placental Communications : Biochemical, Morphological and Cellular Aspects. *Communications placentaires : aspects biochimique, morphologique et cellulaire.*
Edited by L. Cedard, E. Alsat, J.C. Challier, G. Chaouat, A. Malassiné
ISBN : John Libbey Eurotext 0 86196 227 3
INSERM 2 85598 401 7

204 Pharmacologie Clinique : Actualités et Perspectives. (6e Rencontres Nationales de Pharmacologie clinique).
Edited by J.P. Boissel, C. Caulin, M. Teule
ISBN : John Libbey Eurotext 0 86196 225 7
INSERM 2 85598 454 8

207 Thyroperoxidase and Thyroid Autoimmunity. *Thyroperoxydase et auto-immunité thyroïdienne.*
Edited by P. Carayon, T. Ruf
ISBN : John Libbey Eurotext 0 86196 277 X
INSERM 2 85598 440 8

210 Hormones and Cell Regulation (15th European Symposium). *Hormones et Régulation Cellulaire (15e Symposium Européen).*
Edited by J.E. Dumont, J. Nunez, R.J.B. King
ISBN : John Libbey Eurotext 0 86196 279 6
INSERM 2 85598 443 2

Reproduction photomécanique
IMPRIMERIE LOUIS-JEAN
BP 87 — 05003 GAP Cedex
Tél. : 92.51.35.23
Dépôt légal : 44 — Janvier 1991
Imprimé en France